Homelessness and Mental Health

Homelessness and Mental Health

Edited by

João Mauricio Castaldelli-Maia
Assistant (Aux.) Professor of Psychiatry,
Department of Neuroscience, FMABC University Center, Brazil

Antonio Ventriglio
Honorary Researcher, Department of Clinical and
Experimental Medicine, University of Foggia, Italy

Dinesh Bhugra
Professor Emeritus of Mental Health and
Cultural Diversity, Kings College London, UK

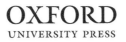
OXFORD
UNIVERSITY PRESS

OXFORD
UNIVERSITY PRESS

Great Clarendon Street, Oxford, OX2 6DP,
United Kingdom

Oxford University Press is a department of the University of Oxford.
It furthers the University's objective of excellence in research, scholarship,
and education by publishing worldwide. Oxford is a registered trade mark of
Oxford University Press in the UK and in certain other countries

© Oxford University Press 2022

The moral rights of the authors have been asserted

First Edition published in 2022

Published in the United States of America by Oxford University Press
198 Madison Avenue, New York, NY 10016, United States of America

British Library Cataloguing in Publication Data

Data available

Library of Congress Control Number: 2021943292

ISBN 978–0–19–884266–8

DOI: 10.1093/med/9780198842668.001.0001

Printed and bound in the UK by
TJ Books Limited

Contents

Section 6 **Special groups**

Section 7 **Conclusions**

Abbreviations

ACT	assertive community treatment		IQ	intelligence quotient
AHDH	attention deficit and hyperactivity disorder		LGB	lesbian, gay, and bisexual
			LGBT	lesbian, gay, bisexual, and transgender
ASD	autism spectrum disorder		LGBTQ+	lesbian, gay, bisexual, transgender, and questioning plus
CAPS	Centro de Atenção Psicossocial [psychosocial care center]		MATRICS	Measurement and Treatment Research to Improve Cognition in Schizophrenia
CES-D	Center for Epidemiologic Studies–Depression			
CI	confidence interval		MI	motivational interviewing
CM	contingency management		MMSE	Mini-Mental State Examination
DIS	Diagnostic Interview Schedule		MoCA	Montreal Cognitive Assessment
DSM	*Diagnostic and Statistical Manual of Mental Disorders*		MRI	magnetic resonance imaging
EIPP	Early Intervention in Psychosis Programme		NGO	non-governmental organization
ETHOS	European Typology of Homelessness and Housing Exclusion		NHS	National Health Service
			PTE	potentially traumatic experience
EU	European Union		PTSD	post-traumatic stress disorder
FEP	first-episode psychosis			
FrSBe	Frontal Systems Behavior Scale		SUD	substance use disorder
			TBI	traumatic brain injury
HEARTH	Homeless Emergency Assistance, and Rapid Transition to Housing		UBS	Unidades Básica de Saúde [basic health centre]
			UK	United Kingdom
HIV	human immunodeficiency virus		UPSA	University of California, San Diego Performance-based Skills Assessment
HMI	homeless mentally ill			
HY	homeless youth		US	United States
ICD-10-CM	International Classification of Diseases, Tenth Revision, Clinical Modification		USICH	United States Interagency Council on Homelessness
			WAIS	Wechsler Adult Intelligence Scale
ID	intellectual disability			
IDD	intellectual and developmental disability		WASI	Wechsler Abbreviated Scale of Intelligence
IDEAS	Indian Disability Evaluation and Assessment Scale			

Contributors

Amal Abdel-Baki
Professor, Department of Psychiatry, Centre Hospitalier de l'Université de Montréal (CHUM), Université de Montréal, Canada

Debanjan Banerjee
Postdoctoral Researcher in Geriatric Psychiatry, Department of Psychiatry, National Institute of Mental Health and Neurosciences (NIMHANS), India

Prama Bhattacharya
Assistant Professor at Jindal School of Psychology and Counselling, Department of Humanities and Social Sciences (HSS), Indian Institute of Technology Kanpur (IITK), India

Dinesh Bhugra
Professor Emeritus of Mental Health and Cultural Diversity, Kings College London, UK

Eszter Braun
Junior Doctor, Department of Psychiatry and Psychotherapy, Germany

Mario A. Brondani
Associate Professor, Director, Dental Public Health Graduate Program, Chair, Division of Dental Public Health, Associate Editor, Gerodontology, Dentistry, Oral Health Sciences The University of British Columbia, Point Grey Campus, Canada

Joshua D. Brown
Clinical Associate of Psychiatry, Tufts University School of Medicine Center, USA

Michael J. Brown
Professor, School of Nursing & Midwifery, Queen's University Belfast, UK

João Mauricio Castaldelli-Maia
Assistant (Aux.) Professor of Psychiatry, Department of Neuroscience, FMABC University Center, Brazil

Hubert Côté
Department of Psychiatry, Université de Montréal Pavillon Roger-GaudryFaculté, Canada

Charles Abrantes Coura
Psychologist, Pontifical Catholic University of São Paulo, Brazil

Anamika Das
Assistant Divisional Medical Officer, India

Sarbani Das Roy
Co-Founder and Director of Iswar
Sankalpa, India

Lucas C. Davanso
Medical School (FMABC), ABC
Health University Center, Santo
André, São Paulo, Brazil

Julie Marguerite Deschênes
School of Social Work, Université de
Montréal, Faculté des arts et sciences
Pavillon Lionel-Groulx, Canada

Virginie Doré-Gauthier
Assistant Clinical Professor,
Department of Psychiatry and
Addiction of the Faculty of
Medicine, Hôpital en santé mentale
Albert Prévost, Université de
Montréal, Canada

Isabel Bernardes Ferreira
Social Worker, Department of
Psychology, Pontifícia Universidade
Católica de São Paulo, Brazil

Marcos Roberto Vieira Garcia
Professor, Department of Psychology,
Federal University of São Carlos
(UFSCar), Brazil

Gábor Gazdag
Clinical Professor, Department
of Psychiatry and Psychotherapy,
School of Medicine, Centre for
Psychiatry and Addiction Medicine,
Jahn Ferenc South Pest Hospital,
Hungary

Priscila Dib Gonçalves
Department of Epidemiology,
Mailman School of Public Health,
Columbia University, USA

Israel Gonzalez-Urbieta
Department of Psychiatry—Hospital
de Clínicas, National University
of Asunción, Mariscal López and
Cruzada de la Amistad, UK

Guru S. Gowda
Assistant Professor, Department
of Psychiatry, National Institute
of Mental Health And Neuro
Sciencesand Neurosciences
(NIMHANS), India

Stefan Gutwinski
Department of Psychiatry
and Psychotherapy, Charité
Universitätsmedizin Berlin, Germany

Stephen W. Hwang
Professor, MAP Centre for Urban
Health Solutions, St. Michael's
Hospital, Canada

Erhabor Sunday Idemudia
Clinical Psychologist, Full Professor
of Research, Faculty of the
Humanities and Health Sciences,
North-West University, South Africa

Sujita Kumar Kar
Associate Professor, Department of
Psychiatry, King George's Medical
University, Chowk, India

Nick Kerman
Postdoctoral Fellow, Centre
for Addiction and Mental
Health, Canada

Channaveerachari Naveen Kumar
Professor of Psychiatry and Adjunct
Professor, Centre for Psychosocial
Support in Disaster Management,
National Institute of Mental
Health and Neuro Sciencesand
Neurosciences (NIMHANS), India

Henry Chi-Ming Leung
Honorary Associate Professor,
Department of Psychiatry, Chinese
University of Hong Kong

Isabelle Sarah Lévesque
Psychiatrist, Jean-Talon
Hospital, Clinique Jean-Pierre
Mottard, Canada

Michael I. MacEntee
Professor Emeritus, Faculty of
Dentistry, University of British
Columbia, Canada

Luiz Gustavo Maestrelli
Biological Sciences, Positivo
University, and Medicine at Pontifical
Catholic University of Parana, Brazil

Anjali Mago
Interim Director, Department of
Health at Keewaytinook Okimakanak
(KO) First Nation Tribal Council in
Thunder Bay, Canada

Narayana Manjunatha
Associate Professor, Department
of Psychiatry, National Institute of
Mental Health and Neurosciences
(NIMHANS), India

Suresh Bada Math
Professor of Psychiatry, Head of
Forensic Psychiatry Services, Tele-
medicine Centre and In-charge
of Legal-Aid Clinic, National
Institute of Mental Health And
Neuro Sciencesand Neurosciences
(NIMHANS), India

Edward McCann
School of Nursing and Midwifery,
Trinity College Dublin, Ireland

Raphaël Morisseau-Guillot
Psychiatry Resident, Department of
Psychiatry, Université de Montréal
Pavillon Roger-GaudryFaculté de
médecine, Canada

Graham Pluck
Director, Institute of Neurosciences,
Universidad San Francisco de
Quito, UK

Wulf Rössler
Psychiatric University Hospital,
Switzerland

Hans-Joachim Salize
Mental Health Services Research
Group, Central Institute of Mental
Health, Germany

Stefanie Schreiter
Assistant Physician, Department
of Psychiatry and Psychotherapy,
Charité—Universitätsmedizin Berlin,
Germany

Christian G. Schütz
Professor, Department of
Psychiatry, University of British
Columbia, Canada

Neha Sharma
Assistant Professor, Tufts University
School of Medicine, Program
Director, Child & Adolescent
Psychiatry Fellowship, Tufts Medical
Center, USA

Anderson Sousa Martins da Silva
Psychiatrist and Professor of
Psychiatry, Medical School,
Universidade Nove de Julho, Brazil

Etienne de Miranda e Silva
Clinical Psychiatrist, Baeta Neves,
São Bernardo do Campo, Brazil

Angela Bianco Smith
Clinical Social Worker, San
Diego, USA

Cara A. Struble
Graduate Student, Department
of Psychology, Wayne State
University, USA

Paul Summergrad
Professor and Chairman,
Department of Psychiatry and
Professor of Psychiatry and
Medicine, Tufts University School of
Medicine and Psychiatrist-in-Chief,
Tufts Medical Center, USA

John Sylvestre
Professor, Centre for Research
on Educational and Community
Services, University of
Ottawa, Canada

Philip Timms
National Psychosis Unit, Bethlem
Royal Hospital, UK

Julio Torales
Professor, Department of Psychiatry
and Medical Psychology, Head of
the Mental Health Department, and
Head of the Social Anthropology
Department, National University
of Asunción School of Medical
Sciences, Paraguay

Paul A. Toro
Professor, Department of Psychology,
Wayne State University in
Detroit, USA

Adarsh Tripathi
Additional Professor, Department
of Psychiatry, King George's Medical
University, Lucknow, India

Gabor S. Ungvari
Clinical Professor, Department of
Psychiatry, University of Western
Australia; Adjunct Professor,
Department of Psychiatry, Notre
Dame Australia, Australia

Antonio Ventriglio
Honorary Researcher, Department of
Clinical and Experimental Medicine,
University of Foggia, Italy

Marc Vogel
Specialist in Addiction Psychiatry,
University of Basel, Psychiatric
Services of Thurgovia, Switzerland

Larina Chi-Lap Yim
Department of Psychiatry, The
Chinese University, Hong Kong

Section 1

Background

Chapter 1

Introduction

João Mauricio Castaldelli-Maia,
Antonio Ventriglio, and
Dinesh Bhugra

Background

The contemporary definition of homelessness has to be seen as a multifaceted societal issue with specific factors at play in different settings. Relative poverty, insecure housing, unemployment, and insecure unemployment can all contribute to homelessness and it is worth noting that these factors will vary across cultures. This definition differs from other definitions (1). Often, homeless individuals are blamed for their homelessness as a result of their own actions. They are labelled as criminals, alcoholics, druggies, spiritually fragile, and/or mentally ill—all stigmatizing and discriminatory terms. Whereas these deep-rooted ideas about homelessness still persist, statements that most of the homeless might be affected by psychotic disorders are obsolete (1). However, there is little doubt that homelessness and mental disorders are interlinked with bi-directional causality. A majority of the investigators support the idea of such a complex relationship. Mental disorder can instigate homelessness, although the latter may likewise influence the former's development, exacerbation, and continuance (1).

Homelessness is often expressed as a crisis—a break in the typical, cultured means of civilizations. In addition, severe mental disorders have been noted and reported in homeless populations for a considerable period of time. Individuals with severe mental illness often experience a range of housing settings depending on their personal and financial conditions or the available rehabilitation programmes, which will depend upon healthcare systems (2), in addition to societal conditions and local policies on social care, employment housing, and so on. Due to various deinstitutionalization programmes and developments in the middle of the last century (i.e. mental health patients were discharged from old-fashioned asylums, sometimes without any clear post-discharge plans), individuals with mental disorders were referred to the care of their families, supervisory houses, and assisted lodgings, depending on the type of rehabilitation programme available (2) but, in many cases, these were temporary measures and did not work out for many individuals. Initiation of community care was often not supported by adequate financial resources, thereby adding to the pressures on individuals who then ended up on the streets.

International perspective

European researchers have been investigating the relationship between homelessness and mental health disorders since the beginning of the nineteenth century. More recently, in Germany, observations have indicated that the growing numbers of homeless people are related to increasing poverty and a shortage of affordable accommodation, leading to an increased scientific and political interest (3). The prevalence of mental disorders among homeless people in many countries of Europe is similar to that in other continents, thereby suggesting a consistent relationship. In Eastern European countries, homelessness has become a bigger concern since the end of the communist system. In 2014, a survey was conducted in Budapest, Hungary, to assess the psychiatric conditions of homeless people and the impact of their psychiatric illness on social relations, employment, and substance use, and found that rates of psychiatric disorders were higher than expected (4). The vast majority (86%) of homeless people living in a shelter had a diagnosis of a psychiatric disorder, predominantly alcohol and personality disorders (4).

Recent estimates from the 2018 US Housing and Urban Development survey indicate that 17.3% of homeless individuals surveyed during a single night had a serious mental illness (5). This estimate is similar to a study conducted in the late 1990s (6), where 15% of a probability sample of homeless adults in Buffalo, New York, were identified as having a severe mental disorder during their lifetime. That estimate increased to almost three-quarters of the sample when assessing rates for any mental disorder (6). These findings were also replicated by several other studies in the Americas. However, it would appear that, in South America, mental health and substance use disorders are more prevalent in the homeless population compared to the general population. The majority of the Brazilian studies are concentrated in the wealthier regions (Southeast and South) and show a higher prevalence of men in the surveys. Among the mental health disorders, psychotic and affective disorders were the most prevalent in this group (7).

Cannabis and alcohol were the substances most used in the adult homeless population, followed by cocaine (crack) (8). There are few studies on tobacco smoking and injectable drugs, although these do show significant rates (8). Latin-American street children are at higher risk of having post-traumatic stress, anxiety, and depressive disorders. Substance use is also a significant issue in this group. Because of ease of local availability, cocaine use is particularly associated with street children in Latin America. Inhalant use is also common but, as with other substances, this may be more associated with homeless street children as compared to domiciled ones (9). Overall, street children in Latin America face a great number of challenges and risks to their mental health, most of which are consequences of the various correlates of extreme poverty, including lack of available mental healthcare, vulnerability to physical, sexual, and emotional abuse, and family dysfunction (9).

There is a vicious cycle of poverty, ill health, and homelessness in some Asian countries too. These cultures in transition are struggling with rapid industrialization and urbanization. For example, in India, although relative poverty is variable, psychotic disorders are the most common psychiatric illnesses in the homeless, followed by mood disorders, substance use disorders, and intellectual disabilities (10). Lack of rehabilitation services; impaired ability to self-care; illness factors such as untreated mental disorder, scarcity of mental health resources, and a higher level of comorbidities; and social factors such as poverty and low literacy, stigma, lack of employment, rapid urbanization, and other housing barriers are the primary reasons in India contributing to homelessness in the mentally ill population (10). More developed areas in Asia are also experiencing similar phenomena. The number of homeless people in Hong Kong is rising, mainly because of the high cost of rental housing and other economic factors. In a study conducted there (11), approximately half of the homeless subjects were mentally ill at the time of the interview. Although 41% of the subjects with mental illness had previously undergone a psychiatric assessment, only 13% were receiving psychiatric care at the time of interview. As the authors note, these figures are likely to be an underestimate (11).

Clinical issues

There is an important interface among homelessness, mental disorders, and physical conditions. In that sense, some key clinical conditions could play an important contributory role in the genesis of mental ill health among the homeless population. We illustrate these here by selecting a couple of exemplars. For example, in common physical conditions such as chronic pain in homeless populations, research data are rare, but where undertaken, data show consistently higher rates compared to the general population. In the UK, a study with 150 shelter users found a chronic pain prevalence of 59%, with a mean duration of more than 6 years (12). Similarly, a Canadian study (13) found a higher prevalence (52%) in a similar sample, persisting for 10 years on average.

Oral health is equally important and increasingly evidence is emerging that poor oral health can contribute to poor physical and mental health and homeless individuals often find it very difficult to access appropriate dental treatment (14). However, it is apparent that once offered such interventions, they are willing to accept these services.

The world is now facing a public health crisis due to the coronavirus disease 2019 (COVID-19) pandemic. It has been described as a 'public health emergency of international concern' by the World Health Organization (15). During any such health outbreak, homeless individuals are much more vulnerable due to ongoing challenges to their physical, psychological, and social well-being. Indeed, homeless people are one of the populations at risk. The impact of the infection may well last longer than the pandemic itself.

Psychiatric issues

As mentioned earlier, homeless individuals have a higher incidence of drug and alcohol use (16) and approximately 20–25% of homeless people have psychiatric problems (17). High rates of substance abuse, schizophrenia, bipolar disorders, personality disorders, and major depression are found in the homeless group in comparison with the general population (17). Anxiety was reported in 20.5% of the homeless and substantial levels of depressive disorders (18).

There is also a reported high prevalence of post-traumatic stress disorder among the homeless, especially refugees and migrants. Both pre-migration and post-migration stressors were shown to predict post-traumatic stress disorder (19). However, the diagnosis of post-traumatic stress disorder must be carried out carefully. Studies also point out that homelessness is an important issue experienced by migrants at both reception and the post-migration period. Accommodating refugees may constitute a major burden to new countries at reception. In some countries, refugees are left to take shelter in insecure and often crowded places, thereby putting their physical and mental well-being at risk. Studies further found that the homelessness problem does not end for refugees even after being granted asylum status (19).

Cognitive competence influences individual functioning in all areas, such as social, emotional, academic, and occupational functioning. Understanding the mechanisms through which cognitive impairment can influence an individual's susceptibility to homelessness is essential to providing effective services for improving health outcomes among this population (20). As noted previously, this is important because of the bidirectional relationship between homelessness and cognitive impairment, especially when psychiatric disorders such as schizophrenia, bipolar disorder, intellectual disability, autism spectrum disorder, organic disorders, and substance abuse are concerned (21).

Services

Providing care for homeless individuals with mental disorders is a crucial challenge to mental health professionals. The clinical outcome and recovery are likely to be subject to multiple factors such as occupation, public support, stable accommodation, assertive social treatment, physical and mental healthcare integration, community-based care, and inclusive health policies (22), among other factors. In some countries, specialized mental healthcare services for the homeless population began in the 1980s. These were a response to the increased awareness of the relationship between homelessness and mental health disorders (23). They have established means of working in non-clinical situations, such as the street, day centres, and hostels for the homeless, with close collaborations with voluntary sector services and housing and social services (23). More recently, these services have developed more sophisticated outreach models (24) which require evaluation and duplication.

Homeless individuals require a variety of social, health, and community facilities to meet their basic needs. However, some of these individuals may have had negative experiences with services, which may lead them to avoid using these services, thereby worsening health problems and resulting in further entrenchment in homelessness (25). Like the general population, several specific factors contribute to positive and negative service experiences among people who are homeless, such as accessibility and availability of services, personal beliefs and explanatory models, organizational policies and procedures, previous interactions with service providers, sense of safety and welfare, service environment, and quality of services, among other factors (25). The complexity of psychosocial care for the homeless includes specific features such as extreme poverty, social susceptibility, being itinerant, and also the struggle with the bureaucracy of health systems. Treating this population thus involves a day-to-day multimodal approach from teaching basic self-care to guaranteed subsistence and access to the available resources within the local context. The social support and security safeguards, dialogue about the possible mental health and substance use problems, and the possible treatments of detected disorders are crucial (26).

Conclusion

The numbers of individuals who can be classified as being homeless are affected by a variety of reasons which include economic factors such as poverty and unemployment, which may or may not be a result of rapid urbanization. Migration from rural to urban areas and across countries and scarcity of secure accommodation and employment will affect rates of homelessness. Some groups, such as those with psychiatric disorders, are more vulnerable to homelessness than others. Rates of psychiatric disorders are shown to be consistently higher in homeless individuals, although in some cases, psychiatric illnesses may lead to homelessness.

References

1. **Foster A, Gable J, Buckley J.** Homelessness in schizophrenia. Psychiatr Clin North Am. 2012;**35**(3):717–734.

2. **Nelson G, Aubry T, Hutchison J.** Housing and mental health. In: International Encyclopedia of Rehabilitation. Center for International Rehabilitation Research Information and Exchange (CIRRIE); 2010. Available from: http://cirrie.buffalo.edu/encyclopedia/en/article/132/.

3. **Schreiter S, Bermpohl F, Krausz M,** et al. The prevalence of mental illness in homeless people in Germany—a systematic review and meta-analysis. Dtsch Arztebl Int. 2017;**17**(40):665–672.

4. **Braun E, Gazdag G.** Pszichiátriai zavarok előfordulása hajléktalanok között [Prevalence of psychiatric disorders in homeless population]. Psychiatr Hung. 2015;**30**(1):60–67.

5. **US Department of Housing and Urban Development.** HUD 2018 Continuum of Care Homeless Assistance Programs Homeless Populations and Subpopulations. 2018.

6. **Toro PA, Wolfe SM, Bellavia CW,** et al. Obtaining representative samples of homeless persons: a two-city study. J Community Psychol. 1999;**27**(2):157–177.

7. **Heckert U, Andrade L, Alves MJ, Martins C.** Lifetime prevalence of mental disorders among homeless people in a southeast city in Brazil. Eur Arch Psychiatry Clin Neurosci. 1999;**249**(3):150–155.

8. **Brunini SM, Barros CVL, Guimarães RA,** et al. HIV infection, high-risk behaviors and substance use in homeless men sheltered in therapeutic communities in Central Brazil. Int J STD AIDS. 2018;**29**(11):1084–1088.

9. **Pluck G.** The 'street children' of Latin America. Psychologist. 2015;**28**(1):20–23.

10. **Tripathi A, Nischal A, Dalal PK,** et al. Sociodemographic and clinical profile of homeless mentally ill inpatients in a north Indian medical university. Asian J Psychiatr. 2013;**6**(5):404–409.

11. **Homeless Outreach Population Estimation (H.O.P.E.) Hong Kong 2015.** Research report. City University of Hong Kong; 2016. Available from: http://www.cityu.edu.hk/youeprj/hopehk2015_chi.pdf.

12. **Fisher R, Ewing J, Garrett A, Harrison EK, Lwin KK, Wheeler DW.** The nature and prevalence of chronic pain in homeless persons: an observational study. F1000Res. 2013;**2**:164.

13. **Hwang SW, Wilkins E, Chambers C, Estrabillo E, Berends J, MacDonald A.** Chronic pain among homeless persons: characteristics, treatment, and barriers to management. BMC Fam Pract. 2011;**12**:73.

14. **Wallace BB, MacEntee MI, Pauly B.** Community dental clinics in British Columbia, Canada: examining the potential as health equity interventions. Health Soc Care Community. 2015;**23**(4):371–379.

15. **World Health Organization.** Coronavirus disease 2019 (COVID-19): situation report, 72. 2020. Available from: https://apps.who.int/iris/handle/10665/331685.

16. **Keogh C, O'Brien KK, Hoban A, O'Carroll A, Fahey T.** Health and use of health services of people who are homeless and at risk of homelessness who receive free primary health care in Dublin. BMC Health Serv Res. 2015;**15**:58.

17. **Coohey C, Easton SD, Kong J, Bockenstedt JKW.** Sources of psychological pain and suicidal thoughts among homeless adults. Suicide Life Threat Behav. 2014;**45**(3):271–280.

18. **Notaro SJ, Khan M, Kim C, Nasaruddin M, Desai K.** Analysis of the health status of the homeless clients utilizing a free clinic. J Community Health. 2012;**38**(1):172–177.

19. **Chen W, Hall BJ, Ling L, Renzaho AM.** Pre-migration and post-migration factors associated with mental health in humanitarian migrants in Australia and the moderation effect of post-migration stressors: findings from the first wave data of the BNLA cohort study. Lancet Psychiatry. 2017;**4**(3):218–229.

20. **Adair CE, Holland AC, Patterson ML,** et al. Cognitive interviewing methods for questionnaire pre-testing in homeless persons with mental disorders. J Urban Health. 2012;**89**(1):36–52.

21. **Depp CA, Vella L, Orff HJ, Twamley EW.** A quantitative review of cognitive functioning in homeless adults. J Nerv Ment Dis. 2015;**203**(2):126–131.

22. **Fazel S, Geddes JR, Kushel M.** The health of homeless people in high-income countries: descriptive epidemiology, health consequences, and clinical and policy recommendations. Lancet. 2014;**384**(9953):1529–1540.

23. **Craig T, Timms P.** Out of the wards and onto the streets? Deinstitutionalization and homelessness in Britain. J Ment Health. 1992;**1**(3):265–275.

24. **Queen AB, Lowrie R, Richardson J, Williamson AE.** Multimorbidity, disadvantage, and patient engagement within a specialist homeless health service in the UK: an in-depth study of general practice data. BJGP Open. 2017;**1**(3):bjgpopen17X100941.

25. **Kerman N, Gran-Ruaz SM, Lawrence M, Sylvestre J.** Perceptions of service use among currently and formerly homeless adults with mental health problems. Community Ment Health J. 2019;**55**(5):777–783.

26. **Londero MFP, Ceccim RB, Bilibio LFS.** Consultation office of/in the street: challenge for a healthcare in verse. Interface. 2014;**18**(49):251–260.

Chapter 2

Homelessness and mental illness in the UK: Some historical fragments

Philip Timms

Introduction

When I originally wrote on this topic, over 20 years ago, the issue of psychiatric disorder and homelessness was viewed as a contemporary phenomenon without historical precedent. Discussions at the time revolved around two bogey men: the recent mental hospital closures and the introduction of 'care in the community' policies. Both of these factors were held to be responsible, at least in the US and UK, for the large numbers of visible homeless people on the streets of major cities. There was some disagreement about how much this was a mental health issue and how much simply to do with lack of appropriate housing (1). But there was also a more general discussion about how health services should respond to indigent populations (2).

More recently, the UK has experienced the economic policies of austerity. These have resulted in reductions, across the board, of health, social, and housing services. Homelessness, not just of people with mental health problems, has been transformed from a temporary phenomenon that appeared to be slowly disappearing, to an increasingly familiar, uncomfortable, and embarrassing feature of our streets.

There is some evidence for historical antecedents to our contemporary situation with homelessness and mental illness, although it is fragmentary and poorly documented. And this issue extends beyond the provision, or non-provision, of psychiatric services. The presence of homeless people with a severe mental illness is deeply embedded in the wider context of poverty and homelessness in the UK.

The homeless people of past centuries were, in the main, without a voice and deemed worthy either of condemnation or (perhaps) charitable attention. One exception was Charles Dickens. He created a gang of homeless children in

Oliver Twist, like the children he saw in his *Night Walks* (3), and wrote a short account of the Wapping workhouse. Otherwise, most of the materials that have survived are details of legislation, court proceedings, crude occupancy statistics, and contemporary mythologies of vagrancy, with the mentally ill mentioned usually only in passing. There have, however, been two common threads running through the centuries. One has been the visibility of the street homeless, leading to the construction of strange mythologies about Mafia-like underworld societies of vagrants (4, pp. 123–145). The other has been the institution established by the state to deal with the poor and indigent—the workhouse.

Law and the workhouse

Both homelessness, and society's responses to it, have followed changing social conditions since the late thirteenth century. In pre-Reformation England, there still flourished large numbers of monasteries and houses of religion that provided a widespread system of relief to the poor. However, the theological landscape was in flux. St Francis had taught that the total renunciation of possessions was part of a spiritual ideal. This had produced a relatively benevolent view of both poverty and the reliance on others through begging (5). However, the subsequent growth of monastic orders, and their acquisition of starkly worldly elements of wealth and power, had produced a more cynical view of their motives.

Around the middle of the fourteenth century, the nature of the wandering homeless had also changed. Prior to this period, charity had been extended to the old, the infirm, and those on pilgrimages. Now, large numbers of destitute industrial workers appeared on the scene as a rising population and falling wages drove peasants off the land. At the same time, the feudal contractual relationship between landlord and villein, which tied the peasant to his land and his lord, had begun to break down. This was possibly due to an over-supply of labour, which meant that the local lords were less worried by local workers moving around (6). This social dislocation was subsequently exacerbated by the profound social disruption of many areas of the country caused by the Black Death (7).

The wandering poor, once seen as pilgrims or deserving objects of Christian charity, came to be seen at best as immoral idlers, at worst as a threat to the very fabric of society. And this was reflected in legislation.

The first statute that mentioned indigent people, albeit as part of a wider project to limit wage rises, was passed in 1349 (8). In response to the dearth of labourers created by the Black Death, the Ordinance of Labourers attempted to impose a universal condition of work for those under 60 years of age—and to enforce price controls on labour. To further its aim of universal employment, it specifically forbade the giving of alms to 'able-bodied beggars'. This was ineffective and was bolstered by the Statute of Labourers in 1351, which bemoaned 'the malice of servants who were idle and not willing to serve after the pestilence [Black Death] without excessive wages'.

The Statute of Cambridge, in 1388, followed the Peasants' Revolt in 1381. This forbade servants to move out of their 'hundred' (the administrative area of the time) without permission, and so restricted their ability to travel in search of work. It did, however, introduce a formal geographic basis for accountability for the poor. Each 'hundred' became responsible for housing and keeping its own paupers—but there was no special provision for maintaining the sick or disabled. And, for the first time, this act differentiated beggars as 'sturdy', capable of work, or 'impotent', incapacitated by age or infirmity.

Punishment was the mainspring of policy set out in these acts, with the penalty of the stocks for able-bodied beggars. However, despite the rigours of legal sanctions, the numbers of homeless continued to increase. And with Henry VIII's dissolution of the monasteries in the first half of the sixteenth century, even the limited provision of religious charity disappeared. The problem, however, remained. So, from 1531 to 1601, the Tudors and Elizabeth I initiated a system of local relief in which the main provider of care was the local church parish, a secular institution. New institutions, 'Houses of Correction', or bridewells, were established, the first being chartered in London in 1553. A subsequent act of 1576 ordered their establishment in all counties and corporate towns (9).

> [T]o the intent youth may be accustomed and brought up in labour and work, and then not likely to grow up able rogues, and to the intent that such as already be grown up in idleness and so rogues at this present, may not have any just excuse in saying that they cannot get any service of work. (10)

These were the first workhouses. As the preceding extract from the act suggests, they were supposed to train and rehabilitate through work. However, the aim of punishment was also stated within this and subsequent acts.

The advantage of devolving responsibility to the local level was that any provision would be responsive to local need and would be locally accountable. On the other hand, no allowance was made for the ability of a given parish to respond to the demands placed upon it. The funds allocated were often insufficient. By the seventeenth century, most of these institutions had become little better than gaols. The workhouses built later, in the eighteenth century, faced similar problems and became similarly squalid and punitive.

The next major development of these institutions was the Poor Law Amendment Act of 1834, which combined all but the larger parish workhouses into so-called unions, each union combining the functions of several smaller workhouses. This reduced the number of workhouses from 15,000 to 650 and resulted in the building of large, custodial institutions that persisted well into the twentieth century.

The test of destitution, and eligibility, was merely the willingness to enter the workhouse. It was specified that no resident should be better off than any independent labourer, so conditions were made as unpleasant as possible. The works of Dickens and Hardy are eloquent testament to the rigour with which this policy was applied and the dread of the workhouse became a fixed part of the psychological landscape of the English working classes.

The report of the Royal Commission (11), which preceded that act, noted that, in many existing workhouses, one would hear 'the incessant ravings of some neglected lunatic'. Their account of the Dover workhouse identified seven such people living there, two of whom were chained to their beds for the protection of the other inmates. The report goes on to address the needs of vulnerable groups such as 'the aged and impotent' and 'children'. It stated that 'both the requisite classification and the requisite superintendence may be better obtained in separate buildings than under a single roof'. In other words, separate institutions—or at least buildings—should be set up for such vulnerable groups.

In terms of the mentally ill, the Royal Commission noted that 'The principle of separate and appropriate management has been carried into imperfect execution, in the cases of lunatics, by means of lunatic asylums'. So, in terms of the 'impotent', or unfit to work, the workhouse would deal with children, the physically unwell, and the aged, in separate units. The emergent asylums would accommodate those with mental illness. In reality, with few exceptions, general mixed workhouses were the rule (12). The notion of some separation of functions did, however, persist. In 1864, the Metropolitan Houseless Poor Act ordered the unions to segregate the vagrant, mobile poor from the local poor of the parish into what was called a 'casual ward'. In 1882, a 2-day detention system was introduced, whereby any vagrant inmate was obliged to give a day's labour for every 2 nights' board.

The first formal link between the workhouses and health provision was initiated by the 1867 Metropolitan Poor Act which mandated that all London workhouses had to have hospital facilities that were separate from the general workhouse. This, effectively, established the first state hospitals in the UK.

In spite of such provision, the rapid urban expansion of the mid-nineteenth century overwhelmed a system of poor relief that had been established, after all, for predominantly rural areas. Organizations such as the Salvation Army, spurred by the appalling conditions of the workhouses (13), began to see themselves as providers of superior accommodation for the poor that was supportive rather than punitive. Lord Rowton, an exemplar of Victorian notions of both philanthropy and hard-nosed commerce, wanted to do good—and saw a niche in the market. His first Rowton Hotel, in Vauxhall, London, was a dormitory-style hostel, which charged rates that the working man could afford. But it also provided luxuries such as clean sheets, footbaths, hot water, washing facilities, and space to dry clothes. The model proved popular enough to justify six more Rowton Houses (as they came to be known) in London, and the model was even exported to Milan in the shape of the Albergo Popolare (14).

In tandem with this increasing concern for the living conditions of working men, punitive attitudes towards homeless people began to change, at least in law. In 1909, the Minority Report of the Royal Commission on the Poor Law finally accepted the principle that society's duty was to help the vagrant rather than to punish him (or her). In 1919, the new Ministry of Health assumed responsibility for supervising Poor Law administration but the individual institutions remained under the direct control of local Boards of Guardians. Conditions in the casual wards continued to be grim and punitive. A Departmental Committee estimated that a quarter of the users of casual wards were suffering from mental illness, mental handicap, or alcoholism. The subsequent Poor Law Act of 1930 transferred administration of poor relief to elected local authorities. Again, separate facilities were recommended for some groups such as women, the sick, and the young—but none for the mentally ill (15).

The advent of the Second World War in 1939 proved to be a watershed for the casual wards. Able-bodied men were recruited for the war effort and their numbers dropped to a few thousand from a peak of 16,911 in May 1932. Post-war social optimism led not only to the establishment of the National Health Service, but also to the desire to eradicate 'vagrancy'. This led to the establishment of the National Assistance Board in 1948. Its aim was 'to make provision whereby persons without a settled way of living may be influenced to lead a more settled way of life'. The casual wards were taken over and renamed 'reception centres' to provide just temporary accommodation. However, occupancy had dropped to levels that rendered most of them redundant. This was probably due to high levels of employment at the time and to the welfare state's newly introduced provisions for ameliorating poverty and preventing destitution. So, the National Assistance Board promptly closed 136 of the 270 centres it had taken over. In 1968, the new Department of Health and Social Security took over the reception centres and, by 1970, there were just 17 left. However, echoes of the workhouse remained. Instead of a day's work there was a 'work task' that had to be completed before an individual could leave after an overnight stay. Living conditions were still miserable. A study of reception centres as late as 1968 revealed that residents were suffering from severe malnutrition (16). Sick bays were established, visiting medical officers appointed, and referrals increasingly made to local services (17). However, this seemed to have little impact on the high levels of psychiatric morbidity in such establishments (18).

The 'lunatic paupers'

A stock character of the Elizabethan and Jacobean period was the wandering lunatic, the Tom O'Bedlam or Abram Man. Shakespeare gives King Lear a short speech bemoaning the fate of those with 'houseless heads and unfed sides' and chastises himself, as sovereign, for having 'ta'en too little care of this'. Edgar then enters, disguised as a madman who calls himself 'poor Tom ... whom the foul fiend vexes' (*King Lear*, Act III, Scene IV). However, the documentary evidence is scant concerning the real-life patterns for this archetypal character. The names seem to have derived from the Bethlem hospital, Abram possibly referring to the name of one of the wards. By the early seventeenth century, it had just 20–30 beds to serve the whole country (19), so it is perhaps not surprising that ex-patients were to be found wandering country lanes and city streets. According to different accounts, they either made marks on their arm or carried a tin plate on their arm to identify them as ex-patients. This has been interpreted as amounting to a licence to beg, and there is, indeed, a recorded case of a false licence having been bought to facilitate begging in 1598. However, by 1675 the practice had presumably died out as the governors of Bethlem had announced that people presenting themselves in this way were frauds (4, pp. 115–117). Licence or not, in Elizabethan England the standard method of dealing with them seems to have been that described by Edgar in *King Lear*: 'Whipped from tithing to tithing, and stock-punish'd and imprison'd.'

One of the first specific legislative mentions of the homeless mentally ill is to be found in an Act of Parliament of 1714 concerned with the management of vagrancy in general (20). The 'Act for ... the More Effectual Punishing of such Rogues, Vaga-bonds, Sturdy Beggars, and Vagrants, and Sending them Whither They Ought to be Sent' was pretty coercive but, at least, it specifically forbade whipping for lunatics. These were described as 'Persons of little or no Estates, who, by Lunacy, or otherwise, are furiously mad, and dangerous to be permitted to go abroad'. It empowered two or more Justices of the Peace to confine such persons 'safely locked up in such secure place' while 'such lunacy or madness shall continue'. The costs for any such confinement for paupers would be met by the parish concerned. The act also empowered Justices to return to their home parish anyone so confined. An amendment in 1744 (21, p. 118) was only notable in providing for 'keeping, maintaining and curing'—the idea of cure being mentioned for the first time.

There is little evidence of the numbers confined as a result of this act, or of the situations in which they were to be confined. There was still, after all, only one public asylum in the whole country, Bethlem (22). Some workhouses, such as St Peter's in Bristol, separated the 'pauper lunatics' from those of sound mind (21). Others did not. In 1812, the philanthropist Sir George Onesiphorus Paul found individuals deemed mad 'chained in the cellar or garret of a workhouse'. More often they would be 'fastened to the leg of a table, tied to a post in an outhouse, or perhaps shut up in an uninhabited ruin; or if his lunacy be inoffensive, left to ramble half naked and half-starved through the streets and highways, teased by the scoff and jest of all that is vulgar, ignorant and unfeeling'. His observations formed part of an argument for the establishment of separate institutions for the mentally ill (23).

Throughout the nineteenth century, some 20–25% of all known pauper lunatics in England and Wales were accommodated in workhouses (24). A House of Commons committee of 1807 reported that there were 1765 pauper lunatics in Poor Houses, Houses of Industry, and Houses of Correction (21). Further evidence that workhouses continued to serve as repositories for the mentally ill comes from a comment in a Poor Law Commissioners report of 1842:

> From the express prohibition of the detention of dangerous persons of unsound mind in a workhouse ... combined with the prevalent practice of keeping insane persons in a workhouse before the passing of the Poor Law Amendment Act, it may be inferred that persons of unsound mind, not being dangerous, may be legally kept in a workhouse. It must, however, be remembered that with lunatics, the first object ought to be their cure by means of proper medical treatment. This can only be obtained in a well-regulated asylum; and therefore the detention of any curable lunatic in a workhouse is highly objectionable on the score both of humanity and economy.

Again, the possibility of cure is mentioned, with the optimistic notion that what could not be achieved by the workhouse could be achieved by the asylum. This disapproval of the use of the workhouse as accommodation for the mentally ill was echoed in 1859 by the Lunacy Commission, who stated that 'the stringent conditions [to deal with able bodied paupers of sound mind] are not only unnecessary for the insane but are obviously very unjust and detrimental to them'. A further tangential reference is found in the observations made by a foreign visitor in 1871:

> The workhouse purports at one and the same time to be: (i) a place where able-bodied adults who cannot or will not find employment can be set to work; ... (vi) an asylum for those of unsound mind not being actually dangerous. (25)

The general feeling that the workhouse was not a good place for the mad resulted, in 1875, in a weekly grant to all unions in England and Wales from the Poor Law Board. Four shillings per person, per week, was offered towards the extra cost of maintaining pauper lunatics in county asylums (26). As the entire cost would otherwise fall upon the local parish rates, this was a powerful inducement to transfer such individuals to an asylum. It could help a local metropolitan union to reduce its expenditure on such people by 60%. However, in 1889, 14% (11,827) of pauper lunatics in England and Wales outside London were still confined in workhouses, while 8% remained at home, and 78% were placed in county asylums. A vigorous programme of asylum building meant that, in London, only 2% (275) were accommodated in workhouses. The majority (96%) were placed in asylums. So, outside London at least, the workhouse continued to be a substantial provider of shelter for the mentally ill up until the First World War.

From then until the Second World War very little seems to have been written on the subject. Even George Orwell does not seem to have noticed any madness in his perambulations through the world of the destitute in the London and Paris of the 1930s. To be fair, he was at pains to stress the ordinariness of destitute men who found themselves the victims of a callous economic system. However, he does seem to have noticed that 'there is an imbecile in every collection of tramps' (27)—presumably those who would today be regarded as having learning/intellectual difficulties.

The closure of hostels in London

Much was written both for, and against, the closure of mental hospitals from the 1960s to the 1980s. Over the years from 1970 to 1995, a parallel (but silent) process of institutional dissolution occurred, the closure of the traditional hostels for the homeless. These included not only the Department of Health and Social Security reception centres/resettlement units but also Salvation Army Hostels, Rowton Houses, and night shelters. There was no overall plan and the closures took place for a variety of reasons, similar in many ways to those leading to the closures of mental hospitals. Standards had obviously slipped in the Rowton Houses since their Victorian heyday. Three such hostels precipitated a crisis in 1983 (28) when local authorities had started to pressure owners into improving the conditions in their squalid establishments. The company owning the Rowton Houses promptly threatened to evict all the residents. The situation was resolved when the local authorities responsible bought up the three hostels in their area, planning to close them within 5 years.

Nationally, the Department of Health and Social Security had had a policy of closing resettlement units for some time (29). It was felt that centrally funded institutions were inappropriate in the age of local social service and housing departments. Large institutions were also seen as unsuitable places for influencing people 'to lead a more settled way of life'. So, national policy changed. It was decided to close all resettlement units and to replace them with local initiatives.

In London in 1981 there were 9751 bed spaces in the wider network of direct access hostels, with 6000 in large, traditional hostels for the homeless. The London Boroughs Association described them as 'at once a resource and a problem' (30). A resource because of the shelter provided, a problem because of the often-appalling physical conditions and catastrophically inadequate staffing. This same report recommended the opening of 600 beds yearly to replace the old hostels but noted that such schemes faced financial and planning difficulties. Belated enforcement of fire regulations led to the contraction of some hostels and the closure of others. By 1985, the numbers of direct access bed spaces had declined to 4885 and by 1990 to around 2000 (31). In September 1995, the closure of the Camberwell Spike alone, the largest of the old National Assistance Board reception centres, resulted in the loss of 900 bed spaces. Direct access reprovision for this institution amounted to only 62 bed spaces, the rest being in specialist, referral-only, units. The result was a 75% loss of direct access hostel spaces during the 1980s.

A system of grants was offered to alternative providers, which included the voluntary sector and local authorities. There was to be no overall reduction in funding, but potential service providers were slow in coming forward. Eight such schemes had been approved by 1989, but none had sufficient bed spaces to replace the units due for closure. The resettlement agency thus found itself double funding and the closure policy stalled (32). There now remained 1796 beds in resettlement units, 670 of which were in London, the national focus of the homelessness problem.

Psychiatry and the homeless mentally ill

The first to address the issue directly was a German psychiatrist, K. Wilmanns (33). Vagrancy was an offence and those who could not demonstrate that they had a home to go to could be arrested and confined in the police workhouse. He noticed that many of the homeless so detained were transferred to his hospital from the local workhouse. In his survey of these patients, he found 120 homeless men and women who had been committed with a diagnosis of schizophrenia. American workers (34) suggested in 1939 that the prevalence of mental illness was higher in what they called 'the disorganized community'.

Two roughly equivalent descriptive classifications of the homeless were constructed, both breaking down the population into itinerant workers, itinerant non-workers, and non-itinerant non-workers. Anderson, an American sociologist, called these, respectively, hobos, tramps, and bums (35). Thirty years later, a French psychiatrist, described such groups as 'errants, vagabonds and clochards' (36). Neither of these somewhat arbitrary classifications served to clarify matters to any helpful degree and indeed may well have contributed to further stigmatizing attitudes.

A more grounded approach was taken by the redoubtable Mrs Solenberger, the director for the central district of Chicago's Bureau of Charities in the early twentieth century. Her 'One thousand homeless men' study represents data collected in the South Side of Chicago in the course of the daily work of her charitable office. She worked tirelessly accumulating information about those homeless lodging house residents who applied to her bureau for assistance (37)—and even sought advice from Adolf Meyer, the professor of psychiatry at Johns Hopkins University. This study was prompted by the awareness of an increase in the numbers of homeless men, and the explosion of cheap lodging houses for their accommodation 'in every large city in the country'. There were certainly a lot in Chicago—nearly 80,000 men in lodging houses during the winter months of 1908. She created her own typology of homelessness, which was more descriptive and, to my mind, more helpful than those mentioned previously:

- Self-supporting—those who were able to work, usually in seasonal work, and were, effectively, using lodging houses as cheap hotels for short periods.
- Temporarily dependent—runaways, victims of accidents, sudden unemployment, or recent immigrants with no command of the language.
- Chronically dependent—those disabled by chronic health problems, alcoholism, leaning difficulties, or mental illness.
- Parasitic—'criminals; impostors; begging letter writers; confidence men, etc.'

Those with 'insanity' were deemed to be part of the chronically dependent group and she devoted an entire chapter of her study to 'the insane, feeble-minded and epileptic'. They constituted 89 out of her total of 1000 men. Among other themes that persist to the present day, she asked 'whether they are homeless and vagrant because of their insanity, or insane because of their vagrancy'. She concluded, on the basis of her experiences, that 'insanity acts as a cause of vagrancy more often than vagrancy as a cause of insanity'. And, interestingly, that half of her group of men with insanity were 'men of refinement'. She did, however, add the reservation that as her interviewers at the bureau were not medically or psychologically trained, consequently they had probably missed a number of men with mental health problems, significantly underestimating the problem.

She also gave a clear account of what, in more recent times, has been called 'Greyhound therapy'—the practice of buying a mentally ill person a ticket for travel so that they don't stay in your area, where you would otherwise have to make provision for them. She notes 'one lad who had wandered about the country for 3 months—frequently travelling on tickets furnished by county poor relief agents who were anxious to avoid the expense of his care'. He had, after a few days in Chicago, became agitated and paranoid and had to be committed to an institution. Indeed, the fact that she seems to have been quite familiar with the process of involuntary hospitalization suggests a significant incidence of severe mental health problems within her homeless clientele.

She also noted the unpleasant propensity of the imposition of laws against homelessness in certain areas prompting the relocation of homeless people to adjacent areas, without any alleviation of the problem for the homeless people concerned.

Thirty years later, another Chicago study found that one in twenty of a random sample of homeless men was recommended for immediate transfer to 'the Psychopathic Hospital', with another 10% classified as 'pre-psychotic, potentially psychotic or question of psychosis' (38). Even given the vagueness of these quasi-diagnostic groupings, these findings again suggest a high rate of psychosis for this group of homeless men. And this study is, I think, the first that mentions the process of 'shelterization'—when someone becomes so used to the habits of the homeless shelter and its associated routines that, however unpleasant their situation, they find it hard to leave.

Bogue, a sociologist, looked at the inhabitants of Chicago's skid row in 1956 (39). Although alcoholism was his main focus (and, indeed, he found a very high rate of alcoholism), his non-psychiatric researchers noted that roughly one in five of the men he interviewed were suffering from 'mental illness' or 'mental and nervous trouble' of some description. He commented that voluntary agencies should be able to 'recommend a psychiatric examination' in order to provide this section of the destitute population with an appropriate service.

In the UK, post-war interest started with a review by Stuart Whiteley of a series of acute male admissions to a South London observation ward (40). Eight per cent were of no fixed abode, a much higher proportion than would be expected from the numbers of homeless men in the local area. Around a third were diagnosed as suffering from schizophrenia, mostly with delusional ideas—and those suffering from schizophrenia tended to be living in the most impoverished circumstances, such as night shelters, rather than common lodging houses. His view was that, for his patients, 'the main cause [of homelessness] is the personality defect which does not allow him to form relationships'. He went on to recommend that:

> When he falls ill, the down and out should, ideally, be treated in a separate institution … where his environment was as near his normal habitat as possible. He would then be more likely to stay … it would be an advantage if he could be committed to the institution for a definite period, and as so many appear in court, this should be possible.

By the time a pair of Birmingham psychiatrists conducted a survey of admissions in 1966 (41), 23% of their acute male admissions were of no fixed abode and this proportion was rising fast compared with non-urban hospitals in their region. Of these homeless patients, 74% had had previous hospital admissions, prompting the authors to comment that 'Their plight is evidence that the initial enthusiasm evoked by the new act [1959 Mental Health Act] for the discharge of psychotics into the community was premature and has resulted in the community services being overwhelmed'. However, they also recognized that this was not the whole story, and that there was also a housing deficit created by the closure of 'lodgings available for persons of no fixed abode'. Their description of the themes of inadequate community care and lack of low-cost housing was prescient, but their recommendation of further research did not bear fruit. These first studies of those who had actually managed to come to the attention of hospital services were followed by more epidemiological surveys of hostel populations. Griffith Edwards' team interviewed the entire population of the Camberwell Reception Centre (18). He found 25% had been admitted to a mental hospital—equal to the proportion of those with alcohol problems. This was the first epidemiological evidence to challenge the stereotype of the homeless man as necessarily a drinker.

This evidence for a high prevalence of mental illness in the homeless population was confirmed by a doorstep survey of two Salvation Army hostels for men (42): 15% were diagnosed with schizophrenia and 50% as being personality disordered. Hospital and community care was blamed: 'The small number of schizophrenics who were receiving treatment suggests both a failure of community care and inappropriately early discharge.' These sentiments were echoed by Crossley and Denmark (43) in another survey of a Salvation Army hostel with a high prevalence of psychotic illness: 'It is surely not right to unload onto a voluntary organization, whose function is not to act as a therapeutic agency, patients who still need community care.'

Robin Priest's 1976 Edinburgh survey approached the problem in a more sophisticated fashion, comparing a general survey of the homeless population with those who were actually admitted to hospital (44).

He confirmed an unusually high prevalence of schizophrenia in the homeless population (32%) but, surprisingly, found that this prevalence was greater

Table 2.1 British hostel surveys

Survey (reference)	Diagnosis (%)			
	Schizophrenia	Alcoholism	Affective disorder	Personality disorder
Edwards et al. (1968) (18)	24	25	N/K	N/K
Crossley and Denmark (1969) (43)	20	N/K	N/K	66
Priest (1976) (44)	32	18	5	18
Lodge Patch (1971) (42)	15	N/K	8	31
Tidmarsh (1972) (17)	~25	25	5	17
Timms and Fry (1989) (45)	37	9	14	11

N/K, not known.

in the general homeless population than in the subgroup that had presented to psychiatric services for treatment. The population outside hospital were more likely to suffer from schizophrenia than those in hospital. This finding suggested that, compared with men with other diagnoses, those with schizophrenia tended not to find their way to treatment (Table 2.1).

In fact, over the majority of the post-war period, successive surveys in British hostels, night shelters, and prisons have demonstrated the presence of large numbers of homeless men with schizophrenia and alcohol problems. There has been a curious absence of those anxiety and depressive disorders that characterize the bulk of the psychiatric symptomatology presenting in a general practice setting. This may have been due to more extreme psychopathology tending to mask more affective complaints. My own survey of a Salvation Army Hostel in 1989 (45) suggested that nothing very much had changed over the preceding 30 years.

Epilogue

Homeless people, and thus the homeless mentally ill, have been a constant feature of the English social landscape since the fourteenth century—and for at least a century in the US. The mechanisms for dealing with the problem have been moulded by the changing tempers of the times, but have swung between ideas of punishment and ideas of help. Although sparsely documented, the presence of the mentally ill in those institutions set up to deal with the homeless and indigent has been a recurrent theme since the latter part of the seventeenth century. Disquiet about this situation was intermittently expressed by various committees from the mid-nineteenth century. Even during this period, the heyday of the Victorian asylum, it appears that substantial numbers of the mentally ill were still accommodated in Poor Law institutions rather than psychiatric ones. What evidence there is suggests that the essentials of the situation have remained substantially unchanged over the 150 years of the asylum's ascendancy, the era of psychiatric deinstitutionalization, and latterly the era of 'community care'. Even when its resources were apparently greater, certainly in terms of bed numbers, psychiatry never really got to grips with the substantial numbers of people with severe, long-term psychiatric illness who were accommodated in institutions for the indigent and homeless (46).

The setting up of the Central London Homeless Mentally Ill Initiative in 1995 (47) (a number of dedicated mental health services for homeless people), was prompted by the increasing visibility of homeless people with mental illness on the streets. Although many felt that this was a consequence of the closure of psychiatric units (which had been going since 1955), it almost certainly had more to do with the hostel closures of the 1980s, described previously. Homeless people with severe mental illness are clearly vulnerable both to shortfalls in healthcare and to inadequacies in other systems, such as housing. And, historically, public sympathy has been counter-balanced by both a sense of intimidation and the wish to place such people away, out of sight. Whether it is in an asylum, a workhouse, or a prison has not really seemed to matter.

Over the last 20 years, the efforts to bring psychiatric and social care to a range of homeless milieux has produced a range of high-quality and effective projects. However, the experience of the last 10 years suggests that their effectiveness has been severely limited by the reductions of generic provisions for social housing and financial benefits, exemplified in the UK by more stringent tests of incapacity for work (48). As in previous historical eras, economics has been a determining factor in this field. Decent mental (and physical) healthcare for homeless people should, indeed, be an obligation for all health services. But, on its own, it is often not enough to resolve the homelessness that, all too frequently, has resulted from severe mental illness.

References

1. Cohen CI, Thomson KS. Homeless mentally ill or mentally ill homeless? Am J Psychiatry. 2002;149(6):816–823.
2. Roderick P, Victor C, Connelly C. Is housing a public health issue? BMJ. 1991;302(6769):157–160.
3. Dickens C. Night Walks. London: Penguin Books Ltd; 2010.
4. Beier AL. Masterless Men: The Vagrancy Problem in England 1560–1610. London: Methuen; 1987.
5. Southern RW. Western Society and the Church in the Middle Ages. London: Penguin; 1970.

6. **Briggs C.** English serfdom, c.1200–c.1350: towards an institutionalist analysis. In: **Cavaciocchi S** (Ed), Schiavitù e servaggio nell'economia europea secc. XI–XVIII [Serfdom and Slavery in the European Economy 11th–18th Centuries]. Florence: Firenze University Press; 2014:13–32.

7. **Trevelyan GM.** English Social History. London: Penguin; 1986.

8. **Clark, G.** The long march of history: farm wages, population and economic growth, England 1209–1869. Available from: https://www.econstor.eu/bitstream/10419/31320/1/50512257X.pdf.

9. **Power E, Tawney RH** (Eds). Tudor Economic Documents, Vol. II. London: Longmans; 1924.

10. **De Schweinitz K.** England's Road to Social Security. Pittsburgh, PA: University of Pennsylvania Press; 1943.

11. **Senior NW.** Poor Law Commissioners' Report of 1834. Copy of the Report made in 1834 by the Commissioners for Inquiring into the Administration and Practical Operation of the Poor Laws. Presented to both Houses of Parliament by Command of His Majesty. London: Printed for H.M. Stationery Office by Darling and Son, 1905. Available from: https://oll.libertyfund.org/titles/1461.

12. **Leach J, Wing J.** Helping Destitute Men. London: Tavistock; 1980:2–4.

13. **Booth W.** In Darkest England and the Way Out. New York: Funk & Wagnalls; 1890.

14. **Higginbotham P.** Rowton Houses. 2019. Available from: http://www.workhouses.org.uk/Rowton/.

15. **Tidmarsh D, Wood S.** Report to DHSS on research at Camberwell Reception Centre (Unpublished report). London: Institute of Psychiatry; 1986.

16. **Ollendorff RJV, Morgan A.** Survey of residents in Camberwell Reception Centre (Unpublished report to the National Assistance Board). London; 1968.

17. **Tidmarsh D.** Services for the destitute: Camberwell reception centre. In: **Wing J, Hailey AM** (Eds), Evaluating a Community Psychiatric Service: The Camberwell Register, 1964–1971. Oxford: Oxford University Press; 1972:73–76.

18. **Edwards G, Williamson V, Hawker A, Hensman C, Postoyan S.** Census of a reception centre. Br J Psychiatry. 1968;**114**(513):1031–1039.

19. **MacDonald M.** Mystical Bedlam. Cambridge: Cambridge University Press; 1981.

20. **Allderidge P.** Hospitals, madhouses and asylums: cycles in the care of the insane. Br J Psychiatry. 1979;**134**:321–333.

21. **Porter R.** Mind-Forged Manacles: A History of Madness in England from the Restoration to the Regency. London: Penguin; 1989.

22. **Parry-Jones WL.** The Trade in Lunacy: A Study of Private Madhouses in England in the Eighteenth and Nineteenth Centuries. London: Routledge & Kegan Paul Ltd; 1971.

23. **Paul GO.** Observations on the Subject of Lunatic Asylums. Gloucester: Private Publication; 1812.

24. **Myers ED.** Workhouse or asylum: the nineteenth century battle for the care of the pauper insane. Psychiatr Bull. 1998;**22**(9):575–577.

25. **Webb S, Webb B.** English Poor Law History: Part 2: The Last Hundred Years. London: Longmans, Green & Co; 1929.

26. **Cochrane D.** 'Humane, economical, and medically wise': the LCC as administrators of Victorian lunacy policy. In: **Bynum WF, Porter R, Shepherd M** (Eds), The Anatomy of

Madness: Essays in the History of Psychiatry. Volume 3, The Asylum and its Psychiatry. London: Routledge; 1988:247–272.

27. **Orwell G.** Down and Out in Paris and London. London: Victor Gollanz; 1933.

28. **Greater London Council.** Four Victorian Hostels. London: Greater London Council; 1986.

29. **Hewetson J.** Homeless people as an at-risk group. Proc R Soc Med. 1975;**68**(1):9–13.

30. **Greater London Council, London Boroughs Association.** Report of a Joint Working Party on Provision in London for People Without a Settled Way of Living. Hostels for Single Homeless in London. London: London Boroughs Association; 1981.

31. **Harrison M, Chandler R, Green G.** Hostels in London: A Statistical Overview. London: Resource Information Service; 1992.

32. **The Resettlement Units Executive Agency.** Annual Report and Financial Statement 1990/91. London: HMSO; 1991.

33. **Wilmanns K.** Zur psychopathologie des landstreichers: eine klinishe studie. Leipzig: Johann Ambrosius Barth; 1906.

34. **Faris RE, Dunham HW.** Mental Disorders in Urban Areas: An Ecological Study of Schizophrenia and Other Psychoses. Chicago, IL: University of Chicago Press; 1959.

35. **Anderson N.** The Hobo: The Sociology of the Homeless Man. Chicago, IL: University of Chicago Press; 1923.

36. **Vexliard A.** Le Clochard: Etude de Psycholgie Sociale. Paris: Desclee de Brouwer; 1953.

37. **Solenberger AW.** A Thousand Homeless Men. New York: Charities Publication Committee; 1911.

38. **Sutherland EH, Locke HJ.** Twenty Thousand Homeless Men: A Study of Unemployed Men in the Chicago Shelters. Chicago, IL: JB Lippincott; 1936.

39. **Bogue DJ.** Skid Row in American Cities. Chicago, IL: Community and Family Study Centre, University of Chicago; 1963.

40. **Whiteley JS.** Down and out in London: mental illness in the lower social groups. Lancet. 1955;**2**(6890):608–610.

41. **Berry C, Orwin A.** No fixed abode: a survey of mental hospital admissions. Br J Psychiatry. 1966;**112**(491):1019–1025.

42. **Lodge Patch IC.** Homeless men in London. I. Demographic findings in a lodging house sample. Br J Psychiatry. 1971;**118**(544):313–317.

43. **Crossley B, Denmark JC.** Community care—a study of the psychiatric morbidity of a Salvation Army hostel. Br J Sociol. 1969;**20**(4):443–449.

44. **Priest RG.** The homeless person and the psychiatric services: an Edinburgh survey. Br J Psychiatry. 1976;**128**:128–136.

45. **Timms P, Fry A.** Homelessness and mental illness. Health Trends. 1989;**21**(3):70–71.

46. **Craig T, Timms PW.** Out of the wards and onto the streets? Deinstitutionalisation and homelessness in Britain. J Ment Health. 1992;**1**(3):265–275.

47. **Craig T, Bayliss E, Klein O,** et al. The Homeless Mentally Ill Initiative: Evaluation of Four Clinical Teams. London: Department of Health; 1995.

48. **Abdul-Hamid WK, Bui K.** Psychiatry, homeless patients and welfare reforms: Historical links and chains. Int J Soc Psychiatry. 2014;**60**(1):71–74.

Section 2

International perspective

Chapter 3

Continental European experience: Germany

Stefanie Schreiter, Stefan Gutwinski,
Hans-Joachim Salize, and Wulf Rössler

Prevalence and development of homelessness in Germany

Historical background

For many centuries, wayfarers, mendicants, vagabonds, and artisans and merchants on the road were part of different cultural groups in European societies (1). At the turn of the twentieth century, increasing industrialization, urbanization, and the growing impact of the psychiatric belief system changed society's view on homeless people and put homelessness in the context of mental illnesses such as 'dementia praecox' (2). The German researcher Wilmanns (2–6) interpreted homelessness as a multifactorial phenomenon influenced by other factors such as mental illness and substance use. In the 1920s, homelessness was integrated into the concept of psychopathy as a 'characterological inferiority' (7). Kurt Schneider characterized homeless people as suffering from an 'inner restlessness' and an 'addiction to change and new things' and called them 'unsteady psychopaths' (8). These developments cleared the way for the Nazi prosecution of homeless people in the 1930s and 1940s, who were now categorized as 'asocial' (9). In this period, at least 10,000 homeless people were sterilized or taken to concentration camps, and many were executed or died under terrible living conditions (10,11, p. 61). Even in the first years of the German post-war period, some scientific publications still characterized homelessness as a defect of character (10,12,13).

In the 1970s, the interpretation of homelessness changed in that it was seen rather as a result of poverty and social exclusion (1). Additionally, during this period, psychiatric institutions in Germany experienced a far-reaching transformation from a system of hospitalization of patients in large institutions to community-based psychiatry (14). Homelessness became increasingly accepted as a 'chosen form of living' by institutions rather than seen as a complex societal problem (14).

In the 1990s, the increasing rates of unemployment and the rise of rental fees as well as developments caused by the German reunification led to a rapid increase of homeless people in Germany (1). This process was followed by an increasing scientific interest in the field of psychiatric and epidemiological research in Germany. Fichter, among others, conducted mostly descriptive studies among homeless populations in different German cities such as Munich (15–22). These developments were supported by the process of 'deinstitutionalization' as a result of the reform of the mental healthcare system after 1975 and the increasing influence of social psychiatry (14). After a decreasing interest in the research community after the turn of the century, increasing numbers of homeless people in psychiatric hospitals and emergency departments have led again to growing research attention on the social problem of homelessness in Germany by other research groups (23–28).

Current developments of homelessness in Germany

Unfortunately, there is no official register, survey, or statistic of homeless people in Germany. Initiatives to promote a homeless census failed with respective governments due to reasons of high cost and workload. Because of increasing political pressure, a first homeless count will be conducted solely in the city of Berlin 2020 (29). Therefore, the numbers of homeless people in Germany are based on estimation by the non-governmental working group on help for the homeless (Bundesarbeitsgemeinschaft Wohnungslosenhilfe). For the year 2018, an estimated number of 678,000 people were considered as homeless, including 441,000 approved asylum seekers, which is an estimated increase of 4% compared to 2017 (Fig. 3.1) (30). Excluding asylum seekers (for reasons of missing sociodemographic data), 41,000 people in Germany were living rough or on the streets (30); 30% were living with a homeless partner and/or children (30). The number of children and homeless youth under the age of 18 years is estimated to be 19,000 (8%) (Fig. 3.2) (30). Additionally, 27% (59,000) of all homeless people in Germany (excluding approved asylum seekers) are estimated to be female, which represents an increase in homeless women and families living on the streets (30).

For the year 2017, homeless people from other European Union countries accounted for 15% (400,000) of the total, many of them living rough or on the streets. Most notably in urban areas such as Berlin, around 50% of people living on the streets were born in other European Union countries (31), which often leads to the misinterpretation that homelessness is a result of increased immigration from mainly eastern European Union countries. Leading structural

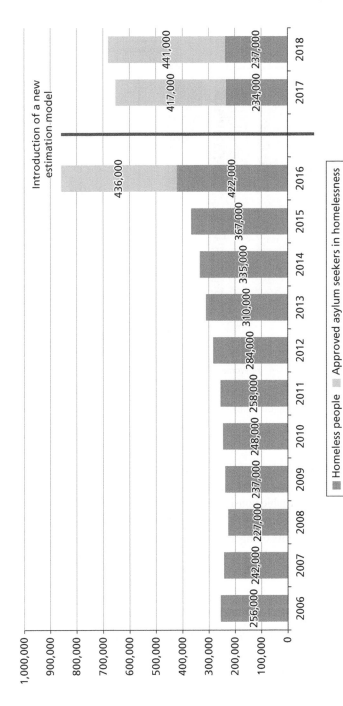

Fig. 3.1 Estimated numbers of homeless people in Germany by the Federal Working Group on Homelessness. Adapted from Bundesarbeitsgemeinschaft Wohnungslosenhilfe e.V., copyright (2021) www.bagw.de.

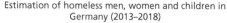

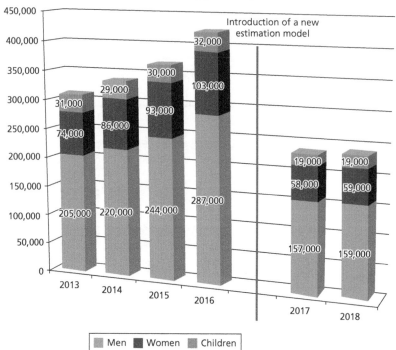

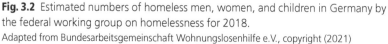

Fig. 3.2 Estimated numbers of homeless men, women, and children in Germany by the federal working group on homelessness for 2018.
Adapted from Bundesarbeitsgemeinschaft Wohnungslosenhilfe e.V., copyright (2021) www.bagw.de.

causes of growing numbers of the homeless in Germany are the shortage of affordable housing space, a shortage of welfare housing, and the consolidation of poverty (31). Affordable housing for low-income households and people receiving welfare payments in urban areas is especially scarce (31). In the year 2015, the rate of tenants living at the risk of poverty was 29%, which affected mainly young adults under 35 years (31). In particular, housing for single-person households (17.2 million) is more and more needed (31).

Mental health and homelessness in Germany

Studies on prevalence rates of mental illness among homeless people in Germany were firstly conducted in the 1980s and mostly in the 1990s; Table 3.1 gives a detailed description of studies among homeless people in Germany. Based on a recent meta-analysis on the prevalence of mental illness among homeless people in Germany, the pooled 1-month prevalence of any mental

Table 3.1 Details of included studies

Study	When data collected	Where data collected	Sample type	Definition of homelessness	Recruitment strategy	Sample size	Tools	Diagnostic criteria	Mean age (years)	Women (%)	Professional interviews	Participation rate (%)
Fichter, 1996, 1997, 1999 (32, 37, 39); Meller, 2000 (29)	1989 to 90	Munich	Representative random sample	No home for at least 30 days before interview	Common locations for the homeless	146	DIS-III, MMSE	DIS-III	43	0	No[+2]	85
Greifenhagen 1997, (31); Mesller,. 2000 (29)	1989 to 90	Munich	Representative random sample	No home for at least 30 days before interview	Common locations for the homeless	32	DIS-III, MMSE	DIS-III	35.5	100	No[+2]	89
Reker, 1997 (26)	1990	Munster	Data collected on all residents of a shelter for homeless men	>3 months living in city shelter	City shelter for homeless men	52	Semi-structured interview, GAF	ICD-10	45.0	0	Yes	78.8
Podschus, 1995 (28); Dufeu, 1996 (40)	1993 to 94	Berlin	Random smaple	Section 72 of the German FWA	City mission soup kitchen	72	CIDI[+1]MMSE, GAF	ICD-10	45.0	0	Yes	78.8

(continued)

Table 3.1 Continued

Study	When data collected	Where data collected	Sample type	Definition of homelessness	Recruitment strategy	Sample size	Tools	Diagnostic criteria	Mean age (years)	Women (%)	Professional interviews	Participation rate (%)
Podschus, 1995 (28); Dufeu, 1996 (40)	1993 to 94	Berlin	Random sample	Section 72 of the German FWA	City mission soup kitchen	72	CIDI[+1], MMSE, GAF	ICD-10	40.5	0	Not stated	85
Fichler, 2006 (36); Quadieg, 2007 (27)	1994 to 96	Munich	Data collected longitudinally on all homeless people	(1) Accommodation in home of friends or relatives, (2) accommodation at emergency shelter, (3) accommodation in unusual places	Recruitment in line with accommodation	129	SCUD, MMSE, FPI-R, GAF, SCL-90-R	SCUD, MMSE, DSM-IV	44.4	15.5	Not stated	Not stated
Fichter, 1999, 2000, 2001, 2003, 2005, (11, 33 to 35, 38)	1994 to 96	Munich	Representative random sample	No home fo atleast 30 days before interview	Common locations for the homeless	265	SCID, MMSE	DSM-IV	44.7	0	No[+2]	88

Study	Year	City	Sampling	Definition of homelessness	Recruitment location	N	Instruments	Classification	ICD-10 / DSM-IV %	%	Representative	%
Vollum 2004 (12, 21)	1996	Dontmund	Representative random sample	Literally homeless as difined by Rossi (e2)	Adivice centers and city shelters	82	CID+1, AMDP	ICD-10	41.4	0	Yes	81.5
Salize, 2001, 2002 (23, 24, e3)	1997 to 99	Mannheim	Representative random sample	No room or home	Common locations for the homeless	102	SCID, MLDL	DSM-IV	40.0	13.7	Not stated	Not stated
Torchalla, 2004 (22)	2001	Tubingen	Data collected on al homeless women	Section 72 of the German FWA	Advice centers, recruitment workers	17	SCID, BeLP	DSM-IV	29	100	Not stated	77.3
Lagnle, 2005 (30)	2002 to 03	Tubingen	Data collected on all appropriate individuals	Section 72 of the German FWA	Common locations for the homeless	91	SCID, BML, MMSE, MWT-B, WAIS-R, GAF, BeLP	ICD-10	40.0	0	Yes	60.3
Bronner, 2013 (e1); Jahn 2014 (2)	2010 to 12	Munich	Representative random sample	Residents of homeless shellers	Facilities for the homeless	232	SCID, MALT, BDI, mmini ICF, APP, SF-36, B-L, CGI, MMSE, WAIS	DSM-IV	48.1 20.7	20.7	Not stated	55

[1]+Parts on dependency disorders and psychosomatic disorder +²Trained Lyapeople

AMDP, Working Group for Methods and Documentation in Psychiatry (Arbetsgemenischaftfur Mthods and Dokumentation in der Psychatre); BDI: Beck Depression in wentory: BeLP: Berlin Quality of Life Profile (Berliner Lebens qualifiat profil): B-L Complaints

List (Beschwerderlist): BML: Brunswick List of Feature (Braunschwe Markimalista) for chronic, multiply-impaired alcoholics FQA: Federal Welfare Act: CGI: Clinical Global Impression Scale; CIDI: Composite International Diagnostic Interview; DIS: Diagnostic Interview Schedule; FPI-R: Freiburg Personality Interveory (Frieburger Personlickisnestar) – Rewision; GAF: Global Assesment of Functioning; WAIS-R; Wechster Adult Inteligence Scale – Revision; MALT: Munich Alcoholism Test (Muncher Alcoholism mushetest); Mini-CF-APP: Mini-ICF-APP Social Functiong Scale; MLDL Munich Quality of Life List (Munchener Lebensqualits-Dimensionen-Laste); MMSE: Mini-Mental Status Examination; MWT-B Multiple-choice Vocabulary Test (Mehrfachwahl-Wortschatztest), version B; SCID: Structured Clinical Interview for DSM; SCL 90-R: Symptom checklist 90 – Revised; SF-36; Short Form Health Survey; WAIS: Wecher Adult Intelgence Scale.

illness was 77.5% (95% confidence interval (CI): 72.4%; 82.3%), which is 3.8 times higher than Germany's general population (19.8% 1-month prevalence rate of *Diagnostic and Statistical Manual of Mental Disorders*, fourth edition, disorders according to the German Health Interview and Examination Survey for Adults, Studie zur Gesundheit Erwachsener in Deutschland (DEGS1)) (23,32). Substance-related disorders were the most common type of mental illness with a pooled prevalence of 60.9% (95% CI: 53.1%; 68.5%) and 21 times higher than in the general population (2.9%) (23,32). The authors reported a prevalence of alcohol dependency 1.5 times higher than in other Western countries (including the US, the UK, and Australia) (55.4% (95% CI: 49.2%; 61.5%) versus 37.9% (95% CI: 27.8%; 48.0%)) (23,33). High rates of alcohol use among homeless people in Germany are partly rooted in a social support or healthcare system which is often based on abstinence in contrast to evidence-based Housing First concepts (34), making it difficult for those particularly at risk to access the mental healthcare system (e.g. people with missing health insurance, people with experienced stigma or negative attitudes towards the mental healthcare system). Additionally, the availability and the price regulation of drugs in Germany result in comparatively low prices for alcoholic beverages. These structural barriers negatively add to the individual risk of being drawn towards substance use as a major coping strategy among those who are marginalized (35). Prevalence rates of psychotic illnesses (8.3%) were similar and drug dependency (13.9%) lower than in other Western countries (23).

Homeless women constitute an especially neglected subgroup in the field of research as well as models of care in Germany. Only 131 (10.7%) of the total of 1220 homeless people in German studies were female (Table 3.1) (23). A meta-analysis found particularly high prevalence rates in German studies involving only female homeless people for all mental disorders (83.3% (95% CI: 56.9%; 100.0%) versus male: 76.6% (95% CI: 68.7%; 83.7%)), psychotic illnesses (23.1% (95% CI: 5.0%; 47.7%) versus male: 7.6% (95% CI: 5.8%; 9.7%)), and drug dependency (24.6% (95% CI: 17.4%; 32.6%) versus male: 10.1% (95% CI: 4.8%; 16.9%)). Homeless women are a subgroup who may be confronted with particular difficulties: estimated numbers of unreported homeless women are particularly high, as women are less likely to live directly on the streets but to find passing shelter in apartments of friends or acquaintances. As a consequence, their homelessness is more likely to go undetected, and they often do not use the available support system (36). As a result, homeless women are more frequently confronted with difficulties such as dependency on others and lack of safeguards (36). Because study sampling focused mainly on homeless people on the streets or in homeless shelters, homeless women have not yet been sufficiently focused on in the field of research.

In the most recent German study among a homeless population in Germany (Seewolf Studie, 2012), the lifetime prevalence of any mental disorder was 93.3%, which equals the rate from earlier studies from Munich in the 1990s (28,37); the 1-month prevalence rate was 74.0% (28). Thus, the psychiatric healthcare system has been increasingly confronted with homeless people with mental illness. A recent survey conducted among psychiatric inpatients in one of the largest psychiatric centres in Berlin showed a rate of homeless patients of 13.0%, and 18.3% living in some form of socio-therapeutic facility (38). Patients without their own apartment were more likely to be male, younger, and have a lower level of education (38). Homeless patients were diagnosed with a substance use disorder significantly more often (74.2%); psychotic disorders were the highest among homeless patients (29.0%) (38). In contrast to numbers from North America and other Western countries, length of hospital stay was significantly shorter in homeless patients compared to stably housed patients (39,40). In a prospective cohort study among psychiatric inpatients across European countries, homelessness predicted a length of hospital stay in opposite directions in different countries: compared to other patients, homeless patients stayed a longer time in hospitals in Belgium, the UK, and Italy, but a shorter time in Germany (40). Homeless patients might not have the resources and support to seek help and benefit from hospital-based care, especially if barriers are high such as in Germany, which might explain differences in length of hospital-based treatment.

System of care for homeless people with mental illness in Germany

Germany has an elaborate and statutory social security system, including a public healthcare system, unemployment security system, and a pension system. Additionally, Germany has a long tradition of social support by the Catholic and Protestant Churches, with a broad network of social support, especially for unemployed people, the elderly, and children.

The healthcare system in Germany is a universal multipayer system, in which approximately 85% of citizens pay public health insurance (Gesetzliche Krankenversicherung) and others have private health insurance. Membership in health insurance is mandatory for the population. The healthcare insurance contribution is 50% paid by employees and 50% by employers. For people with no income, such as homeless people, the municipalities contribute to health insurance. All citizens are entitled to benefit from the public healthcare system (including European Union migrants). This includes a broad range of specific medical psychiatric care including outpatient services from psychiatrists and psychotherapists in office practice, psychiatric outpatient departments, hospital treatment, and other mental health services. Additionally, there are a wide range of specialized forms of accommodation and occupation services for people with severe mental illness financed by social welfare.

The German system of social support offers a minimum of social benefits, which include rent for a (cheap) flat, a basic income (e.g. Arbeitslosengeld, Grundsicherung (41,42)) in case of unemployment, chronic illness, or disability, and monetary support for children (e.g. Kindergeld). This social support system is financed by the contribution of employees and employers and state taxes. Contributions are obligatory for both employees and employers.

The pension insurance is also a mandatory system for all employees and employers. It is based on a generation agreement, which comprises the pension payment for the elderly financed by the working population, who themselves will receive a pension from the contribution of the next generation. The amount of pension relies on the amount of contribution from each person, although there is a minimum pension for all, including people with disabilities or lifelong unemployment.

Although the social support system seems to cover and reach all citizens, there are still people not receiving health insurance or social benefits (e.g. Grundsicherung or pension). There are various reasons which lead to exclusion from the social welfare system, such as a complicated administrative application process (especially for social benefits), mental disorders (intelligence deficits, substance use, etc.), rejecting the support of institutions (mostly due to traumatic experience with state institutions in the past), immigration status, and others (43,44). One crucial institutional reason for exclusion lies in responsibilities not being clearly defined among institutions (43,45). One example is the lack of clarity concerning obligations for people with mental disorders, who are eligible to receive support according to the common law codebook 5, sections §67 or §53—but who are sometimes sent from one agency to another, finally not receiving any support. Therefore, a considerable number of people fall through the cracks of the social welfare system and are at risk of becoming homeless. Still, even in case of homelessness, the respective federal state is obliged to provide a 'sufficient' housing substitute, mostly comprising homeless shelters. Due to the previously mentioned lack of clarity regarding responsibilities, often people with mental illness end up in homeless shelters instead of specialized housing. Other reasons are barriers in the form of restrictions regarding behaviour or lifestyle or substance use and the shortage of available housing in urbanized areas. Furthermore, specialized housing for people with severe mental illness in Germany is generally broadly available, but not always in line with internationally accepted concepts of supported housing, which provides housing independently from additional support adapted to the individual's needs and resources (46). Internationally accepted and positively evaluated concepts regarding care models for homeless people with mental health problems such as assertive community treatment (47) are difficult to establish due to complex and different responsibilities among various providers, agencies, and institutions.

For people excluded from the social system, there is a broad range of social support with shallow barriers from non-governmental providers, especially offered by the social welfare agencies of the Catholic and Protestant Churches. This support system comprises mostly direct help such as free soup kitchens, shelters, or free medical outreach treatment. In most of the larger German cities, there are well-organized systems, such as the 'Berliner Kältehilfe' (48) which collects and publishes a list of homeless support facilities in Berlin including healthcare, sleeping, food, and social contact for homeless people. This information is available through booklets or online, as well as via a mobile app (48). The 'Kältehilfe' also provides a bus offering support for homeless people during winter times in cooperation with shelters in Berlin. Still, there are a large number of homeless people particularly with additional challenges such as mental health problems or language barriers who are not receiving adequate support.

Current research activities in the field of housing for homeless people with mental illness in Germany

Historically, there is a long-standing support system for homeless people as well as research interest in Germany. In line with certain social developments, research interest peaked in the 1990s and mainly consisted of descriptive studies on homeless people and prevalence rates of mental disorders among sociodemographic factors (16–19). Studies on housing or therapy interventions are scarce. Between 2010 and 2013, an intervention trial on motivational case management (MOCA) was conducted among people at risk of losing accommodation in the German cities of Mannheim and Freiburg (49). During a 6-month follow-up period, quality of life and social support was improved (partly statistically significant) and psychosocial needs for care decreased (49). Possibly, due to a long-standing and therefore complex social support system, research on interventions for homeless people with mental disorders in Germany is limited. Internationally approved concepts like Housing First, mainly developed in North America, are just recently being implemented (50). Still, there is a long list of low-barrier institutions such as the Jenny De la Torre–Stiftung (51) offering (anonymous) medical care for homeless people or individual projects like the 'Mainz Model', which operates according to the principle, 'if the patient doesn't come to the doctor, the doctor must go to the patient' (52).

Conclusion—homelessness and mental health in Germany

German psychiatrists and researchers have recognized the phenomenon of homelessness since the nineteenth century. Despite a wide-ranging social welfare system, the number of homeless people has increased in the last decade. In line with international studies, homeless people in Germany often suffer from mental disorders with a lifetime prevalence of 93.3% (28) and a 1-month prevalence of 77.5% (23). Substance use disorders (60.9%), affective disorders (15.2%), and psychosis (8.3%) are the most common mental illnesses among homeless people in Germany (23). The German mental healthcare system still suffers from structural barriers, such as abstinent-orientated institutions, a lack of outreach social work or healthcare and Housing First programmes, and complex, administrative procedures. Future research needs to focus on so-far neglected subgroups such as homeless women and children and adolescents, migrants, and people with severe mental illness; future models of care should more strongly focus on access barriers and patient preferences.

References

1. **Greifenhagen A, Fichter** M. Psychiatrische Obdachlosenforschung. Nervenarzt. 1996;**67**(11):905–910.
2. **Wilmanns K.** Zur Psychopathologie des Landstreichers. Eine klinische Studie. Leipzig: Barth; 1906.
3. **Garcia C.** Karl Wilmanns und die Landstreicher. Nervenarzt. 1986;**57**(4):227–232.
4. **Wilmanns K.** Bekämpfung des Landstreichertums. Munch Med Wochenschr. 1904;**46**:2068.
5. **Wilmanns K.** Das Landstreichertum, seine Abhilfe und Bekämpfung. Monatsschr Kriminol. 1904/1905;**1**:605–620.
6. **Wilmanns K.** Das Vagabundentum in Deutschland. Z Gesamt Neurol Psychiatr. 1940;**196**(1):65–112.
7. **Carls H.** Vagabondage und Berufsleben und ihre Bedeutung für die Entwicklung von Psychopathien. In: **Carls H** (Ed), Die Wanderer-Fürsorge. Caritas, Elberfeld; 1930:XX–XX.
8. **Schneider K.** Die psychopathischen Persönlichkeiten, 3rd extended ed. Leipzig: Deuticke; 1934.
9. **Lechler KL.** Erkennung und Ausmerze der Gemeinschaftsunfähigen. Dtsch Ärztebl. 1940;**71**:293–297.

10. **von Treuberg E.** Mythos Nichtseßhaftigkeit. Zur Geschichte des wissenschaftlichen, staatlichen und privat-wohltätigen Umgang mit einem diskriminiertem Phänomen. Dissertation, Gießen; 1989.

11. **Ayaß W.** 'Asoziale' im Nationalsozialismus. Überblick über die Breite der Maßnahmen gegen soziale Außenseiter und die hieran beteiligten Stellen. In: **Sedlaczek D, Lutz T, Puvogel U, Tomkowiak I** (Eds), 'Minderwertig' und 'asozial': Stationen der Verfolgung gesellschaftlicher Außenseiter. Zurich: Chronos; 2005:51–64.

12. **Bock H.** Die Psychologie der Obdachlosigkeit. Wanderer. 1962;**2**:17–24.

13. **Merkle G.** Eine soziopsychiatrische Untersuchung an 120 Stadtstreichern. Medical Dissertation, Universität München; 1974.

14. **Armbruster J, Dieterich A, Hahn D, Ratzke K.** 40 Jahre Psychiatrie-Enquete: Blick zurück nach vorn. Köln: Psychiatrie Verlag; 2015.

15. **Schreiter S, Bermpohl F, Schouler-Ocak M,** et al. Bank account ownership and access among in-patients in psychiatric care in Berlin, Germany—a cross-sectional patient survey. Front Psychiatry. 2020;**11**(Jun):508.

16. **Fichter M, Quadflieg N, Greifenhagen A, Koniarczyk M, Wolz J.** Alcoholism among homeless men in Munich, Germany. Eur Psychiatry. 1997;**12**(2):64–74.

17. **Greifenhagen A, Fichter M.** Mental illness in homeless women: an epidemiological study in Munich, Germany. Eur Arch Psychiatry Clin Neurosci. 1997;**247**(3):162–172.

18. **Salize HJ, Horst A, Dillmann-Lange C,** et al. Needs for mental health care and service provision in single homeless people. Soc Psychiatry Psychiatr Epidemiol. 2001;**36**(4):207–216.

19. **Dufeu P, Podschus J, Schmidt LG.** Alkoholabhängigkeit bei männlichen Wohnungslosen. Häufigkeit, Ausprägung und Determinanten [Alcoholism among homeless men: prevalence, clinical features, and determinants]. Nervenarzt. 1996;**67**(11):930–934.

20. **Salize HJ, Dillmann-Lange C, Stern G,** et al. Alcoholism and somatic comorbidity among homeless people in Mannheim, Germany. Addiction. 2002;**97**(12):1593–1600.

21. **Rössler W, Salize HJ, Biechele U.** Psychisch kranke Wohnsitzlose—die vergessene Minderheit. Psychiatr Prax. 1994;**21**(5):173–178.

22. **Salize HJ, Horst A, Dillmann-Lange C,** et al. Wie beurteilen psychisch kranke wohnungslose ihre lebensqualität? Psychiatr Prax. 2001;**28**(2):75–80.

23. **Schreiter S, Bermpohl F, Krausz M,** et al. The prevalence of mental illness in homeless people in Germany—a systematic review and meta-analysis. Dtsch Arztebl Int. 2017;(17):665–672.

24. **Salize HJ, Werner A, Jacke CO.** Service provision for mentally disordered homeless people (PSYNDEXshort). Curr Opin Psychiatry. 2013;**26**(4):355–361.

25. **Hoell A, Salize HJ.** Die psychiatrische Versorgung von wohnungslosen Menschen mit psychischen Problemen. Spectr Psychiatr. 2018;**2**:8–12.

26. **Hoell A, Franz M, Salize HJ.** Die gesundheitliche Versorgung von wohnungslosen Menschen mit psychischen Problemen Übersichtsarbeit zu aktuellen Interventionen und deren Ergebnisse. Die Psychiatr. 2017;**2**:1–11.

27. **Salize HJ, Hoell A.** Soziale Ungleichheit und psychische Gesundheit. Nervenarzt. 2019;**90**(11):1187–1200.

28. Bäuml J, Brönner M, Baur B, Pitschel-Walz G, Jahn T. Die SEEWOLF-Studie Seelische Erkrankungsrate in den Einrichtungen der Wohnungslosenhilfe im Großraum München. Freiburg: Lambertus Verlag; 2017.

29. Nacht der Solidarität. Homepage. Available from: https://www.berlin.de/nacht-der-solidaritaet/.

30. Bundesarbeitsgemeinschaft Wohnungslosenhilfe e.V. Wohnungslosigkeit: Kein Ende in Sicht. 2019. Available from: https://www.bagw.de/fileadmin/bagw/media/Doc/2019/PRM_2019_11_11_Schaetzung_Zahl_der_Wohnungslosen.pdf.

31. Bundesarbeitsgemeinschaft Wohnungslosenhilfe e.V. Pressemitteilung: BAG Wohnungslosenhilfe: 650.000 Menschen in 2017 ohne Wohnung. 2019. Available from: http://www.bagw.de/de/themen/zahl_der_wohnungslosen/index.html.

32. Jacobi F, Wittchen HU, Holting C, et al. Prevalence, co-morbidity and correlates of mental disorders in the general population: results from the German Health Interview and Examination Survey (GHS). Psychol Med. 2004;34(4):597–611.

33. Fazel S, Khosla V, Doll H, Geddes J. The prevalence of mental disorders among the homeless in Western countries: systematic review and meta-regression analysis. PLoS Med. 2008;5(12):1670–1681.

34. Patterson M, Palepu A, Frankish CJ, Somers JM. Housing First improves subjective quality of life among homeless adults with mental illness: 12-month findings from a randomized controlled trial in Vancouver, British Columbia. Soc Psychiatry Psychiatr Epidemiol. 2013;48(8):1245–1259.

35. Khantzian EJ. Self-regulation and self-medication factors in alcoholism and the addictions. Similarities and differences. Recent Dev Alcohol. 1990;8:255–271.

36. Riege M. Frauen in Wohnungsnot. Erscheinungsformen—Ursachenanalyse—Lösungsstrategien—Forderungen. Kinder und Frauen zuletzt?! Frauen Wohnungsnot VSH Verlaug für Soz Hilfe. 1994;25:9–24.

37. Fichter M, Koniarczyk M, Greifenhagen A, et al. Mental illness in a representative sample of homeless men in Munich, Germany. Eur Arch Psychiatry Clin Neurosci. 1996;246(4):185–196.

38. Schreiter S, Heidrich S, Zulauf J, et al. Housing situation and health care for patients in a psychiatric centre in Berlin, Germany—a cross-sectional patient survey. BMJ Open. 2019;9(12):e032576.

39. Salit SA, Kuhn EM, Hartz AJ, Vu JM, Mosso AL. Hospitalization costs associated with homelessness in New York City. N Engl J Med. 1998;338(24):1734–1740.

40. Dimitri G, Giacco D, Bauer M, et al. Predictors of length of stay in psychiatric inpatient units: does their effect vary across countries? Eur Psychiatry. 2018;48:6–12.

41. Federal Employment Agency. Brochure: Unemployment Benefit II/Social Assistance Basic Security Benefits for Jobseekers. 2017. Available from: https://www.proarbeit-kreis-of.de/site/assets/files/1170/sgb2-merkblatt-en_ba013347.pdf.

42. Bundesministerium für Soziales. Grundsicherung im Alter und bei Erwerbsminderung. 2018. Available from: https://www.bmas.de/DE/Themen/Soziale-Sicherung/Sozialhilfe/grundsicherung-im-alter-und-bei-erwerbsminderung.html.

43. Keicher R, Gillich S. Ohne Wohnung in Deutschland Armut, Migration und Wohnungslosigkeit. Freiburg: Lambertus Verlag; 2017.

44. **Dillmann R, Schiffer-Nasserie A.** Der soziale Staat: Über nützliche Armut und ihre Verwaltung Ökonomische Grundlagen. Politische Maßnahmen. Historische Etappen. Hamburg: VSA Verlag; 2018.

45. **von Paulgerg-Muschiol L.** Wege In Die Wohnungslosigkeit. Eine qualitative Untersuchung. Doctoral Thesis, Universität Siegen; 2009.

46. **Gühne U, Weinmann S, Riedel-Heller SG, Becker T** (Eds). S3-Leitlinie Psychosoziale Therapien bei schweren psychischen Erkrankungen. Berlin: Springer; 2019.

47. **Coldwell CM, Bender WS.** The effectiveness of assertive community treatment for homeless populations with severe mental illness: a meta-analysis. Am J Psychiatry. 2007;**164**(3):393–399.

48. **Berliner Kältehilfe.** Homepage. Available from: https://www.kaeltehilfe-berlin.de/.

49. **Salize HJ, Arnold M, Uber E, Hoell A.** Verbesserung der psychiatrischen Behandlungsprävalenz bei Risikopersonen vor dem Abrutschen in die Wohnungslosigkeit. Psychiatr Prax. 2017;**44**(1):21–28.

50. **Housing First Berlin.** What does Housing First do? Available from: https://housingfirstberlin.de/projekt/.

51. **Jenny de la Torre–Stiftung.** Homepage. Available from: http://www.delatorre-stiftung.de/.

52. **Trabert G.** Medizinische Versorgung für wohnungslose Menschen—individuelles Recht und soziale Pflicht statt Exklusion. Gesundheitswesen. 2016;**78**(2):107–112.

Chapter 4

Research on homelessness and mental health: What we've learned from the United States and nations in Europe

Cara A. Struble and Paul A. Toro

Introduction

Homelessness, once thought to be an isolated problem in developing nations, has now been recognized as a major social issue throughout the developed world (1). As a result, homelessness has become a major research focus in the US and most other developed nations (2–6). Literature on this topic has flourished in recent decades (7). Research on homelessness has extended to mental health professionals. Clinical and community psychologists are especially interested in capturing the extent of mental illness among the homeless. Since researchers typically implement diverse methodology, estimated rates of mental illness among the homeless vary substantially across studies, both within and between nations. This variation across studies might be due to differing methodologies or to true cross-national differences. An international understanding of mental health characteristics within the homeless population would enhance learning and broaden the perspectives of those studying homelessness in developed nations. After a brief review of methodological issues relevant to the study of mental disorders among the homeless, we will compare and contrast prevalence estimates obtained across the US and Europe. We will then suggest recommendations for future research.

Methodological issues in research on homelessness

A complete review of the literature comparing homelessness research in the US and Europe is beyond the scope of this chapter and has been considered elsewhere (8,9). However, there are noteworthy differences that affect our ability to synthesize findings and improve our understanding of mental illness among the homeless. Research in the US diverges from European research in numerous ways, including theoretical perspectives on homelessness, definitions of homelessness, sampling methodology, and mental health measures (10). We will now review each of these differences in more detail.

Theoretical perspectives on homelessness

US and European researchers typically diverge on explanations for homelessness, leading to differences in the scope of research and policy reform. These differences affect how researchers attempt to understand, prevent, and treat homelessness. In the US, homelessness researchers are predominantly clinical and community psychologists (9). Studies in the US are often person-centred, focusing on individual factors that might make an individual vulnerable to experiencing homelessness (10,11).

In contrast, this particular approach to understanding homelessness can be considered as over-pathologizing in Europe, where research is primarily headed by political scientists and sociologists (1,10). European researchers instead focus on the effects of economic and social factors on homelessness such as limited housing (9,10). Nations emphasizing structural elements as the causes of homelessness tend to implement stronger policies to aid individuals with economic burdens in hopes of reducing the rates of homelessness (8). Alternatively, when causes of homelessness are attributed to individual characteristics, as is often seen in the US, fewer economic or structural resources might be available. Over time, such differences could lead to a true variation in the size and composition of homeless populations across nations.

Defining homelessness

Researchers differ in their conceptualizations of homelessness, utilizing unique definitions to classify individuals. Toro and Warren (12) noted that definitions vary in both the quality of housing and duration of homelessness. Researchers in the US generally make a distinction between those who are literally homeless and are sleeping in shelters, the streets, or similar settings (e.g. abandoned buildings, cars) versus those who are precariously housed (e.g. doubled up, couch surfing, experiencing extreme poverty) but at high risk of becoming homeless (12). Much of the homelessness literature conducted in the US comes from studies on the literally homeless. European researchers take a broader perspective in defining homelessness, often studying individuals with inadequate or unstable housing arrangements rather than 'rough sleepers' who lack housing entirely (e.g. literally homeless) (8,13). These international differences in defining homelessness contribute to distinct research samples, each with unique characteristics. Directly comparing these samples might lead to an inaccurate understanding of international homelessness.

Sampling methodology

Failure to obtain a representative sample is a commonly cited problem among homelessness research (14,15). Many options for sampling participants exist, with the most primitive method being single-location or single-site recruitment (16). Recent large-scale studies have implemented sophisticated probability sampling procedures for selecting representative groups from shelters, food programmes, and other sites across large geographical areas (16–18). Sampling most commonly occurs at service locations (e.g. shelters, soup kitchens, outpatient programmes), but not all homeless people utilize these resources. Failure to obtain a representative sample that includes individuals who do and do not utilize services would lead to biased results. Studies suggest that differences do exist between sheltered versus unsheltered homeless individuals, with those on the street reporting longer durations of homelessness (19). To date, studies have failed to identify significant differences in mental health characteristics across both groups, but available research has been limited by small sample sizes (19,20).

There appear to be three distinct subgroups within the homeless population, including single adults, families, and youth (1). In the US, single adults are typically males (70–80%) between the ages of 18 and 50, with a history of alcohol or drug abuse/dependence (60–80%) (2,21). Homeless families, which are less common in Europe, tend to include a single mother with young children often under 5 years old (22). Homeless youths are minors or young adults under age 25 who are away from home without parental consent. Much of this subgroup has spent little or no time on the streets, but research on homeless youth focuses on street youth (1).

Similar to the general population, men, women, and youth display distinct psychiatric characteristics. For instance, homeless mothers and youth have been found to demonstrate less substance abuse compared to single adults (5). Roll et al. (23) investigated the characteristics of single men, single women, and women with children and found that women overall reported more psychological distress compared to single men, while these men were more likely to report a history of substance abuse (23). When attempting to compare studies, researchers must consider which subgroup(s) are recruited and analysed, as large variation in estimates might be due to how heavily each typology is represented within the sample.

Measurement

Controversies exist in the best ways to assess mental illness among the homeless. Complicating the issue further, US and European researchers might utilize different diagnostic systems to classify mental health disorders (*Diagnostic and Statistical Manual of Mental Disorders* (*DSM*), fifth edition, versus the International Classification of Diseases, 11th revision). Researchers can utilize numerous indicators of mental illness throughout their studies, including (a) standardized clinical interviews, (b) cut-off scores on a symptom checklist, (c) psychiatric hospitalization history, and (d) observer assessments (14). In homelessness research, each method may have merits in terms of reliability, validity, and/or practicality.

A standardized clinical interview, such as the Diagnostic Interview Schedule (DIS), tends to yield more conservative estimates while less rigorous methods including symptom checklists and psychiatric hospitalization yield higher estimates of mental illness. For example, in a study of 76 homeless adults in Buffalo, New York, the DIS revealed that 74% of the sample met criteria for a lifetime diagnosis of any *DSM-III* disorder. Within this sample, 53% and 37% met criteria for alcohol and drug abuse/dependence, respectively. Only 15% met lifetime criteria for serious mental illness including major affective or schizophrenia spectrum disorders. The proportion of the sample with any psychiatric diagnosis reduced when focusing on symptoms in the past 6 months, with only 58% reporting recent symptoms (35% substance abuse, 15% serious mental illness). The rate of serious mental illness was 33% based on prior psychiatric hospitalizations. More problematically, there were participants with a history of psychiatric hospitalizations who did not meet lifetime criteria for any psychiatric disorder via the DIS. The highest estimate of current serious mental illness was found using a symptom checklist, with 41% of the sample surpassing a cut-off score on the SCL-90-R (20).

This study revealed many nuances relevant to operationally defining and measuring mental illness. Researchers should be aware of whether they are estimating current or lifetime mental illness, as assessment of current symptoms (e.g. symptoms present within the last 6–12 months) might yield lower estimates compared to lifetime prevalence. Researchers must decide whether they are examining serious mental illness (e.g. affective and schizophrenia spectrum disorders) versus any psychiatric diagnosis (i.e. anxiety or personality disorders). Further, researchers must determine whether to combine substance abuse/dependence in their conceptualization of mental illness or examine alcohol and drug abuse/dependence separately. Given the high lifetime prevalence of substance use in the homeless population, this distinction could greatly impact estimates obtained across studies. Given the impact these methodological considerations have on interpretation of findings, it is unsurprising that a wide range of estimates for mental illness have been obtained within and across nations.

Comparing homelessness and mental health internationally

The literature suggests that both the extent of homelessness and the composition of the homeless population vary across developed nations. We have examined prevalence estimates of homelessness in a multi-nation study, and recently extended upon previous findings (24). We now present lifetime prevalence estimates of literal homelessness throughout the US, Canada, and eight European countries via telephone surveys. Countries with the highest rates of lifetime literal homelessness, based on random samples of fixed phones called, included the UK (7.7%,), Canada (8.2%), and the US (6.1%). Poland (4.2%), Belgium (3,4%), and Italy (3.6%) were found to have moderate prevalence estimates, while Portugal (2.8%), Germany (2.3%), the Czech Republic (2.4%), and France (2.0%) had the lowest rates of literal homelessness.

Prevalence of mental illness among homeless people in the US and Europe

Although mental illness is one risk factor for homelessness, many homeless people do not report a history of mental illness, nor do all individuals with mental illness, serious or otherwise, become homeless. As discussed previously, research on mental illness in the homeless population might be restricted by the operationalization of homelessness and sampling. Measures can yield vastly different estimates of mental illness, under- or over-identifying individuals with a mental illness. Updated rates of mental illness (e.g. overall, affective, psychotic, and substance abuse disorders) in the US and Europe will be compared, highlighting the effects of inconsistent sampling and measurement.

Overall estimates of mental illness

United States

Researchers estimate that the overall prevalence of mental illness within the homeless population is quite high but variable, ranging from 2% to 91% (25). Recent estimates from the 2018 US Housing and Urban Development survey found that 95,680 (17.3%) of homeless individuals surveyed during a single night had a serious mental illness (26). This recent estimate is consistent with our previously mentioned finding from the late 1990s, where 15% of a probability sample of homeless adults in Buffalo, New York, were identified as having lifetime histories of serious mental illness using the DIS-III. That estimate increased to 74% when estimating rates for any mental illness (e.g. anxiety, personality, and substance abuse disorders) (16).

Similar estimates using the DIS have been found by researchers in other cities over the years including Baltimore, Maryland (approximately 15.7% seriously mentally ill, 78.4% any mental illness) (27) and Detroit, Michigan (20% seriously mentally ill) (28). In St. Louis, Missouri, North and Smith found comparable estimates for any lifetime psychiatric diagnosis in men (76.7%), while only 47.7% of women reported lifetime symptoms to warrant a diagnosis (29). There is even greater variance when diagnoses are made by clinical examination without diagnostic instruments such as the DIS. For instance, in Westchester County, New York, researchers found that 15% of a sample of men and women met the criteria for a serious mental illness (30) per clinical staff assessment. In contrast, an earlier study on homeless men, women, and children at an emergency department in the US found that staff identified 91% of the sample as having a primary psychiatric diagnosis with 40% having psychoses (31).

Europe

The availability of research on mental health characteristics of the homeless across Europe is much more limited compared to the US. Literature has expanded due to increasing concerns over the growing homeless population, but methodology continues to vary considerably. Estimates ranging from 58% to 100% of samples meeting criteria for psychiatric disorders have been obtained (8). Martens (25) compiled prevalence estimates from available European nations and found that rates of mental illness among European countries are not homogeneous. From lowest prevalence to highest, available estimates include Ireland (32%) (32), Spain (33%) (33), UK (55%) (34,35), France (57.9%) (36), Netherlands (78%) (37), Norway (82%) (38), and Germany (94.5%) (39) although the majority of these estimates are based on single-city studies.

The differences in mental health characteristics of homeless individuals across Europe are likely impacted by sampling and measurement methodologies. For instance, researchers sampled from different populations of homeless individuals, including youth and adolescents (35,37) versus single adults (34). Ireland's low estimate was based on symptom ratings made by staff rather than direct observations of homeless individuals at 12 hostels in Belfast. Estimates in Germany, which utilized the DIS, were considerably higher due in part to the fact that researchers reported any lifetime *DSM-III* Axis I disorder, with relatively high rates of alcohol use considered as a mental disorder (39). Within Europe, it is exceedingly challenging to compare mental health characteristics of the homeless due to these differences.

Affective disorders

Affective disorders consist of depressive and bipolar disorders. Major depressive disorder is relatively common throughout the US and Europe. It is not surprising to find that the prevalence of affective disorders also appears to be high within homeless samples across developed nations. Toro (2) compared estimates from eight studies conducted in various cities in the US (e.g. Baltimore, Maryland; Detroit, Michigan; Los Angeles, California), including representative samples of homeless using similar sampling methodology and measures (DIS for *DSM-III/DSM-III-R* disorders). High rates of affective disorders among homeless adults were uncovered (14–30%) with depressive disorders most common. Bipolar disorders and mania were usually present in less than 5% overall (2,27–29,40–43).

Researchers in Germany conducted a meta-analysis in 2017 on estimates of affective disorders among the homeless in this nation. The pooled estimate across eight studies was 15.2% (44). Though pooled estimates might reduce bias across studies, those included in this meta-analysis were typically based on samples of men or women separately rather than in combination. Follow-up analyses revealed that when interviews were conducted by professionals, estimates ranged from just 11.0% to 15.9% compared to estimates from non-professionals (16.3–46.9%) (44), indicating heterogeneity across studies.

Numerous studies across the US and Europe provide prevalence estimates for major depressive disorder. In a Los Angeles sample, 17.5% reported a 12-month prevalence of major depression, while 21.2% endorsed a lifetime history via the DIS (41). Bellavia and Toro found a relatively high estimate of depression in a sample of 144 homeless adults in Buffalo, New York, in 1999 using the Depression subscale of the SCL-90-R (39.0%) (45). Based on data presented in Martens' (25) review of European nations, the Netherlands (22% of adolescents) (37) and Spain (20% (33); 14.9% (12-month) and 21.0% (lifetime) (46)) demonstrated comparable prevalence estimates of major depression. One study from France reported slightly higher estimates (33.7%) using the Composite International Diagnostic Interview, although this difference may be partly due to seasonal variations as the study was conducted during the winter months (36). Estimates from studies in Germany ranged from 0% to 40.6%, with a pooled estimate of 11.6%, although these findings are limited by the heterogeneity across studies noted earlier (44).

Psychotic disorders

Rates of psychotic disorders among homeless adults have generally exceeded normative rates within the general population; however, schizophrenia and other psychotic disorders are still relatively rare. In the US, studies using the DIS consistently found that under 10% of homeless adults met the criteria for a schizophrenia spectrum disorder (2). Estimates were as low as 2.0% in Baltimore (27), while Koegel et al. (40) identified 13.7% of the homeless sample in the skid row section of Los Angeles met the criteria for schizophrenia using the DIS. US estimates using the Psychoticism subscale from the SCL-90-R, a self-report measure, found that 26.2% of the sample of homeless adults surpassed the cut-off (45).

Estimates for psychotic disorders across Europe tend to be slightly higher than the US, with most studies ranging from 14% to 18% (25). There are some notable exceptions, with 52% of a sample of homeless patients in Denmark diagnosed with schizophrenia by mental health professionals. However, this sample consisted of homeless psychiatric patients, a setting with inflated rates of serious mental illness including psychotic disorders that are not representative of the homeless population overall (47). In Germany, estimates from professional interviewers were under 10% (i.e. 4.9–9.6%) while estimates from non-professionals were as high as 34.4% (44).

Differences in research recruitment sites, diagnostic assessment measures, and diagnostic assessors contribute to differing rates of psychotic disorders among the homeless. Estimates might also vary based on psychotic disorders assessed. Many studies noted earlier focused specifically on schizophrenia. However, the inclusion of related psychotic disorders, including schizoaffective disorder and psychosis, would increase estimated rates and capture a wider range of symptomatology.

Substance use disorders

Substance abuse is prevalent among the homeless in the US and Europe (2,8). Conservative estimates obtained from an annual single-night survey of homeless in the US found that 71,319 (12.9%) of surveyed homeless individuals reported chronic substance abuse (26) while having a history of substance abuse/dependence indicated by the DIS occurs in 60–75% of adult homeless samples (43). As previously mentioned, single men tend to have the highest estimates of substance use problems (68%) (23) compared to women. Large variations exist across nations, as well as across substances. Different diagnostic criteria (i.e. abuse versus dependence versus use disorder), sample (adult men versus women versus youth), and assessment measures will likely result in varied rates of substance abuse across studies. Attitudes and access to substances also differ across nations both in the general population and among homeless, further limiting our ability to understand substance use disorders internationally.

Estimates of alcohol abuse/dependence

Rates of alcohol abuse/dependence are particularly high (2,8,25). Using the DIS in the US, estimates range from 47.5% in St. Louis (29) to 62.9% in the skid row section of Los Angeles (40). Martens (25) presented similar rates from studies in the Netherlands (46% of adolescents) (37) and Russia (60%) (48). In Ireland, women exhibited much lower rates (4.1%), while 46% of men reported alcohol abuse/dependence (49). Rates in Denmark were comparatively low for adults (21%), but data were presented on individuals in psychiatric hospitals (47) which impacts generalizability of findings. In Germany, rates have been quite high, with estimates from structured interviews and pooled analyses ranging from 60% to 82.9% (39,44,50). In context, Germany is known to have the greatest alcohol consumption per capita among western Europe (8).

Estimates of drug abuse/dependence

Rates of drug abuse/dependence also tend to be high in the US, with estimates between 30.8% and 49.0% of homeless adults in Los Angeles (40,41), 34.2% in St. Louis (29), 37.6–48.9% in Buffalo (16,28), 52.2% in Oakland (42), and 53.9% in Detroit (16). In the UK, in London, one study estimated that 68% of homeless participants required services for a drug problem, although this estimate was based on data from rough sleepers (51). European nations previously from the Communist bloc had limited access to illicit substances and have shown low prevalence estimates. For example, the pooled estimate for drug dependency in Germany was 13.9% (44).

Towards an international understanding: recommendations for future research

We have identified two studies to date that have attempted to compare the mental health characteristics of the homeless population across the US and Europe. The first was reported by Muñoz et al. (46). Findings indicated that lifetime prevalence estimates of major depression and schizophrenia were similar across samples. The research was based on two independent studies conducted in Madrid, Spain, and Los Angeles County, California. The authors argued that similarities in measures allowed both studies to be compared. The US sample was given the DIS, while the sample in Spain was administered the Composite International Diagnostic Interview (46), which might have contributed to differences or lack of differences across these nations.

Toro and colleagues (52) compared characteristics of probability samples of homeless adults from two cities in Poland and one city in the US using the same measures with a systematic translation procedure to ensure comparability of measurement. These samples differed significantly in the prevalence of mood disorders (30% in the US versus 16% in Poland) and schizophrenia spectrum disorders (11% in the US versus 4% in Poland). The estimates of substance use disorders also differed significantly across the two nations with higher estimates of alcohol (59.8%) and drug (57.5%) abuse in the US compared to Poland (44.5% and 6.0%, respectively). Rates of mental illness might be lower in Poland since it has a national health system providing psychiatric care, free of charge, to all citizens. The divergent drug estimates are likely due to the easier access to and lower costs of illicit substances in the US (52). Similar methodology allows researchers to propose possible causes for observed differences.

Future directions

It is recommended that researchers move towards an international consensus on the definition of homelessness, sampling procedures, and assessment measures for mental illness. Researchers should explicitly state criteria used to classify the homeless. Findings from those who are homeless and precariously housed should be reported separately rather than aggregated, as these subgroups likely have distinct characteristics, including mental health difficulties. Sampling methods should be documented and utilize sophisticated probability sampling procedures to obtain a representative sample. Researchers should use consistent and multimethod approaches with established psychometric properties to classifying mental illness among homeless people. For instance, diagnostic interviews such as the DIS reveal relatively consistent estimates throughout the US (2) and fairly consistent estimates across nations. However, this interview might provide inaccurate estimates due to the single interview period (15). Thus, research would benefit by providing other estimates in combination, including a symptom count and history of hospitalizations, rather than relying on one particular measure. Thus, a standard battery of measures, translated for applications across different nations, is essential when comparing rates of mental illness across studies. These recommendations would allow researchers to understand similarities and differences in mental health characteristics among the homeless, which would greatly improve our ability to identify plausible explanations for true international differences.

References

1. **Toro PA.** Toward an international understanding of homelessness. J Soc Issues. 2007;**63**(3):461–481.

2. **Toro PA.** Homelessness. In: **Bellack AS, Hersen M** (Eds), Comprehensive Clinical Psychology: Applications in Diverse Populations 9. New York: Pergamon; 1998:119–135.

3. **Fournier L, Mercier C** (Eds). Sans domicile fixe: au-delà du stereotype [Homelessness: Beyond the Stereotype]. Montreal: Méridien; 1996.

4. **Lee BA, Link BG, Toro PA.** Images of the homeless: public views and media messages. Hous Policy Debate. 1991;**2**(3):649–682.

5. **Shinn M, Weitzman BC.** Research on homelessness: an introduction. J Soc Issues. 1990;**46**(4):1–11.

6. **Gore A.** Public policy and the homeless. Am Psychol. 1990;**45**(8):960–962.

7. **Buck PO, Toro PA, Ramos MA.** Media and professional interest in homelessness over 30 years (1974–2003). Anal Soc Issues Public Policy. 2004;**4**(1):151–171.

8. **Philippot P, Lecocq C, Sempoux F, Nachtergael H, Galand B.** Psychological research on homelessness in western Europe: a review from 1970 to 2001. J Soc Issues. 2007;**63**(3):483–504.

9. **Fitzpatrick S, Christian J.** Comparing homelessness research in the US and Britain. Eur J Hous Policy. 2006;**6**(3):313–333.

10. **Christian J.** Homelessness: integrating international perspectives. J Community Appl Soc Psychol. 2003;**13**(2):85–90.

11. **Sosin MR.** Homeless and vulnerable meal program users: a comparison study. Soc Probl. 1992;**39**(2):170–188.

12. **Toro PA, Warren MG.** Homelessness in the United State: policy considerations. J Community Psychol. 1999;**27**(2):119–136.

13. **Shinn M.** International homelessness: policy, socio-cultural, and individual perspectives. J Soc Issues. 2007;**63**(3):657–677.

14. **Robertson MJ.** The prevalence of mental disorder among homeless people. In: **Jahiel RI** (Ed), Homelessness: A Prevention-Oriented Approach. Baltimore, MD: Johns Hopkins University Press; 1992:57–86.

15. **Susser E, Conover S, Struening EL.** Problems of epidemiologic method in assessing the type and extent of mental illness among homeless adults. Hosp Community Psychiatry. 1989;**40**(3):261–265.

16. **Toro PA, Wolfe SM, Bellavia CW,** et al. Obtaining representative samples of homeless persons: a two-city study. J Community Psychol. 1999;**27**(2):157–177.

17. **Burnam A, Koegel P.** Methodology for obtaining a representative sample of homeless persons: the Los Angeles Skid Row Study. Eval Rev. 1998;**12**(2):117–152.

18. **McCaskill PA, Toro PA, Wolfe SM.** Homeless and matched housed adolescents: a comparative study of psychopathology. J Clin Child Psychol. 1998;**27**(3):306–319.

19. **Hannappel M, Calsyn RJ, Morse GA.** Mental illness in homeless men: a comparison of shelter and street samples. J Community Psychol. 1989;**17**(4):304–310.

20. **Toro PA, Wall DD.** Research on homeless persons: diagnostic comparisons and practice implications. Prof Psychol Res Pract. 1991;**22**(6):479–488.

21. **Fischer PJ, Breakey WR.** The epidemiology of alcohol, drug, and mental disorders among homeless persons. Am Psychol. 1991;**46**(11):1115–1128.

22. **Haber M, Toro PA.** Homelessness among families, children and adolescents: an ecological developmental perspective. Clin Child Fam Psychol Rev. 2004;**7**(3):123–164.

23. **Roll CN, Toro PA, Ortola GL.** Characteristics and experiences of homeless adults: a comparison of single men, single women, and women with children. J Community Psychol. 1999;**27**(2):189–198.

24. **Toro PA, Tompsett CJ, Lombardo S,** et al. Homelessness in Europe and the United States: a comparison of prevalence and public opinion. J Soc Issues. 2007;**63**(3):505–524.

25. **Martens WHJ.** Homelessness and mental disorders. Int J Ment Health. 2001;**30**(4):79–96.

26. **US Department of Housing and Urban Development.** HUD 2018 Continuum of Care Homeless Assistance Programs Homeless Populations and Subpopulations. 2018. Available from: https://files.hudexchange.info/reports/published/CoC_PopSub_Natl TerrDC_2018.pdf.

27. **Fischer PG, Shapiro S, Breakey WR, Anthony JC, Kramer M.** Mental health and social characteristics of the homeless: a survey of mission users. Am J Public Health. 1986;**76**(5):519–524.

28. **Toro PA, Rabideau JMP, Bellavia C,** et al. Evaluating an intervention for homeless persons: results of a field experiment. J Consult Clin Psychol. 1997;**65**(3):476–484.

29. **North CS, Smith EM.** A comparison of homeless men and women: different populations, different needs. Community Ment Health J. 1993;**29**(5):423–431.

30. **Haugland G, Siegel C, Hopper K, Alexander MJ.** Mental illness among homeless individuals in a suburban county. Psychiatr Serv. 1997;**48**(4):504–509.

31. **Bassuk EL, Rubin L, Lauriat AS.** Is homelessness a mental health problem? Am J Psychiatry. 1984;**141**(12):1546–1550.

32. **McAuley A, McKenna HP.** Mental disorder among a homeless population in Belfast: an exploratory survey. J Psychiatr Ment Health Nurs. 1995;**2**(6):335–342.

33. **Gonzalez AR, Gonzalez FJ, Fernandez Aguirre MV.** Rehabilitation and social insertion of the homeless chronically mentally ill. Int J Psychosoc Rehabil. 2000;**4**:79–100.

34. **Holland AC.** The mental health of single homeless people in Northampton hostels. Public Health. 1996;**110**(5):299–303.

35. **Craig TK, Hodson S.** Homeless youth in London. I. Childhood antecedents and psychiatric disorder. Psychol Med. 1998;**28**(6):1379–1388.

36. **Kovess V, Mangin-Lazarus C.** The prevalence of psychiatric disorders and use of care by homeless people in Paris. Soc Psychiatry Psychiatr Epidemiol. 1999;**34**(11):580–587.

37. **Sleegers J, Spijker J, van Limbeck J, van England H.** Mental health problems among homeless adolescents. Acta Psychiatr Scand. 1998;**97**(4):253–258.

38. **Dyb E, Johannessen K.** Bostedsløse I Norge 2012 – En kartlegging (Homeless in Norway 2012 – A survey). NIBR-report 2013:5. English summary available from: http://www.nibr.no/filer/tekstfiler/2013_5_English_summary

39. **Fichter MM, Quadflieg N, Koniarczyk M,** et al. Mental illness in homeless men and women in Munich. Psychiatr Prax. 1999;**26**(2):76–84.

40. **Koegel P, Burnam A, Farr RK.** The prevalence of specific psychiatric disorders among homeless individuals in the inner city of Los Angeles. Arch Gen Psychiatry. 1988;**45**(12):1085–1092.

41. **Koegel P, Sullivan G, Burnam A, Morton SC, Wenzel S.** Utilization of mental health and substance abuse service among homeless adults (Unpublished manuscript). Santa Monica, CA: RAND Corporation; 1990.

42. **Robertson MJ, Zlotnick C, Westerfelt A.** Drug disorders and treatment contact among homeless men and women in Almeda County, California. Am J Public Health. 1997;**87**(2):221–228.

43. **Toro PA, Goldstein MS, Rowland LL,** et al. Severe mental illness among homeless adults and its association with longitudinal outcomes. Behav Ther. 1999;**30**(3):431–452.

44. **Schreiter S, Bermpohl F, Krausz M,** et al. The prevalence of mental illness in homeless people in Germany: a systematic review and meta-analysis. Dtsch Arztebl Int. 2017;**114**(40):665–672.

45. **Bellavia CW, Toro PA.** Mental disorder among homeless and poor people: a comparison of assessment methods. Community Ment Health J. 1999;**35**(1):57–67.

46. **Muñoz M, Vázquez C, Koegel P, Sanz J, Burman MA.** Differential patterns of mental disorders among the homeless in Madrid (Spain) and Los Angeles (United States). Soc Psychiatry Psychiatr Epidemiol. 1998;**33**(10):514–520.

47. **Nordentoft M, Knudsen HC, Jessen-Petersen B,** et al. Copenhagen Community Psychiatric Project (CCPP): characteristics and treatment of homeless patients in the psychiatric services after introduction of community mental health centers. Soc Psychiatry Psychiatr Epidemiol. 1997;**32**(7):369–378.

48. **Spence J.** Homeless in Russia: a visit with Valéry Sokolov. Share International Archives, June 1997. Available from: https://www.share-international.org/archives/social-justice/sj_Russian-hmless.htm.

49. **Robertson MJ, Greenblatt M.** Homelessness: A National Perspective. New York: Plenum Press; 1992.

50. **Fitcher MM, Quadflieg N.** Prevalence of mental illness in homeless men in Munich, Germany: results from a representative sample. Acta Psychiatr Scand. 2001;**103**(2):94–104.

51. **Fountain J, Howes S, Strang G.** Unmet drug and alcohol service needs of homeless people in London: a complex issue. Subst Use Misuse. 2003;**38**(3–6):377–393.

52. **Toro PA, Hobden KL, Durham KW, Oko-Riebau M, Bokszczanin A.** Comparing the characteristics of homeless adults in Poland and the United States. Am J Community Psychol. 2014;**53**(1–2):134–145.

Chapter 5

Street children in Latin America

Graham Pluck

Introduction

In many cities around the world, particularly those with lower economic development, children can be observed seemingly unsupervised in the urban environment. They are sometimes working, for example, shining shoes or selling newspapers, or they may be involved in petty crime, street gangs, or sex work, among many other contexts. The heterogeneity of the population is such that all that links them is their youth, their presence in urban environments, unsupervised by adults, and the context of poverty (1). They are frequently referred to as 'street children' in English, or several related terms such as 'street-connected youth'. The term 'street children' clearly encompasses young people in an extensive range of life contexts and unfairly lumps children working hard to help their families together with petty criminals and street gangs. Nevertheless, a street child is the commonly understood expression used by researchers and non-governmental organization workers alike (2).

Considering the heterogeneity within the concept of 'street children', a further distinction is useful. Some street children are described as being *of-the-street*, that is, those who are living independently in the urban environment with little contact with families and support services. Such children are homeless and, in fact, may be roofless, for example, rough sleeping in public places. The homeless of-the-street children can be contrasted with children *in-the-street*—those who spend much time unsupervised in the urban environment, but who do have family-based or other adult-supervised places to return to. Many working children in Latin American cities fall into this latter category. There appear to be far more in-the-street children than of-the-street children in Latin American countries (3).

Due to the extreme informality of street children's lives, and their preponderance in countries with limited census and social welfare services, estimates of the numbers of street children have tended to be mere guesswork. A figure of 100 million globally for the prevalence of street children (broadly defined), and growing, is sometimes given. However, this is acknowledged as being so unreliable as to be described as a myth by the Consortium for Street Children (4). More recently, a regression-based approach using reliable studies from select countries has estimated the worldwide prevalence of children of-the-street (e.g. literally homeless) aged 10–14. This estimated that there are between 10 and 15 million globally (5), with a significant number of these in Latin American countries. This is probably the most reliable estimate of the overall prevalence, but only estimates the most severe form of youth street-connectedness, and only within a relatively narrow age range.

Poverty, family dysfunction, and abuse

At a gross socio-geographical level, street children are mainly associated with what is sometimes referred to as the Global South, meaning low- and middle-income countries in Asia, Africa, the Caribbean, and Latin America. The factors contributing to street involvement of youth in these countries are similar to those in developed countries, where they would commonly be referred to as runaway or homeless youth. Although multifactorial, the most important factors appear to be poverty, family discord, and abuse, suggesting that whether in developed or developing countries, children use street connectedness to escape unfavourable domestic conditions (6). Nevertheless, there are some differences between the phenomena of non-domiciled youth in developing and developed countries. In the latter, runaway or homeless youth tend to be older, to be a balance of boys and girls, and are more likely to come from non-poverty backgrounds. In comparison, in-the-street children in developing countries (7) are usually younger children, boys, and from extreme poverty backgrounds (8). Nevertheless, escaping from family discord appears to be a common feature to both.

Indeed, there is ample evidence that street-connected youth in developing countries suffer high levels of mental illness, substance dependence, and are vulnerable in general to victimization (8). It is tempting to blame the street context for the high levels of psychopathology, and although that is almost certainly part of the picture, the socioeconomic background is also of great relevance. Research conducted with street-connected youth in several areas of Brazil (mean age 14.2) suggested that physical abuse, poverty, and family dysfunction are closely linked (9). Indeed, psychiatric assessments of 351 street-connected youth (mean age 12.5) in Sao Paulo, Brazil, most of whom were living in supervised group homes, found that virtually all had been neglected by their parents. In contrast, about 58% had experienced early physical or sexual abuse (10). Another study of 260 male and 15 female homeless street children in Ecuador (mean age 13.7), found that all of the females and 29% of the males had left home to avoid sexual abuse, with an additional 30% of the males citing phys-ical abuse as the reason for leaving (11). Mental health was not measured in the Ecuadorian sample, but almost all of the children were daily users of in-halant, marijuana, and cocaine-based products, indicating significant psycho-logical problems. In the Sao Paulo sample, 89% were diagnosed with psychiatric disorders.

Abuse also seems to be relevant for domiciled street children living with their families. Another large study in Sao Paulo, this time of 126 street-working chil-dren (mean age 10.5), compared them to non-working siblings. As expected, scores on scales measuring psychopathology were high in the street workers. However, so were levels of reported childhood traumas, including sexual and physical abuse. When parental abuse was taken into account statistically, being a street worker was unrelated to levels of psychopathology (12). This suggests that for many street-working children, dysfunctional family conditions are more psychologically toxic than the street connectedness. Further analysis from the same sample reported that there were very few differences between exposure to urban violence between the working children and the non-working children, but that the working children were more maltreated at home com-pared to their non-working siblings (13). Over the longer term, childhood exposure to physical and sexual abuse is linked to adult homelessness and mal-adaptive psychosocial traits (14). Therefore, this can hinder attempts to escape street connectedness.

Indeed, it is likely that many children in Latin America who move fully into street-living (i.e. homelessness), progress from being children in-the-street (e.g. street workers) (8), and do so to avoid poverty, abuse, and violence in their homes, families, or neighbourhoods. Ethnographic work with street children in Rio de Janeiro, Brazil, supports this, with children describing a gradual pro-cess in which they would spend time in the street situation, but return home at night. This allowed them to adapt to the street situation step by step before spending most of their time effectively homeless in the streets. In most cases, there was no individual crisis in which they became 'runaways' (15).

Nevertheless, the progression to street connectedness necessarily exposes children to victimization in other forms. In general, attitudes to street children among the public are unsympathetic and often hostile and stigmatizing (2). Further, state violence against street children is well recognized. In one no-torious case, armed men opened fire on a group of 50 street children sleeping rough in front of the Candeleria in Rio de Janeiro, Brazil. Many were injured, and three died instantly, while three others were abducted and driven away to be shot elsewhere. The gunmen were later discovered to be military policemen (16). Such extreme cases are rare, but harassment and violence against street children by police officers are frequently reported in several Latin American countries (17). A study of 124 of-the-street youths (mean age 14.4) in La Paz, Bolivia, found that 21% reported assaults by police officers, including some sexual assaults, and almost all reported generally tricky relationships with the police, involving derogatory statements, assaults, and financial extortion (18). However, it should also be noted that security forces are by no means the only perpetrators of assaults on street-connected youth. In the La Paz study, 36% of the children also reported being assaulted by other street children. In general terms, those children living in the streets are vulnerable to abuse and assault from many different sources, including vigilantes, older gang members, and sex-trade clients.

In addition, working in the urban environment, unsupervised by adults, is a form of street connectedness that exposes children to abuse. A large study of 584 children (mean age 11.9) working in four Latin American cities (Bogota, Lima, Quito, and Sao Paulo) reported on the patterns of work and risks. A majority of the children were selling items in the streets, helping to park vehicles, or begging, and worked an average of 39 hours per week. Two-thirds were attending school in addition to their jobs. A quarter of the sample reported being physically or mentally abused while working (defined as being beaten, stabbed, choked, or humiliated) (3). About 40% had suffered an injury while working (defined as cuts, burns, traffic accidents, etc.) severe enough to prevent them from continuing to work for the day (19).

Post-traumatic stress

Given the high levels of exposure to potentially traumatic events among Latin American street children, it should not be surprising that high levels of post-traumatic stress have also been reported. In an institute-based sample of street children in Mexico City (mean age 14.9), about 50% were considered to have at least moderate levels of post-traumatic stress and exposure to traumatic events (20). Similarly, an institution-based sample of former street children (mean age 13.5) in Quito, Ecuador, found a prevalence of probable post-traumatic stress disorder (PTSD) of 60% (21). These prevalence estimates are much higher than generally found in homeless adolescents in developed countries (22).

Nevertheless, one other study in Latin America has reported lower levels of PTSD in a street child sample. This study of children of-the-street (mean age 13.9) in Port-au-Prince, Haiti, reported a prevalence of 15% for probable PTSD, in association with high levels of psychometrically measured resilience (23). This is a relatively low level considering that all the children reported significant traumatic experiences, including the Haitian earthquake of 2010, and the levels of PTSD were said to be lower than in non-street-connected Haitian children (24).

The differences in prevalence estimations between Mexico, Ecuador, and Haiti, are likely partly due to the different measurement methods used. However, the resilience suggested in the Haitian research may also be a contributing factor. The samples in Mexico and Ecuador, which revealed high prevalence, were of institution-based street children. It is possible that the most resilient children remain on the street and do not seek out assistance from charitable services. In support of this, there is a significantly lower prevalence of PTSD in Haitian youths who are living in the streets because of extreme poverty (often born to parents who were themselves homeless), compared to similar youths living in the streets because of family breakdown, or from having left domestic service (24). Unfortunately, there are no other studies from Latin America on post-traumatic stress in street-connected youth. However, studies from other parts of the world do tend to suggest high levels of PTSD in street children (25,26). A study in Burundi (Africa) revealed that current street children had significantly higher severity scores for PTSD than children who had lived in families but now resided in a care centre for vulnerable youth. Former street children displayed intermediate levels, and children living with their families had the lowest levels of severity (26). This suggests that youth street connectedness is indeed a risk factor of PTSD. Interestingly, in the same study, it was suggested that appetitive aggression (i.e. an interest in and pleasure from violence) by street-connected and other at-risk youth may have protective effects for the development of mental illness and may even be seen as a resilience strategy. This is equivalent to suggestions that involvement in extreme violence by soldiers 'inoculates' them against the development of trauma-related psychopathology (27).

Cognitive development and cognitive reserve

In contrast, street-connected youth may be at a relatively increased risk of the development of post-traumatic stress due to cognitive factors. Many street children have limited access to education, and in combination with other challenges to their psychological and neurological development, tend to develop poor cognitive skills, in comparison to more privileged children. A review of this phenomenon reported a relatively consistent pattern of low intelligence test performance in street child samples, equivalent to performing about one standard deviation below normative data (28). This may increase the risk for post-traumatic stress among street children as a low cognitive function is consistently found to be a pre-trauma risk factor for the development of post-traumatic stress (29). However, it should also be noted that research in Ecuador and Bolivia suggests that although street children score below the levels of non-street children, the critical factor appears to be poverty in general, not homelessness per se (30,31).

Nevertheless, the low cognitive ability probably provides less cognitive reserve, which, in addition to being a risk factor for post-traumatic stress, is also a risk for the development of depression in adolescents (32). To this, we can add high levels of childhood traumas experienced by street-connected youth that contribute to the development of multiple psychiatric disorders through increasing externalizing and internalizing behaviours (33). These factors may put street-connected youth at enhanced risk of developing mental disorders. Indeed, high levels of psychopathology, including hopelessness, depression, self-harm, and suicide, have been described in street children samples from around the world (8).

Affective disorders

Despite this, the evidence for psychopathology among populations of street children in Latin American has been somewhat equivocal until recently. Although medically orientated reports have implied poor mental health of street-connected youth, few have used established assessment tools. Further, ethnographic-orientated research has tended to emphasize the strength and resilience of street children, rather than illnesses, suggesting surprisingly good psychological health. Notable in this respect, in the Latin American context, has been highly influential work published by Lewis Aptekar on his research with Colombian street children. He described 56 of-the-street children in the city of Cali (mean age 11.6), reporting that they were surprisingly emotionally healthy (34). However, the projective tests used to decide this, human figure drawing to derive a measure of emotional functioning, and the Bender–Gestalt test to obtain measures of ego strength, are of dubious validity (35). This may be why Aptekar failed to detect mental illness in his sample. The few studies using accepted psychiatric assessments have tended to show the opposite, that is, significant levels of affective and other disorders in Latin American street children.

A previously mentioned study of 351 street-connected youth in Sao Paulo, Brazil, included psychiatrist-administered assessments for International Classification of Diseases, tenth revision, behavioural and mental disorders. The children and adolescents were all referred from group homes or the courts to a day centre that also provided psychiatric outreach. Of all the referrals, 89% were positive for at least one psychiatric disorder, including 35% positive for mood disorders, 16% positive for attention deficit hyperactivity disorder, and

9% positive for anxiety disorders (10). A large sample of street-working youths (mean age 10.5), also previously mentioned, in Sao Paulo, Brazil, was screened with the Strengths and Difficulties Questionnaire, and those who scored positive (at a low threshold) were assessed with the Schedule for Affective Disorders and Schizophrenia for School-age Children, which is designed to identify probable psychopathology according to *Diagnostic and Statistical Manual of Mental Disorders* (*DSM*)-*III-R* and the *DSM-IV* criteria. Using this procedure, it was estimated that around 31% of the overall sample were positive for at least one *DSM* psychiatric disorder (12).

Depression and anxiety were also measured in the sample described previously in Haiti. In that research, validated self-report scales of affective disorder were used: the Child Depression Inventory (based on the Beck Depression Inventory) and the Beck Anxiety Inventory. Overall, using standard cut-off scores for psychopathology, 13% of the street children were positive for anxiety, and 30% were positive for depression (24). These are seemingly high-prevalence figures, although the authors downplay them, suggesting that they may be lower than in youth in general in Haiti, considering the research was conducted 4 years after the 2010 earthquake, which devastated the country.

Overall, there is minimal reliable data on the mental health status of street-connected youths in Latin American countries. But what does exist, suggests high levels of diagnosable psychiatric disorders, in particular, PTSD, depression, and anxiety.

Substance abuse

Another important feature of the mental health of street-connected youth is substance abuse. A globally focused systematic review of substance abuse by street children reported generally high levels, with the most common substances being tobacco, inhalants, alcohol, and marijuana (8). The pathways to substance abuse by street-connected youth are complex, but research from Brazil mainly associates history of sexual abuse with increased risk (9).

Within Latin American countries, cocaine-based substances are also frequently associated with street-connected youth (11,36,37), probably more so than in other parts of the world. This reflects easy availability and lower purchase costs due to widespread cocaine production in several Latin American countries. A study of 310 street-connected youth in Sao Paulo, Brazil, recently estimated that, after tobacco, crack cocaine was the most frequently abused substance (38). It was used by about 44% of their sample. In some cases, street children may become involved with cocaine use by working in the actual production of the drug (11).

However, inhalant use is also prevalent, and it is considered to be at epidemic levels in low- and middle-income countries (8), including those in Latin America. The use of inhalants and glue sniffing is particularly attractive to street-connected youth due to the ready accessibility and low cost. A study of substance use patterns among in-the-street children (mean age 14.4) in La Paz, Bolivia, reported that 40% were glue sniffing, and the majority had been doing so for several years. Even more of the children reported the abuse of paint thinner as an inhalant, with 88% reporting its use, again the majority had been using it over several years (18). A study in Tegucigalpa, Honduras, reported similarly high levels of glue sniffing. In that study, the prevalence of glue sniffing was 53% in of-the-street children (mean age 13.1), but was very low (<1%) in a sample of in-the-street working children (mean age 9.9) (39).

It is likely that substance abuse is most consistently associated with children in the direst socioeconomic situations, those who are literately homeless (i.e. of-the-street), and less frequently associated with in-the-street children such as street workers. A study in Ecuador with of-the-street children (mean age 13.7) who lacked almost any adult supervision reported a rate of solvent abuse at 98% (11). A different study in Ecuador of former street children (mean age 13.5), mainly former street workers, reported that only 19% reported ever having tried glue sniffing (21). Nevertheless, this is still a high figure considering their ages. In comparison, rates of solvent abuse among Ecuadorian secondary school children are generally quite low, with rates for past-year usage of comparable age groups being less than 3% (40). In fact, in general, across Latin America, the rates of solvent abuse in school children are considerably lower than those observed in street-connected youths (40).

Sniffing glue and other inhalants likely has an element of self-medication, given the high rates of trauma and mental illness associated with street connectedness in Latin American youth. However, it has been proposed that solvent and glue abuse has other functions, such as providing activities to aid cohesion within peer groups, as well as providing a way to fend off hunger and make users feel less vulnerable, which may make it easier to deal with conflict or criminal encounters (41). Hence, in some cases, substance abuse can be seen as a response to the extreme poverty situation faced by street-connected youth.

Access to mental healthcare

Street children in Latin America clearly have complex mental health needs, often in fact potentially dual diagnoses involving both mental health and substance abuse issues. Unfortunately, they are often the least likely to receive the care they need. This is partly due to their informal lives, often unknown to public health agencies and charitable services, and without the means to pay for private medical care. It is worth noting here the inverse care law proposed by Tudor Hart in 1971, which proposes that the availability of health services varies inversely with the needs of the populations served (42). Street children are a particularly potent example, with very high demands, but very little access. The inverse care law is a general feature of healthcare provision, and according to the proposer, is exacerbated by market-driven medical services; such systems are the predominant healthcare models in Latin American countries (43). Due to the wide wealth gap in most Latin American countries, the extremely poor, including street children, often find healthcare inaccessible.

Conclusion

In summary, street children in Latin America, like those in other parts of the world, are a very diverse group of youths. Common themes concerning their mental health are high exposure to potentially traumatic events, including sexual and physical abuse, and related to this, high levels of PTSD. In addition, levels of other disorders, particularly depression and substance abuse, are observed. However, it should also be recognized that due to the huge variety of life contexts, most generalizations about the problems of 'street children' should be avoided. Some street-connected youths in Latin American countries are involved with gang activity, crime, and substance abuse. On the other hand, many are not, and are defined as street children mainly because of their need to work at a young age, as a consequence of their families' low socioeconomic status. As young people in the urban environment, the only thing that links the various 'street children' is extreme poverty, which can be seen as the fundamental source of the high rates of observed psychopathology.

References

1. Pluck G. The 'street children' of Latin America. Psychologist. 2015;**28**(1):20–23.
2. Makofane M. A conceptual analysis of the label 'street children': challenges for the helping professions. Soc Work. 2014;**50**(1):134–145.
3. Pinzon-Rondon AM, Botero JC, Benson L, Briceno-Ayala L, Kanamori M. Workplace abuse and economic exploitation of children working in the streets of Latin American cities. Int J Occup Environ Health. 2010;**16**(2):162–169.
4. Thomas de Benitez S. State of the World's Street Children: Research. London: Consortium for Street Children; 2011.
5. Naterer A, Lavrič M. Using social indicators in assessing factors and numbers of street children in the world. Child Indic Res. 2016;**9**(1):21–37.
6. Embleton L, Lee H, Gunn J, Ayuku D, Braitstein P. Causes of child and youth homelessness in developed and developing countries: a systematic review and meta-analysis. JAMA Pediatr. 2016;**170**(5):435–444.

7. **Aptekar L, Stoecklin D.** Street Children and Homeless Youth: A Cross-Cultural Perspective. Dordrecht: Springer; 2014.

8. **Woan J, Lin J, Auerswald C.** The health status of street children and youth in low- and middle-income countries: a systematic review of the literature. J Adolesc Health. 2013;**53**(3):314–321.

9. **Raffaelli M, Santana JP, de Morais NA, Nieto CJ, Koller SH.** Adverse childhood experiences and adjustment: a longitudinal study of street-involved youth in Brazil. Child Abuse Negl. 2018;**85**:91–100.

10. **Scivoletto S, da Silva TF, Rosenheck RA.** Child psychiatry takes to the streets: a developmental partnership between a university institute and children and adolescents from the streets of Sao Paulo, Brazil. Child Abuse Negl. 2011;**35**(2):89–95.

11. **Schlaefer K.** Voices from the Shadows: Documenting the Human Rights Abuses of Street Youth in Ecuador. Berkeley, CA: School of Public Health, University of California; 2005.

12. **Maciel MR, Mello AF, Fossaluza V,** et al. Children working on the streets in Brazil: predictors of mental health problems. Eur Child Adolesc Psychiatry. 2013;**22**(3):165–175.

13. **Mello AF, Maciel MR, Fossaluza V,** et al. Exposure to maltreatment and urban violence in children working on the streets in Sao Paulo, Brazil: factors associated with street work. Braz J Psychiatry. 2014;**36**(3):191–198.

14. **Pluck G, Lee KH, David R, Macleod DC, Spence SA, Parks RW.** Neurobehavioural and cognitive function is linked to childhood trauma in homeless adults. Br J Clin Psychol. 2011;**50**(1):33–45.

15. **Rizzini I, Butler UM.** Life trajectories of children and adolescents living on the streets of Rio de Janeiro. Child Youth Environ. 2003;**13**(1):182–201.

16. **Amnesty International.** Rio de Janiero 2003: Candelária and Vigário Geral 10 Years On. London: Amnesty International; 2003.

17. **Thomas de Benitez S.** State of the World's Street Children: Violence. London: Consortium for Street Children; 2007.

18. **Huang CC, Barreda P, Mendoza V, Guzman L, Gilbert P.** A comparative analysis of abandoned street children and formerly abandoned street children in La Paz, Bolivia. Arch Dis Child. 2004;**89**(9):821–826.

19. **Pinzon-Rondon AM, Koblinsky SA, Hofferth SL, Pinzon-Florez CE, Briceno L.** Work-related injuries among child street-laborers in Latin America: prevalence and predictors. Rev Panam Salud Publica. 2009;**26**(3):235–243.

20. **Shein-Szydlo J, Sukhodolsky DG, Kon DS, Tejeda MM, Ramirez E, Ruchkin V.** A randomized controlled study of cognitive-behavioral therapy for posttraumatic stress in street children in Mexico City. J Trauma Stress. 2016;**29**(5):406–414.

21. **Pluck G, Banda-Cruz DR, Andrade-Guimaraes MV, Ricaurte-Diaz S, Borja-Alvarez T.** Post-traumatic stress disorder and intellectual function of socioeconomically deprived 'street children' in Quito, Ecuador. Int J Ment Health Addiction. 2015;**13**(2):215–224.

22. **Stewart AJ, Steiman M, Cauce AM, Cochran BN, Whitbeck LB, Hoyt DR.** Victimization and posttraumatic stress disorder among homeless adolescents. J Am Acad Child Adolesc Psychiatry. 2004;**43**(3):325–331.

23. **Cenat JM, Derivois D, Hebert M, Amedee LM, Karray A.** Multiple traumas and resilience among street children in Haiti: psychopathology of survival. Child Abuse Negl. 2018;**79**:85–97.

24. **Derivois D, Cenat JM, Joseph NE, Karray A, Chahraoui K.** Prevalence and determinants of post-traumatic stress disorder, anxiety and depression symptoms in street children survivors of the 2010 earthquake in Haiti, four years after. Child Abuse Negl. 2017;**67**:174–181.

25. **Atwoli L, Ayuku D, Hogan J,** et al. Impact of domestic care environment on trauma and posttraumatic stress disorder among orphans in western Kenya. PLoS One. 2014;**9**(3):e89937.

26. **Crombach A, Elbert T.** The benefits of aggressive traits: a study with current and former street children in Burundi. Child Abuse Negl. 2014;**38**(6):1041–1050.

27. **Hecker T, Hermenau K, Maedl A, Schauer M, Elbert T.** Aggression inoculates against PTSD symptom severity-insights from armed groups in the eastern DR Congo. Eur J Psychotraumatol. 2013;**4**:1.

28. **Pluck G.** Cognitive abilities of 'street children': a systematic review. Chuo J Policy Sci Cult Stud. 2013;**21**:121–133.

29. **DiGangi JA, Gomez D, Mendoza L, Jason LA, Keys CB, Koenen KC.** Pretrauma risk factors for posttraumatic stress disorder: a systematic review of the literature. Clin Psychol Rev. 2013;**33**(6):728–744.

30. **Dahlman S, Backstrom P, Bohlin G, Frans O.** Cognitive abilities of street children: low-SES Bolivian boys with and without experience of living in the street. Child Neuropsychol. 2013;**19**(5):540–556.

31. **Pluck G, Banda-Cruz DR, Andrade-Guimaraes MV, Trueba AF.** Socioeconomic deprivation and the development of neuropsychological functions: a study with 'street children' in Ecuador. Child Neuropsychol. 2018;**24**(4):510–523.

32. **Goodall J, Fisher C, Hetrick S, Phillips L, Parrish EM, Allott K.** Neurocognitive functioning in depressed young people: a systematic review and meta-analysis. Neuropsychol Rev. 2018;**28**(2):216–231.

33. **Keyes KM, Eaton NR, Krueger RF,** et al. Childhood maltreatment and the structure of common psychiatric disorders. Br J Psychiatry. 2012;**200**(2):107–115.

34. **Aptekar L.** Characteristics of the street children of Colombia. Child Abuse Negl. 1989;**13**(3):427–437.

35. **Miller DN, Nickerson AB.** Projective assessment and school psychology: contemporary validity issues and implications for practice. Calif School Psychol. 2006;**11**(1):73–84.

36. **Avila MM, Casanueva E, Piccardo C,** et al. HIV-1 and hepatitis B virus infections in adolescents lodged in security institutes of Buenos Aires. Pediatr AIDS HIV Infect. 1996;**7**(5):346–349.

37. **de Carvalho FT, Neiva-Silva L, Ramos MC,** et al. Sexual and drug use risk behaviors among children and youth in street circumstances in Porto Alegre, Brazil. AIDS Behav. 2006;**10**(4 Suppl):S57–66.

38. **Oliveira MAF, Gonçalves RMDA, Claro HG,** et al. Profile of homeless children and teens drug users. J Nurse UFPE. 2016;**10**(2):475–484.

39. **Wittig MC, Wright JD, Kaminsky DC.** Substance use among street children in Honduras. Subst Use Misuse. 1997;**32**(7–8):805–827.

40. **Hynes-Dowell M, Cumsille F, Clarke P, Araneda JC, Demarco M, Gonzalez O.** Report on Drug Use in the Americas 2011. Washington, DC: Inter-American Observatory on Drugs; 2011.

41. **Fernandes GT, Vaughn MG.** Brazilian street children: contextual influences in relation to substance misuse. Int Soc Work. 2008;51(5):669–681.

42. **Tudor Hart J.** The inverse care law. Lancet. 1971;1(7696):405–412.

43. **Laurell A, Giovanella L.** Health policies and systems in Latin America. In: Oxford Research Encyclopedia of Global Public Health. Oxford Research Encyclopedias; 2018. Available from: https://oxfordre.com/publichealth/view/10.1093/acrefore/9780190632 366.001.0001/acrefore-9780190632366-e-60.

Chapter 6

Homelessness and mental health in Hungary

Eszter Braun, Gabor S. Ungvari, and Gábor Gazdag

Introduction

Brief history of homelessness in Hungary

Homelessness in Hungary has become a major social issue since the demise of the communist system in 1989. Yet, homelessness is not a new phenomenon as it was ushered in with the period of industrialization when masses of peasants moved to big cities; for instance, the population of Budapest rapidly increased in the nineteenth century. At the time of its foundation in 1880, Budapest's population was 370,000, which nearly doubled to 733,000 by 1900 (1). Housing and other parts of the infrastructure could not keep up with demands, resulting in overcrowded and unhygienic housing conditions. In bed rentals, people even slept in shifts in the same bed (2).

As the number of crime and infectious diseases increased, homelessness was first considered as a matter of public safety and health. With the foundation of the Homeless Shelters Association (Hajléktalanok Menhelye Egylet) in 1879, it became increasingly clear that primarily homelessness is more of a social and housing problem (3).

After the First World War, the housing situation became even worse. Following the Versailles peace treaty, the Austro-Hungarian Monarchy ceased to exist, and Hungary ost a large chunk of its historical territory to the neigh-bouring countries, including Romania and the newly formed Yugoslavia and Czechoslovakia. There was a massive influx of people to Budapest, particularly from the lost regions of Hungary, bringing poverty by increasing unemploy-ment. After a brief, relative consolidation, the economic and social situation further worsened during the economic crisis of the 1930s, necessitating the opening of new shelters and workers' hostels. Charity and religious organiza-tions set up soup kitchens and operated temporary shelters during the harsh

Hungarian winter. By 1936, there were already 11 shelters with about 3200 beds in Budapest; half of which were operated by the city, and more than one-third by the Hungarian Red Cross (4).

During the siege at the end of the Second World War, many shelters in Budapest were destroyed, but their reconstruction and reopening were short-lived. In 1947, the Soviet Union-backed Communist Party came to power, and the profound re-engineering of the whole society began taking place that included social policy. The term 'homeless' was incompatible with the prevailing ideology. Instead of shelters and social welfare, rental housing owned by the state was supposed to solve housing problems. The communist ideology denied the existence of poverty, unemployment, and homelessness in the 'workers' state'. Employment was mandatory, and unemployment illegal and punishable for every citizen and very few people managed to avoid the watchful eye of the state. Homeless people were considered dangerous for the community because they chose to live as an outcast, could escape surveillance, and refused to be 'useful' members of society (5).

Another turning point arrived in 1989. As capitalism returned to Hungary, many labourers from the lower strata of society lost their jobs, while for the rest of the working and middle classes wages stagnated. Homelessness was not illegal, and people were not harassed by the police anymore. The hidden homeless masses suddenly became visible as they filled the streets. In February 1989, the first civil organization, the Societal Committee for the Homeless (Hajléktalanokért Társadalmi Bizottság), was set up to protect the interests of homeless people and attracted publicity. After more than 40 years, the sudden appearance of the huge number of homeless people underscored the scope and gravity of this unsolved social problem (6). With the new legislation introduced in October 2018 (7), history seemed to have repeated itself. Living in public spaces was and became again prohibited, and homeless people could even be prosecuted and imprisoned once again.

Homelessness today

Homeless people are a 'nomadic tribe' because it is almost impossible to track their movements. Therefore it is rather difficult to estimate their numbers (8). The only serious attempt to map the life of the Hungarian homeless population has been made by a non-governmental organization (NGO), called the 3rd of February Working Party of the Shelter Foundation (Február Harmadika Munkacsoport, Menhely Alapitvány). The main purpose of this NGO is to give a picture about the actual living conditions including the number of homeless people in Hungary by surveying the homeless population every year, always on the 3rd of February, starting in 1998. The survey, which is run by social workers

Table 6.1 The number of homeless people on the 3rd February surveys from 2013 to 2018

Year	In a transitional shelter	On the streets	Total
2013	6706	3087	9763
2014	7228	3231	10,459
2015	7239	3689	10,928
2016	6784	3422	10,206
2017	5550	2521	8071
2018	6300	2350	8650

and volunteers, uses a questionnaire that is completed by all consenting people who spent the night in homeless shelters or public spaces. The annual survey covers Budapest and more than 50 country towns and between 2006 and 2012, 32,104 homeless persons responded (9). Table 6.1 details the number of homeless people on the 3rd February from 2013 to 2018 who took part in the survey (10–16).

Homeless care that legislation requires state and civil organizations to deliver

The system of care for the homeless is regulated by the 1/2000. (I.7.) *Governmental Directive on the professional requirements and scope of tasks of social institutions responsible for the well-being of individuals.* Under this legislation, temporary homeless shelters and rehabilitation centres are considered to be specialized institutions, which, in addition to providing food and housing with basic hygiene and health conditions, are also obliged to provide professional social care (17). Residents sign a contract with a designated social worker. An individual care plan must be prepared, which focuses on the physical and mental condition of the resident, and the tasks required or recommended for the improvement or preservation of his/her condition, a time frame for the plan, and other aspects of assistance from the social worker. The care plan must be prepared within 1 month from the commencement of care.

Temporary homeless shelters charge a small fee, which is determined by each shelter. This type of housing is *temporary*, available only up to 2 years. Social care includes individual case management, participation in group sessions, and personalized assistance for moving to a long-term hostel, organizing community life within the institution, and dealing with official affairs. Every resident has the right and access to personalized mental healthcare, including individual and group discussions, intellectually fulfilling leisure time, and psychotherapy, should the latter be deemed necessary. According to the government directive, family and social relationships must be maintained, reflecting the illusionistic view of the legislation, that the homeless have a family and rich social life and the shelter must support these aspects of their life.

Mentally and physically compromised homeless persons, whose needs cannot be met at the shelter, should be cared for in rehabilitation centres. The basic task of these rehabilitation centres is to help mentally ill homeless persons to restore a fulfilling life in the community. This includes returning to work, finding proper accommodation, re-learning to adapt to community standards, developing and maintaining a social life, cultural integration, and finding appropriate recreational activities. Aftercare aims to integrate residents back to their original social environment. The rehabilitation centres' staff are responsible for aftercare, which means securing accommodation, helping develop a social environment, counselling, and maintaining contact with the essential social services. These are the tasks that shelters are supposed to provide according to the government's directive. Still, the directive is merely a guideline and depicts an ideal situation while its implementation has been rarely, if ever, feasible. The directive did not specify how to achieve all these lofty aims and find the resources for them.

For instance, all the shelters have a 'no alcohol' policy. As craving is a very strong and crucial factor of alcohol dependence, addicts have little chance of getting a place in a shelter. Shelters also have very strict house rules. There is a strict curfew, and when someone arrives after that time, the door remains locked. Residents have to report every day where they go and what they do. In most shelters, they can only have visitors once or twice a week, but some shelters forbid visitors. Often 6–12 people live in one room. There is no chance of having a private space or have friends and family there. The counsellor and the rule keeper are almost always the same person. Therefore, the residents do not confide in the counsellor. For example, they cannot admit a relapse into drinking alcohol, because they would lose their place immediately. The government directive is also very contradictory. It promises suitable mental care, yet the residents have to pay for the place in the shelter, which means they have to start to work immediately, regardless of their physical needs and mental state.

There is a widely held consensus in the literature (18–20) that the relationship between psychiatric illness and homelessness is a mutually dependent process that sustains each other, forming a vicious circle. Psychiatric patients often lose their social network, including their family. Living in social isolation, psychotic patients frequently do not receive proper psychiatric help as there is no one to notice their alarming symptoms. In a psychotic state, an adequate relationship with reality is disturbed, the patient's behaviour may become unpredictable, and the consequences of his/her actions cannot be foreseen. In such a state, an accident or suicide attempts could occur, causing permanent damage or death. Psychotic patients can lose or destroy all their belongings and sever their remaining social relationships, which can lead to homelessness. Social workers, who deal with disadvantaged people with complex problems day to day in a homeless shelter, have a higher tolerance for disruptive behaviour, more than family, friends, or neighbours have. This accommodating attitude by their social workers allows mentally ill homeless residents to blend in and integrate into the shelter. At the same time, social workers may miss the underlying psychotic or manic condition causing disruptive and disturbing behaviour, precluding a referral to psychiatric services. People who have become homeless for reasons other than a psychiatric disorder are exposed to traumatic events daily, which, in case of a pre-existing genetic vulnerability, can induce psychiatric disturbances. Such traumatic events include violence (21,22), head injury (23), or substance- and alcohol-related medical and neuropsychiatric conditions (24).

Twenty years of research by the 3rd of February Working Party shows that beyond the existing, meagre services available today, homeless people need adequate housing, mental and social support networks, medical services for addicts and psychiatric patients, support systems for the mentally or physically disabled, and crisis centres (16).

There is compelling research evidence that the traditional care system does not satisfy the psychological–psychiatric needs of homeless people with alcohol and substance dependence and personality disorder. Integrated care is needed, which takes mental status, substance use, financial situation, and housing needs into account. Prospective research is also warranted to create an effective alarm system to identify region-specific needs for the growing homeless population.

Psychiatric disorders in homeless people in Hungary: summary of a recent research project

The following is an overview of the first, and so far the only, survey of psychiatric disorders conducted in a homeless Hungarian cohort (25).

Aims of the survey

In 2014, a survey was conducted in Budapest to assess the psychiatric condition of homeless people and the impact of this condition on social connections, employment status, and substance use.

Participants

The study took place in three homeless shelters run by the Salvation Army: a rehabilitation centre for women, a home for women and children, and a shelter for men.

Assessment

First, all residents in the three shelters received a leaflet informing them about the purpose of the research, and confidentiality. Then they signed the accompanying declaration, accepting participation and consenting to the use of the data acquired during the survey. Those residents who consented to participate completed a questionnaire designed for this survey that enquired about past and current psychiatric treatment, medical conditions, current medications, and criminal offences. This was followed by the completion of the SCID-I and -II interviews. The SCID-I and SCID-II interviews were chosen because they are suitable for establishing the diagnosis of major psychiatric disorders and personality disorders, respectively, and their reliability has also been well established (26–28).

The interviews with the residents took place in a private room in the shelter. The interview lasted about 120 minutes. Residents did not receive any cash or other benefits for participating in the survey. A 3-digit code was randomly generated, to enter the data in an anonymized Excel file. The database contained the following information: age, sex, marital status, level of education, trade/profession, *Diagnostic and Statistical Manual of Mental Disorders (DSM)* diagnosis, medical and psychiatric history including alcohol and substance use, treatment and hospitalization, and criminal record.

Statistical analysis

The statistical analyses were conducted using SPSS for Windows, Version 20.0. Demographic data are presented with means and standard deviations or percentages, as appropriate. Continuous and discrete variables were compared with t-test and chi-square test, respectively. The level of significance was set at $P < 0.05$.

Results

Interest in the survey yielded a participation rate of 36%. Fifty homeless persons, 26 men and 24 women, made up the sample. The mean age of men and women was 49.27 ± 11.7 and 43.54 ± 8.4 years, respectively; 40% were single, 56% divorced, and 70% had two or more children. Only 30% of the participants were currently employed. As eight of the 12 participants with high school qualification also had a trade, altogether 27 (54%) of the participants had some form of a trade qualification.

Forty-three of the 50 participants had a diagnosis of a psychiatric disorder, predominantly personality disorders (50%) and alcohol dependence (44%) on the SCID-I and SCID-II interviews.

Psychiatric diagnoses (42%) were equally frequent in men and women ($P = 0.769$). Men mainly had personality disorders and alcohol dependence, while women mainly suffered from personality and anxiety disorders. Alcohol dependence occurred in both sexes at the same frequency (22%). Sixty per cent of the psychiatrically ill participants had a trade; they were equally distributed between diagnostic groups ($P = 0.450$). Regardless of the level of education, 22% of the participants with a current psychiatric diagnosis had a job.

The age distribution of participants with psychiatric diagnosis was balanced ($P = 0.480$). Thirty-seven percent of the participants with psychiatric diagnosis lived longer than 12 months in shelters or in the streets; participants with bipolar disorder and alcohol dependence were homeless for the longest period. One-third of psychiatrically ill participants had ever attempted suicide. The highest rate was associated with mood disorders and schizophrenia. Only 37% of participants with any psychiatric diagnosis were under psychiatric care; 69% of the participants with major depression were untreated.

Comorbid conditions (i.e. having more than one psychiatric diagnosis) were found in 72% of the cohort. Women had more comorbid conditions than men.

Personality disorders were diagnosed in 58% of the participants. Personality disorders most commonly occurred with drug addiction and anxiety disorders (80%). Comorbid substance-related disorders accompanied 58% of Axis I diagnoses. Comorbid alcohol dependence was more frequent (50%) than drug dependence (33%).

Discussion

The survey revealed that the prevalence of any kind of psychiatric disorder was 86% in the sample. Bipolar disorder, schizophrenia, personality disorder, and addiction were significantly more frequent in the participants than the general population (29–37).

In line with the data collected by the 3rd of February Working Party in 2011, participants came from all over the country. During their lifetime, they had spent a long time in one of the Federation of European Organizations Working with the Homeless (FEANTSA) groups (1, roofless; 2, houseless; 3, insecure accommodation; 4, inadequate housing) (38), so despite its small number ($N = 50$), the sample could be considered fairly representative.

The mean age of the participants was 46.5 years, and as a result of selection, men and women participated in equal number. The mean age in the study was slightly lower than the corresponding figure in Athens (51 years) (19) and higher than in Brazil (39 years) (20). Most participants were middle-aged, single or divorced, with one or more children, on a disability pension or unemployed, with low education.

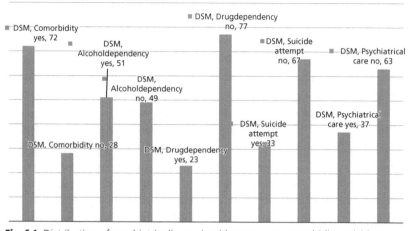

Fig. 6.1 Distribution of psychiatric diagnosis with respect to comorbidity, suicide attempts, and psychiatric care (%).

Psychiatric disorders in this sample were found to be more frequent than in the general population. In contrast to other European surveys where the frequency of psychiatric disorders in women was slightly higher (19,20), the two sexes were equally represented in *DSM* diagnoses in this survey. The higher frequency of anxiety disorders in women in other studies might be due to the higher frequency of post-traumatic stress disorder. The likely reason for the accumulation of post-traumatic stress disorder in women is that psychiatrically compromised women have a higher risk to be victimized than men (39). The sex difference in the Hungarian survey was equalized by the higher rate of addictions and personality disorders in men. Similar to the finding in a comprehensive study (40), 14% of the participants suffered from schizophrenia. An even greater difference from the general population was observed in the prevalence of alcohol dependence, and personality, anxiety, and bipolar disorders. The frequency of personality and bipolar disorders was higher than in the Brazil and Athens samples (19,20), which could be explained by the different climate. Hungary has far harsher autumns and winters, thus even seriously mentally ill homeless people, who otherwise would not accept restrictions, are more inclined to accept accommodation in a shelter.

The frequency of alcohol dependence varied widely across regions; it was 82% in Brazil (20), 5.5% in Athens (19), and 44% in this sample (25). The diversity of findings is due to the variety of consequences of breaking the rules on alcohol consumption.

In this study, comorbidity appeared in similar proportions as in a German (41) and a Brazilian (20) sample. This was mostly a combination of a *DSM* Axis

I disorder and a personality disorder and/or substance abuse. In the Hungarian sample, comorbidity was significantly more frequent in women than in men. Personality disorder was most commonly comorbid with drug dependence and anxiety disorders, while drug dependence was most frequently associated with mood disorders and post-traumatic stress disorder.

The lifetime prevalence of suicide attempts in persons with psychiatric illness was 32% in the Hungarian sample. In another survey of homeless people in Connecticut, US, 51% attempted suicide and half of them were hospitalized (42). The reason for the discrepancy between the two surveys may be due to younger age and the higher proportion of drug dependence in the American sample. In line with the literature (40,42), suicide attempts were most common among people with bipolar disorder and schizophrenia in the Hungarian sample.

The survey also revealed that less than 40% of homeless persons with a diagnosable psychiatric illness are under psychiatric care. Other studies also reported low rates of psychiatric care in the homeless population (43–45). Moreover, psychiatric treatment for the homeless is rarely appropriate. According to a systematic review of the Hungarian psychiatric care system conducted by the Állami Számvevőszék (State Audit Office of Hungary) 'half of the patients [suffering from depression] do not seek help from a doctor (50%); only every second of them is appropriately diagnosed (25%), and only half of the diagnosed patients (12.5%) receive treatment, but only half of them (6.25%) are prescribed the medication in a therapeutically effective dose' (46). The most common cause of avoiding psychiatric care in the homeless population—next to the fact that they did not perceive themselves as mentally ill—is that they had a bad experience while in psychiatric inpatient care (47).

Conclusion

The main finding of the Hungarian survey is that the prevalence of severe psychiatric disorders in homeless people is very high, which is in line with the results of other similar surveys conducted in other countries. Homeless people with psychiatric disorders are a particularly vulnerable group. It would be important to identify early the psychiatrically ill people, particularly the untreated ones and those who have a high risk of suicide or criminal behaviour. It would also be desirable to improve the efficacy of social care and healthcare system for the homeless and to educate social workers and other personnel who care for them.

The low level of engagement of homeless people in psychiatric care indicates that the traditional care model is not appropriate for this particular population.

Homeless psychiatric patients form a special subgroup and looking after them is a complex problem which demands complex solutions. Their care can only be provided by a highly trained interdisciplinary team who follow the person even when they leave the shelter, helping with social integration and providing ongoing mental healthcare even in the face of alcohol and substance use.

References

1. **Csapó K, Kerner K.** Budapest az egyesítéstől az 1930-as évekig. Budapest: Útmutató Tanácsadó és Kiadó Kft; 1999.
2. **Breiter P, Gurály Z, Győri P.** Kérdések és válaszok a hajléktalanságról. Budapest: Menhely Alapítvány; 2002.
3. **Győri P.** A Hajléktalanok Menhelye Egylet. Esély. 1998;5:21–42.
4. **Fehér B.** Hajléktalan emberek Magyarországon: 1989-től napjainkig. Vigilia. 2008;73(6):402–410.
5. **Győri P.** Vannak-e jogaik a hajléktalanoknak? Mozgóvilág. 1996;22(12):96–104.
6. **Oross J.** A hajléktalanság kezelése Magyarországon. In: Kézikönyv a szociális munka gyakorlatához. Budapest: Szociális Szakmai Szövetség; 2001:64–80.
7. 2018. évi XLIV. törvény a szabálysértésekről, a szabálysértési eljárásról és a szabálysértési nyilvántartási rendszerről szóló 2012. évi II. törvény módosításáról.
8. **Homeless World Cup Organization.** Global homelessness statistics. Available from: https://www.homelessworldcup.org/homelessness-statistics/.
9. **Breitner P, Gurály Z, Győri P,** et al. Változó és változatlan arcú hajléktalanság. Budapest: Menhely Alapítvány és Budapesti Módszertani Szociális Központ és Intézményei; 2013.
10. **Győri P, Szabó A.** Gyorsjelentés a hajléktalan emberek 2012 február 3-i kérdőíves adatfelvételéről. Budapest: Menhely Alapítvány—Február Harmadika Csoport; 2012.
11. **Győri P, Gurály Z, Szabó A.** Gyorsjelentés a hajléktalan emberek 2013 február 3-i kérdőíves adatfelvételéről. Budapest: Menhely Alapítvány—Február Harmadika Csoport; 2013.
12. **Győri P, Szabó A, Gurály Z.** Gyorsjelentés a hajléktalan emberek 2014 február 3-i kérdőíves adatfelvételéről. Budapest: Menhely Alapítvány—Február Harmadika Csoport; 2014.
13. **Győri P, Szabó A, Gurály Z.** Gyorsjelentés a hajléktalan emberek 2015 február 3-i kérdőíves adatfelvételéről. Budapest: Menhely Alapítvány—Február Harmadika Csoport; 2015.
14. **Győri P, Szabó A, Gurály Z.** Gyorsjelentés a hajléktalan emberek 2016 február 3-i kérdőíves adatfelvételéről. Budapest: Menhely Alapítvány—Február Harmadika Csoport; 2016.
15. **Győri P, Szabó A, Gurály Z.** Gyorsjelentés a hajléktalan emberek 2017 február 3-i kérdőíves adatfelvételéről. Budapest: Menhely Alapítvány—Február Harmadika Csoport; 2017.
16. **Győri P, Szabó A, Gurály Z.** Gyorsjelentés a hajléktalan emberek 2018 február 3-i kérdőíves adatfelvételéről. Budapest: Menhely Alapítvány—Február Harmadika Csoport; 2018.

17. **Complex Hatályos Jogszabályok Gyűjteménye.** 1/2000. (I. 7.) SzCsM rendelet a személyes gondoskodást nyújtó szociális intézmények szakmai feladatairól és működésük feltételeiről; Available from: http://net.jogtar.hu/jr/gen/hjegy_doc. cgi?docid=A0000001.SCM.

18. **Fazel S, Khosla V, Doll H, Geddes J.** The prevalence of mental disorders among the homeless in western countries: systematic review and meta-regression analysis. PLoS Med. 2008;5(12):e225.

19. **Madianos MG, Chondraki P, Papadimitriou GN.** Prevalence of psychiatric disorders among homeless people in Athens area: a cross-sectional study. Soc Psychiatry Psychiatr Epidemiol. 2013;48(8):1225–1234.

20. **Heckert U, Andrade L, Alves MJ, Martins C.** Lifetime prevalence of mental disorders among homeless people in a southeast city in Brazil. Eur Arch Psychiatry Clin Neurosci. 1999;249(3):150–155.

21. **Bíró G, Vadász A.** A hajléktalan személyek sérelmére elkövetett bűncselekmények egyes kérdései. Esély. 2003;14:31–55.

22. **Kushel MB, Evans JL, Perry S, Robertson MJ, Moss AR.** No door to lock: victimization among homeless and marginally housed persons. Arch Intern Med. 2003;163(20):2492–2499.

23. **Hwang SW, Colantonio A, Chiu S, et al.** The effect of traumatic brain injury on the health of homeless people. CMAJ. 2008;179(8):779–784.

24. **Háberman Z.** 'Ahhoz, hogy elviselje az ember a stresszt, kellett valami oldószer.' H. J. hajléktalan a hajléktalanellátásról. Esély. 2003;14:63–85.

25. **Braun E, Gazdag G.** Pszichiátriai zavarok előfordulása hajléktalanok között. Psychiatr. Hung. 2015;30(1):60–67.

26. **Stuart AL, Pasco JA, Jacka FN, Brennan SL, Berk M, Williams LJ.** Comparison of self-report and structured clinical interview in the identification of depression. Compr Psychiatry. 2014;55(4):866–869.

27. **Gerevich J, Bacskai E, Matuszka B, Czobor P.** The Hungarian adaptation of anxiety disorder module in the SCID-I/NP research version. Psychiatr Hung. 2010;25(5):394–406.

28. **Lobbestael J, Leurgans M, Arntz A.** Inter-rater reliability of the Structured Clinical Interview for DSM-IV Axis I Disorders (SCID I) and Axis II Disorders (SCID II). Clin Psychol Psychother. 2011;18(1):75–79.

29. **A Pszichiátriai Szakmai Kollégium.** Az Egészségügyi Minisztérium szakmai protokollja – a bipoláris affektív betegségek diagnosztikájáról és terápiájáról. 2016. Available from: https://kollegium.aeek.hu/Iranyelvek/Index.

30. **A Pszichiátriai Szakmai Kollégium.** Az Egészségügyi Minisztérium szakmai protokollja: Alkoholbetegség. 2006. Available from: https://kollegium.aeek.hu/Iranyel vek/Index.

31. **A Pszichiátriai Szakmai Kollégium.** Az Egészségügyi Minisztérium szakmai protokollja: Szkizofrénia. 2005. Available from: https://kollegium.aeek.hu/Iranyelvek/Index.

32. **Buda B.** Alkoholpolitikai koncepció. Addictologia Hungarica. 2005;4:204–211.

33. **Davidson JR, Hughes D, Blazer DG, George LK.** Post-traumatic stress disorder in the community: an epidemiological study. Psychol Med. 1991;21(3):713–721.

34. **Kopp M, Szedmák S, Lőke J, Skrabski Á.** A depressziós tünetegyüttes gyakorisága és egészségügyi jelentősége a magyar lakosság körében. Lege Artis Med. 1997;7:136–144.

35. **Sareen J, Cox BJ, Afifi TO, et al.** Anxiety disorders and risk for suicidal ideation and suicide attempts: a population-based longitudinal study of adults. Arch Gen Psychiatry. 2005;62(11):1249–1257.

36. **Alonso J, Ferrer M, Romera B, et al.** The European Study of the Epidemiology of Mental Disorders (ESEMeD/MHEDEA 2000) project: rationale and methods. Int J Methods Psychiatr Res. 2002;11(2):55–67.

37. **Sansone RA, Sansone LA.** Personality disorders: a nation-based perspective on prevalence. Innov Clin Neurosci. 2011;8(4):13–18.

38. **FEANTSA.** ETHOS – European typology of homelessness and housing exclusion. 2017. Available from: https://www.feantsa.org/download/en-16822651433655843804.pdf.

39. **Chapple B, Chant D, Nolan P, Cardy S, Whiteford H, McGrath J.** Correlates of victimization amongst people with psychosis. Soc Psychiatry Psychiatr Epidemiol. 2004;39(10):836–840.

40. **Nilsson SF, Hjorthøj CR, Erlangsen A, Nordentoft M.** Suicide and unintentional injury mortality among homeless people: a Danish nationwide register-based cohort study. Eur J Public Health. 2013;24(1):50–56.

41. **Langle G, Egerter B, Albrecht F, Petrasch M, Buchkremer G.** Prevalence of mental illness among homeless men in the community—approach to a full census in a southern German university town. Soc Psychiatry Psychiatr Epidemiol. 2005;40(5):382–390.

42. **Desai RA, Liu-Mares W, Dausey DJ, Rosenheck RA.** Suicidal ideation and suicide attempts in a sample of homeless people with mental illness. J Nerv Ment Dis. 2003;191(6):365–371.

43. **Kovess V, Mangin Lazarus C.** The prevalence of psychiatric disorders and use of care by homeless people in Paris. Soc Psychiatry Psychiatr Epidemiol. 1999;34(11):580–587.

44. **Rosenheck R, Seibyl CL.** Homelessness: health service use and related costs. Med Care. 1998;36(8):1256–1264.

45. **Henry JM, Boyer L, Belzeaux R, Baumstarck-Barrau K, Samuelian JC.** Mental disorders among homeless people admitted to a French psychiatric emergency service. Psychiatr Serv. 2010;61(3):264–271.

46. **Böröcz I, Federics A, Zachár P.** Jelentés a pszichiátriai betegellátás átalakításának ellenőrzéséről. Budapest: Állami számvevőszék; 2012.

47. **Maness DL, Khan M.** Care of the homeless: an overview. Am Fam Physician. 2014;89(8):634–640.

Chapter 7

Homelessness and mental health in Paraguay

Julio Torales and Israel Gonzalez-Urbieta

Introduction

The modern view of homelessness as a complex social problem and a public health phenomenon involving many social factors stands in contrast with views held in previous periods. In the past, homeless people have been assigned different derogatory labels implying the possible aetiology of their living conditions, including spiritually weak, criminal offenders, alcoholics, or more currently, mentally ill (1). While old notions about mental health and homelessness, such as assertions that up to 50% of homeless people may have schizophrenia, are likely outdated (2,3), we know that these entities are connected. Most researchers agree that this relationship is bidirectional and complex. Mental health problems can cause homelessness, but homelessness can also be a factor in the development, exacerbation, and maintenance of mental health issues (4).

Homelessness and mental health

It is recognized that homeless people constitute a vulnerable population in terms of mental health issues (5). There are undoubtedly multiple factors besides mental illness that contribute to the difficulties homeless people face in obtaining and maintaining stable housing, including involvement in drug or alcohol misuse (6), lack of education or employment (7), and a history of physical, sexual, or emotional abuse (8). Mental illness, however, appears to play a central role in the aetiology of homelessness (9). There is great variability in the reports of the prevalence of mental health results in homeless people, likely due to different sampling strategies and varying definitions of homelessness. Nevertheless, most studies report high levels of depressive symptoms (10), manic episodes (11), and substance use disorders (12). In turn, homelessness can be a predisposing factor for mental disorders; this condition appears to compound the baseline psychological issues, and increase the risk of developing psychopathology (13).

Homelessness in Paraguay

Paraguay is a landlocked country in the middle of South America, with around 30% of the population living below the poverty line, and more than 5% living in extreme poverty. The percentage of people living in the latter category is ten times higher in rural areas (12.17%) than in urban areas (1.63%). There is a deficit of approximately 1.5 million homes in Paraguay, according to the National Secretariat of Housing and Habitat (14). The American Development Bank estimates that 43% of households live in inadequate housing conditions (15). While these numbers can provide an idea about the percentage of the population living in substandard conditions, there are no official numbers regarding the number of homeless people in the country or the percentage distribution among different ethnic populations. It is worth considering, however, that surveys among the homeless are substantially hard to conduct, due to the characteristics intrinsic to their living conditions, such as the lack of a stable home address or a fixed landline. In our experience, the majority of the homeless population in the metropolitan areas correspond to people from native ethnic groups who have been forcibly displaced from their territories due to deforestation, occupation of their land, or lack of economic and social opportunities. These people also have to face specific adversities such as the language barrier, discrimination, and lack of cultural competence of physicians in these areas (16).

Access to mental health services for homeless people in Paraguay

Currently, there are approximately 150 psychiatrists in Paraguay, and most of them distribute their time between working in public hospitals and seeing patients in their private practice. While all doctor visits are free in the public system, the majority of the public hospitals do not have a psychiatrist available. If they do, they only have one professional who has to cover the needs of the entire area, while being contracted for only 1 or 2 days a week. The exceptions to this rule are the Hospital Psiquiátrico and the Hospital de Clínicas, both of which provide free consultations with psychiatrists every day of the week. These hospitals are located in Asunción (the capital city of the country) and San Lorenzo (a city located 15 minutes away from Asunción), respectively, and they are the only hospitals in the metropolitan area that provide free inpatient psychiatry treatment. Another hospital situated in the north of the country also has a psychiatric hospitalization service with six beds available which, at the time of writing, is closed due to issues related to the coronavirus 2019 pandemic.

Despite the availability of some psychiatric services at no cost, there are numerous obstacles or disadvantageous situations for people with limited resources, some of them specific to the homeless. One of these disadvantages is the difficulty in obtaining follow-up with a family psychiatrist. Considering that physicians cover most of these positions in residency training, who frequently move from one rotation to another, patients are seldom followed up by a single psychiatrist. This situation can result in inconsistent management and frequent unnecessary or inappropriate changes of the medication, considering the absence of electronic medical records in the health system that would allow different physicians to easily record the patient's complete medical history and analyse their progress.

The lack of availability of several medications commonly used in psychiatry at no cost is also an impediment to the effective treatment of various disorders that can affect the homeless. At present, the public health system does not cover antidementia medication or medications for attention deficit hyperactivity disorder, and the coverage for other psychopharmacological groups such as antidepressants, mood stabilizers, and antipsychotics is quite limited.

Perhaps the main limiting factor for an adequate approach to the mental health of the homeless is the barrier to access to health services. As mentioned earlier, the attention and availability of psychiatric services are disproportionately centralized in the most important cities of the country, to the detriment of most of the other areas. Thus, many patients must reach the capital to receive the appropriate treatment. Although this factor may constitute a barrier for most people, this can be especially problematic for the homeless, who are almost always in a situation of extreme poverty and, therefore, do not have the means to travel from their region to the metropolitan area. Those who work, in general, do so for a daily salary, which means that taking a day to visit the psychiatrist can represent an economic loss that could result in the absence of food or basic sustenance on that day.

These patients frequently lack basic support systems of family or friends, and the state is absent in this regard. This constitutes a dilemma when treatment requires the use of medications that need to be monitored for their level of toxicity or in patients who come to consult for suicidal ideation or self-injurious behaviour. When patients need inpatient treatment, psychiatric services require that the patients be accompanied by a family member or caregiver throughout the day, due to the lack of infrastructure of the hospitalization centres. This can frequently represent an insurmountable barrier for the homeless, who often lack relatives who can fulfil this function.

A way forward

There are currently no mental health programmes focused on servicing home-less patients. Between May 2017 and June 2018, the National Secretariat of Housing and Habitat developed the National Housing and Habitat Policy (14). It raises among its guiding principles the human right for adequate housing and habitat, social and productive inclusion, and equality of opportunities, but does not explicitly contemplate specific efforts or delineations towards improving access to mental health services for this group. The National Mental Health Policy proposed in 2011 by the Mental Health Direction of the National Health Department included a strategy for promoting equality in the quality of life and health, which constituted a 'set of actions aimed at promoting of the au-tonomy of people, their full and dignified development in the social, political and economic spheres' (17). This document mentions the need to adopt a pro-motional model of care, indicated as 'an approach where the perspective of the promotion is inserted in all actions, whether educational, preventive, pro-tective, diagnostic, treatment and rehabilitation'. It also proposes the adoption of a community care model, as opposed to the assistance and hospital-centric model. Although the policy does not make explicit mention of the homeless, it does emphasize the use of the primary healthcare network to improve access to the mental health of the population, a point that will be discussed in more detail later in this chapter.

The first step in developing policies aimed at improving the mental health of the homeless is to gather reliable information about the sociodemographic data of this group and their specific needs related to mental health, including those associated with barriers to access to health services. This represents a key challenge since this type of information is normally collected through censuses or telephone surveys directed, precisely, to households. This involves designing creative strategies to obtain accurate data. Methods such as indirect estimation, single-contact censuses, and recruitment-reuptake studies have been used in other regions, and each presents its own benefits and disadvantages (18).

From the data obtained, mental health programmes should be developed that are specifically aimed at this population and their needs. These programmes should be implemented in the context of regional or national policies and strat-egies. Programmes should include a holistic approach that aims at the general improvement of the quality of life of these people and that seeks, in addition to providing housing solutions, their complete insertion into the community from the economic, social, educational, and health points of view. It will be essential that these solutions are adapted, and adaptative to the needs of this group, not only in the data collection stage but also those that arise during the implemen-tation of these strategies (19).

One of the deficits that exist in the country is the non-inclusion of mental health services in the general health system. There are numerous health centres and district and even regional hospitals that do not offer psychiatric care due to lack of staff. This omission is quite striking since the simple inclusion of a psychiatrist in these units would significantly improve access to care for populations near these institutions. Moreover, there are now numerous family health units, which are generally the first point of contact for the general population with the health system. These devices are particularly beneficial for the homeless, as they are providing their services within communities, thus eliminating the barrier of the need for transportation to access care. With the creation of the National Mental Health Policy, two protocols were published with guidelines for mental healthcare: Standards and Procedures in Mental Health Care and Clinical Management of Mental Disorders in Primary Health Care. These guides are being socialized through mental health training courses run by the National Department of Public Health and Social Welfare (17). We believe that the training of primary care staff for the diagnosis and basic management of mental disorders will have a significant impact on the care of vulnerable groups such as the homeless (20).

Conclusion

Homelessness and inadequate housing are very prevalent conditions in Paraguay. The relationship between mental health disorders and insufficient living conditions appears to be reciprocal: these disorders are highly prevalent in this population, and homelessness can contribute to the development and exacerbation of mental illness. There are currently no efforts in the country to address the specific needs of the homeless regarding their mental health (21). Several steps are proposed that could improve the mental health and overall standard of living of this vulnerable group.

References

1. **Cook T** (Ed). Vagrancy: Some New Perspectives. London: Academic Press; 1979.
2. **Foster A, Gable J, Buckley J.** Homelessness in schizophrenia. Psychiatr Clin North Am. 2012;**35**(3):717–734.
3. **Folsom D, Jeste DV.** Schizophrenia in homeless persons: a systematic review of the literature. Acta Psychiatr Scand. 2002;**105**(6):404–413.
4. **Institute of Medicine (US) Committee on Health Care for Homeless People.** Health Problems of Homeless People. Washington, DC: National Academies Press; 1988. Available from: https://www.ncbi.nlm.nih.gov/books/NBK218236/.
5. **Hodgson KJ, Shelton KH, van den Bree MBM.** Psychopathology among young homeless people: longitudinal mental health outcomes for different subgroups. Br J Clin Psychol. 2015;**54**(3):307–325.

6. **Hammersley R, Psychol C, Pearl S.** Drug use and other problems of residents in projects for the young, single homeless. Health Soc Care Community. 2007;**4**(4):193–199.

7. **Fry CE, Langley K, Shelton KH.** A systematic review of cognitive functioning among young people who have experienced homelessness, foster care, or poverty. Child Neuropsychol. 2017;**23**(8):907–934.

8. **Giano Z, Williams A, Hankey C, Merrill R, Lisnic R, Herring A.** Forty years of research on predictors of homelessness. Community Ment Health J. 2020;**56**:692–709.

9. **Embry LE, Stoep AV, Evens C, Ryan KD, Pollock A.** Risk factors for homelessness in adolescents released from psychiatric residential treatment. J Am Acad Child Adolesc Psychiatry. 2000;**39**(10):1293–1299.

10. **Bearsley-Smith CA, Bond LM, Littlefield L, Thomas LR.** The psychosocial profile of adolescent risk of homelessness. Eur Child Adolesc Psychiatry. 2008;**17**(4):226–234.

11. **Beijer U, Andréasson S.** Gender, hospitalization and mental disorders among homeless people compared with the general population in Stockholm. Eur J Public Health. 2010;**20**(5):511–516.

12. **Craig TK, Hodson S.** Homeless youth in London: I. Childhood antecedents and psychiatric disorder. Psychol Med. 1998;**28**(6):1379–1388.

13. **Hodgson KJ, Shelton KH, van den Bree MBM, Los FJ.** Psychopathology in young people experiencing homelessness: a systematic review. Am J Public Health. 2013;**103**(6):e24–37.

14. **Secretaría Nacional de la Vivienda y el Hábitat del Paraguay.** Política Nacional de la Vivienda y el Hábitat de Paraguay. Asunción: Secretaría Nacional de la Vivienda y el Hábitat del Paraguay; 2018.

15. **Habitat for Humanity.** Paraguay. 2018. Available from: http://www.habitat.org/lac-es/where-we-build/paraguay.

16. **Tribe R, Morrissey J** (Eds). The Handbook of Professional Ethical and Research Practice for Psychologists, Counsellors, Psychotherapists and Psychiatrists, 3rd ed. Abingdon: Routledge; 2020.

17. **Domingues J, Silva MG da, Nogueira VMR.** A implementação da política de saúde mental no Paraguai: desafios e potencialidades. Rev MERCOSUR Políticas Soc. 2018;**2**:287.

18. **Institute of Medicine (US) Committee on Health Care for Homeless People.** The Methodology of Counting the Homeless. Washington, DC: National Academies Press; 1988. Available from: https://www.ncbi.nlm.nih.gov/books/NBK218229/.

19. **Narasimhan L, Gopikumar V, Jayakumar V, Bunders J, Regeer B.** Responsive mental health systems to address the poverty, homelessness and mental illness nexus: the Banyan experience from India. Int J Ment Health Syst. 2019;**13**(1):54.

20. **Domingues J.** A implementação da Política de Saúde Mental nas cidades gêmeas de Foz do Iguaçu (BR) e Ciudad del Este (PY). Doctoral Thesis. Pelotas: Universidade Catolica de Pelotas, Centro de Ciencias Sociais e Tecnologicas; 2018. Available from: http://pos.ucpel.edu.br/ppgps/wp-content/uploads/sites/5/2018/04/Tese_-_Juliana_Domingues.pdf.

21. **Torales J, Villalba-Arias J, Ruiz-Díaz C, Chávez E, Riego V.** The right to health in Paraguay. Int Rev Psychiatry. 2014;**26**(4):524–529.

Chapter 8

Mental health in Brazilian homeless

Etienne de Miranda e Silva,
Anderson Sousa Martins da Silva, and
João Mauricio Castaldelli-Maia

Introduction

In Brazil, some studies have evaluated mental and substance use disorders in homeless (1–19). These studies show that homeless people have more mental and substance use disorders than the general population. It is a population more exposed to various social vulnerabilities, such as low level of education and socioeconomic status, disruptions in the family, emotional and physical violence, illegal practices, incarceration, and risky behaviours such as unprotected sexual practices with different partners, triggering exposures to sexually transmitted diseases and communicable diseases (20). In this chapter, we review mental and substance use disorders in Brazilian homeless individuals.

Substance use disorders

Several studies point to high rates of drug and alcohol use in homeless people, being around three times more frequent (13). In a study carried out in São Paulo state, rates of 43.2% of alcohol dependence and 30.2% of drug use was found in homeless people. Similar rates were confirmed by studies carried out in the same region (3,12), in which 55.7% and 25.7% of the homeless reported lifetime and frequent use, respectively. Another study carried out in five Brazilian state capitals (10) found that 74.3% of homeless individuals used drugs. These findings demonstrate the alarming rates of substance use in Brazilian homeless people, regardless of the region. In a survey conducted by Van Straaten et al. (21), it was found that the chances of being chronic homeless (>18 months) were twice as high in drug addicts than in non-addicts.

Alcohol

Among all the substances with abuse potential, alcohol is the most prevalent in Brazilian homeless. Studies (1,2,4–8,11,13) found alcohol dependence rates ranging from 25% to 83%. The vast majority found rates above 40% (1,4–8,11,13). Brazilian findings are in line with studies from other countries and regions. According to Fazel et al. (22), 29 surveys, including 5684 homeless individuals in seven countries, found that the most common mental or substance use disorder was alcohol dependence, ranging from 8.1% to 58.5%. They also found that alcohol dependence has increased in recent decades (22).

Concerning the young homeless subpopulation (<18 years old), only one study investigated alcohol use, reporting a rate of regular use of 26%. Thus, it seems that this subpopulation uses less alcohol than adults, but far more than their peers from the general population (23). The high rate of use of this substance among the youth subpopulation can lead to serious damage in the short, medium, and long term, mainly because the neuropsychiatric system is still in the process of maturation (23).

Cannabis

Cannabis is one of the most used drugs by the homeless, with rates of use ranging from 26% to 53.1% (1,2,3,10,12). Surveys carried out in five capitals in Brazil had inhalants and marijuana as the most used illicit drugs during their lives, such as in the general population (24). However, the prevalences of lifetime use were much higher, with 67.6% for cannabis and 53.1% for inhalants among homeless children and adolescents (10). Local studies also found high lifetime prevalences of cannabis use. In the states of São Paulo and Goiás, 50.8% and 37.9% reported cannabis use, respectively (1,3,12). These Brazilian findings are in line with studies conducted abroad. In the cohort conducted by Van Straaten et al. (21), including 344 homeless participants, cannabis use was reported by 43.9%.

Cocaine

Cocaine use disorder in homeless individuals was more prevalent in the Southeastern region, according to a study that investigated mental healthcare services in five Brazilian state capitals (10). The lifetime use of cocaine was 21.2%, and recent use was 10.4% in adult homeless (10). In the state of São Paulo, 34.2% of adult homeless had cocaine use disorder (3,12). A quite similar cocaine use disorder prevalence was found in the state of Góias (38.1%) (1). Cocaine use disorder is more prevalent in the adult population of homeless people than in young people. In the study that investigated mental healthcare services in five Brazilian state capitals, cocaine use disorder prevalence was much lower in the population under 18 years old (10). This was confirmed by a survey carried out in Porto Alegre, in which the values of recent use and last month use were closer to 0% in this subpopulation of homeless people (2).

The use of crack was rarely addressed in studies with a prevalence of use ranging from 25% to 53.1% (2,3,5,13,15), which were performed in the population over 18 years old. These values were much higher than those found in other countries. According to Van Straaten et al. (21), in their analysis of 344 Dutch homeless people, 5.2% had used crack in the last 30 days, and after 18 months of follow-up, 3.5% had used it in the previous 30 days.

Inhalants

The use of inhalants is predominant among children and adolescents living on the streets (2,4,10). The rates of use in this subpopulation were high for lifetime use (67.6%), recent use (41.2%), and heavy use (20.9%) (10). Another study also confirmed the high-prevalence lifetime use (68%), last-month use (58%), and regular use (58%) (2). One study investigated the use of benzydamine in housing institutions for children and adolescents in 27 Brazilian state capitals (11). It found a prevalence of 2.7%, mainly in the state capitals of the Northeast region (85.9% of the users), especially São Luiz, Maceió, and Fortaleza (11). Inhalants also seem to be especially popular among street children in other countries. Embleton et al. (25) conducted a meta-analysis of street children and substance use, including 50 studies in 22 countries. They found a combined prevalence of drug use among children of 60%. In 14 of the 22 countries, 47% of the street children were using inhalants. This meta-analysis found that inhalants were the substances predominantly used by this population, followed by tobacco, alcohol, and marijuana. Inhalant testing can be performed through the collection of urine and blood. In Brazil, studies using these testing methodologies found 88% of urine with an excess of hippuric acid (15) and 91.9% with elevated levels of toluene (16), which could be explained by intentional exposures to toluene.

Tobacco

There was only one study evaluating tobacco smoking in Brazilian homeless individuals (2). The majority reported regular use (58%) (2). This finding is in line with those from other countries. Pettey et al. (26) conducted a study with a sample of 639 with serious mental illness who were homeless or vulnerably housed and receiving community mental health services. The identified smokers completed the Fagerström Test for Nicotine Dependence and additional questions related to smoking behaviour. The prevalence of tobacco

use was 72%, and 62% of smokers had high or very high levels of nicotine dependence. Smoking behaviours included contraband cigarettes (47%) and dis-
carded cigarette butts (25%). It was found that smokers were more than nine
times more likely to have a substance use disorder that co-occurs. This is confirmed by the survey conducted by Guillen et al. (27), with 138 interviewees
from the city of Madrid, Spain. Their results showed that tobacco was the most
consumed substance (70.1%), followed by sedatives (48.6%), alcohol (36.2%),
methadone (13.7%), cocaine (7.2%), cannabis (6.5%), and heroin (5.1%). This
study was conducted with homeless women only.

Injecting drugs

Just a few studies evaluated the use of injectable drugs in homeless people in
Brazil. One study found a rate of use of 5% (8), and another study, 5.6% (3).
The only drug cited was injectable cocaine (3). These rates are quite similar to
the rates found in other countries. However, injectable opioids are the most
popular abroad. Guillén et al. (27) found that the use of heroin in homeless
women in Spain was 5.1%. In the Netherlands, according to Van Straaten et al.
(21), 2.3% of the homeless had used heroin in the last 30 days.

Mental disorders

Mental disorders were associated with the male sex in Brazil (4–7,14). Toro et
al. (28) confirm this in their research in which they evaluated homeless people
in Poland and the US. In both countries, the majority of homeless adults were
male. It also corroborates the European study carried out by Van Straaten et al.
(21) in which the vast majority of the participants who used at least one substance were male.

A minority of the studies with Brazilian homeless investigated mental health
disorders (i.e. assessed substance use disorders only). Most of the studies
which evaluated mental disorders investigated all of them together in a group.
The nomenclature varied, including 'mental problems', 'psychiatric disorders',
'serious mental illnesses', and 'psychiatric problems'. A study conducted in
six state capitals, including 266 adult homeless, found that 51.2% had mental
problems (4). In Rio de Janeiro, a sample of 330 homeless identified that 49.2%
of them had any mental problem, and 19.4% had a mental illness (7). These
results are in line with those from other countries. Fazel et al. (22) stated that
the rates of psychotic diseases ranged from 2.8% to 42.3%, suggesting that in
Western countries, psychotic disorders are greater. In a study carried out by
Schreiter et al. (29) among homeless participants in Berlin, Germany, substance use disorder was diagnosed significantly more frequently (74.2%), and

psychotic disorders were the highest among the mental disorders (29.0%). Regarding serious mental illness in Brazilian homeless, we find prevalences ranging from 9.8% (8) to 22.6% (6). Another Brazilian study conducted in São Paulo reported even higher rates of mental disorders in the homeless under 18 years old (14). They found a prevalence of 88.8% of mental disorders in this subpopulation (14).

Psychotic disorders

The prevalence of psychotic disorders in Brazilian homeless people was found to be 9.6% (5) and 10.7% (6) in two studies. The review by Ayano et al. in 2019 (30) point outs that schizophrenia and other psychotic disorders are the main constituents for disability and premature mortality among homeless people. They included 51,925 homeless in this review, with a notably high rate of psychosis (21.21%), schizophrenia (10.29%), and schizophreniform disorders (2.48%), compared to the general population's usual rates. Developing countries (29.16%) presented higher rates of psychotic disorders compared to the developed countries (18.80%). This was also valid for schizophrenia (22.15% versus 8.83%). Brazil, like other developing countries, has been struggling with a high prevalence of psychotic disorders among the homeless.

Affective disorders

Some studies are evaluating affective disorders in the Brazilian homeless. Both among adult and adolescent homeless, about a third of individuals are affected by these disorders (32.5% (5) in a sample of people over 18 and 35.3% (14) in people under 18 years of age). As for depressive symptoms in adult homeless, a single study showed rates of 58.1% (4) and 49.4% of suicidal ideation (4). At least one suicide attempt was reported by 28.3% (4). Another study evaluated the homeless under 18 years old (10). A lower, but still high, rate was found (9.3%) (10). Again, Brazilian findings are in line with those from other countries. Another review by Ayano et al. focused on suicidal ideation and attempts, including 20 studies with 27,497 homeless people (31). They found prevalences of current and lifetime suicidal ideation of 17.8% and 41.6%, respectively (31). The current and lifetime prevalences of suicide attempts were 9.2% and 28.8%, respectively. According to Fond et al. (32), in their multicentre study with homeless people from four French cities ($n = 700$), 55.4% were diagnosed with major depressive disorder. Thus, Brazil and other countries present high rates of affective disorders in this population, which tends to be underreported. In addition, depressive disorder in this subpopulation tends to be more severe, frequently including suicidal ideation and attempts.

Attention deficit and hyperactivity disorder

Only one study investigated attention deficit and hyperactivity disorder (ADHD) in youth Brazilian homeless (14). The authors found an ADHD prevalence of 16% in a sample of individuals aged 10–18 years (14). In this study, ADHD in childhood was associated with an increased rate of homelessness. This demonstrates the need for more monitoring of ADHD from childhood to adolescence to ease the malfunctioning process that includes homelessness.

Conclusion

The studies presented in this chapter revealed the general scenario of mental health and substance use disorders in homeless people in Brazil. We found different prevalences for different disorders. As a general rule, both in Brazil and worldwide, mental health and substance use disorders are more prevalent in this subpopulation compared to the general population. The majority of the Brazilian studies are concentrated in the South and Southeast regions. No study was found in the North region. Regarding gender, there was a higher prevalence of men in the studies. Only one study had a higher percentage of women.

Among the mental health disorders, psychotic and affective disorders were the most prevalent in this subpopulation. Regarding substance use, cannabis and alcohol were those most used in the adult population, followed by cocaine (crack). Brazilian homeless under 18 years of age report a high prevalence of the use of inhalants. Disorders due to the use of inhalants in homeless people are more associated with children and adolescents, while crack is more associated with the adult population. There are few studies on tobacco smoking and injectable drugs, although the few available show significant rates.

Limitations are noted. Brazil has a lot of socioeconomic and health access differences among its regions. Thus, the findings presented here should not be generalized for the entire country. Some studies were limited to the services frequented by this subpopulation. Several studies rely on small samples. Other studies used non-validated questionnaires. Another important limitation refers to possible memory bias or an attempt to provide socially acceptable answers.

This chapter showed that the presence of mental health and substance use disorders in the homeless is an utmost public health issue. Living on the street already involves a series of limitations, including more precarious health conditions, food, greater exposure to numerous risks, generating increased morbidity, and mortality. It is challenging to approach these individuals, considering that most of them live a 'nomadic life' with little or no attachment. We believe that approaching mental health and substance use disorders in this subpopulation could contribute to a more organized and centred life, making use of all the possible resources available (e.g. housing, healthcare, social networks, and financial incentives). Greater public interventions are needed with a different target and focus for this audience. They should aim to improve basic living conditions, integrating mental health and substance use disorder treatment into social interventions. Brazilian psychosocial care centres (Centros de Atenção Psicossocial (CAPS)) have been playing an essential role in this outcome. CAPS are freely available for all the individuals living in Brazil, legally or not. These Brazilian studies underline the need for more effective early interventions aimed at preventing long-term deleterious, almost unchangeable outcomes in this vulnerable population.

References

1. **Bezerra KF, Gurgel RQ, Ilozue C, Castaneda DN.** Estimating the number of street children and adolescents in two cities of Brazil using capture-recapture. J Paediatr Child Health. 2011;**47**(8):524–529.

2. **Brunini SM, Barros CVL, Guimarães RA,** et al. HIV infection, high-risk behaviors and substance use in homeless men sheltered in therapeutic communities in Central Brazil. Int J STD AIDS. 2018;**29**(11):1084–1088.

3. **de Carvalho FT, Neiva-Silva L, Ramos MC,** et al. Sexual and drug use risk behaviors among children and youth in street circumstances in Porto Alegre, Brazil. AIDS Behav. 2006;**10**(4 Suppl):S57–S66.

4. **Forster LM, Tannhauser M, Barros HM.** Drug use among street children in southern Brazil. Drug Alcohol Depend. 1996;**43**(1–2):57–62.

5. **Grangeiro A, Holcman MM, Onaga ET, Alencar HD, Placco AL, Teixeira PR.** Prevalência e vulnerabilidade à infecção pelo HIV de moradores de rua em São Paulo, SP [Prevalence and vulnerability of homeless people to HIV infection in São Paulo, Brazil]. Rev Saude Publica. 2012;**46**(4):674–684.

6. **Halpern SC, Scherer JN, Roglio V,** et al. Vulnerabilidades clínicas e sociais em usuários de crack de acordo com a situação de moradia: um estudo multicêntrico de seis capitais brasileiras [Clinical and social vulnerabilities in crack users according to housing status: a multicenter study in six Brazilian state capitals]. Cad Saude Publica. 2017;**33**(6):e00037517.

7. **Heckert U, Andrade L, Alves MJ, Martins C.** Lifetime prevalence of mental disorders among homeless people in a southeast city in Brazil. Eur Arch Psychiatry Clin Neurosci. 1999;**249**(3):150–155.

8. **Hoffmann EV, Duarte CS, Fossaluza V,** et al. Mental health of children who work on the streets in Brazil after enrollment in a psychosocial program. Soc Psychiatry Psychiatr Epidemiol. 2017;**52**(1):55–63.

9. **Lovisi GM, Coutinho E, Morgado A, Mann AH.** Social disablement among residents of hostels for the homeless in Rio de Janeiro, Brazil. Int J Soc Psychiatry. 2002;**48**(4):279–289.

10. **Lovisi GM, Mann AH, Coutinho E, Morgado AF.** Mental illness in an adult sample admitted to public hostels in the Rio de Janeiro metropolitan area, Brazil. Soc Psychiatry Psychiatr Epidemiol. 2003;**38**(9):493–498.

11. **Melo APS, Lima EP, Barros FCR, Camelo LDV, Guimarães MDC.** Homelessness and incarceration among psychiatric patients in Brazil. Cien Saude Colet. 2018;**23**(11):3719–3733.

12. **Moura YG, Sanchez ZM, Opaleye ES, Neiva-Silva L, Koller SH, Noto AR.** Drug use among street children and adolescents: what helps? Cad Saude Publica. 2012;**28**(7):1371–1380.

13. **Noto AR, Nappo SA, Galduróz JC, Mattei R, Carlini EA.** Use of drugs among street children in Brazil. J Psychoactive Drugs. 1997;**29**(2):185–192.

14. **Opaleye ES, Noto AR, Sanchez Zv, Moura YG, Galduróz JC, Carlini EA.** Recreational use of benzydamine as a hallucinogen among street youth in Brazil. Braz J Psychiatry. 2009;**31**(3):208–213.

15. **Pinto VM, Tancredi MV, Buchalla CM, Miranda AE.** History of syphilis in women living with AIDS and associated risk factors in São Paulo, Brazil. Rev Assoc Med Bras (1992). 2014;**60**(4):342–348.

16. **Ranzani OT, Carvalho CR, Waldman EA, Rodrigues LC.** The impact of being homeless on the unsuccessful outcome of treatment of pulmonary TB in São Paulo State, Brazil. BMC Med. 2016;**14**:41.

17. **Scivoletto S, da Silva TF, Rosenheck RA.** Child psychiatry takes to the streets: a developmental partnership between a university institute and children and adolescents from the streets of Sao Paulo, Brazil. Child Abuse Negl. 2011;**35**(2):89–95.

18. **Thiesen FV, Barros HM.** Measuring inhalant abuse among homeless youth in southern Brazil. J Psychoactive Drugs. 2004;**36**(2):201–205.

19. **Vernaglia TVC, Leite TH, Faller S,** et al. The female crack users: higher rates of social vulnerability in Brazil. Health Care Women Int. 2017;**38**(11):1170–1187.

20. **Li JS, Urada LA.** Cycle of perpetual vulnerability for women facing homelessness near an urban library in a major U.S. metropolitan area. Int J Environ Res Public Health. 2020;**17**(16):E5985.

21. **Van Straaten B, Rodenburg G, Van der Laan J, Boersma SN, Wolf JR, Van de Mheen D.** Substance use among Dutch homeless people, a follow-up study: prevalence, pattern and housing status. Eur J Public Health. 2016;**26**(1):111–116.

22. **Fazel S, Khosla V, Doll H, Geddes J.** The prevalence of mental disorders among the homeless in western countries: systematic review and meta-regression analysis. PLoS Med. 2008;**5**(12):e225.

23. **Costa MC, Alves MV, Santos CA, C de Carvalho R, P de Souza KE, Lima de Sousa H.** Experimentação e uso regular de bebidas alcoólicas, cigarros e outras substâncias psicoativas/SPA na adolescência [Experimentation and regular use of alcoholic beverages, cigarettes and other psychoactive substances (PAS) during adolescence]. Cien Saude Colet. 2007;**12**(5):1143–1154.

24. **Castaldelli-Maia JM, Martins SS, de Oliveira LG, van Laar M, de Andrade AG, Nicastri S.** Use transition between illegal drugs among Brazilian university students. Soc Psychiatry Psychiatr Epidemiol. 2014;**49**(3):385–394.

25. **Embleton L, Mwangi A, Vreeman R, Ayuku D, Braitstein P.** The epidemiology of substance use among street children in resource-constrained settings: a systematic review and meta-analysis. Addiction. 2013;**108**(10):1722–1733.

26. **Pettey D, Aubry T.** Tobacco use and smoking behaviors of individuals with a serious mental illness. Psychiatr Rehabil J. 2018;**41**(4):356–360.

27. **Guillén AI, Marín C, Panadero S, Vázquez JJ.** Substance use, stressful life events and mental health: a longitudinal study among homeless women in Madrid (Spain). Addict Behav. 2020;**103**:106246.

28. **Toro PA, Hobden KL, Wyszacki Durham K, Oko-Riebau M, Bokszczanin A.** Comparing the characteristics of homeless adults in Poland and the United States. Am J Community Psychol. 2014;**53**(1–2):134–145.

29. **Schreiter S, Heidrich S, Zulauf J,** et al. Housing situation and healthcare for patients in a psychiatric centre in Berlin, Germany: a cross-sectional patient survey. BMJ Open. 2019;**9**(12):e032576.

30. **Ayano G, Tesfaw G, Shumet S.** The prevalence of schizophrenia and other psychotic disorders among homeless people: a systematic review and meta-analysis. BMC Psychiatry. 2019;**19**(1):370.

31. **Ayano G, Tsegay L, Abraha M, Yohannes K.** Suicidal ideation and attempt among homeless people: a systematic review and meta-analysis. Psychiatr Q. 2019;**90**(4):829–842.

32. **Fond G, Tinland A, Boucekine M,** et al. Improving the treatment and remission of major depression in homeless people with severe mental illness: the multicentric French Housing First (FHF) program. Prog Neuropsychopharmacol Biol Psychiatry. 2020;**99**:109877.

Chapter 9

Indian perspectives on homelessness and mental health

Adarsh Tripathi, Anamika Das, and
Sujita Kumar Kar

Introduction

The home or domicile is considered as the place of living but it has a deeper
concept as a place which is enriched with affection, love, belongingness, care,
and security. Article 25 of the Universal Declaration of Human Rights states
that 'Everyone has the right to a standard of living adequate for the health and
well-being of himself and of his family, including food, clothing, housing and
medical care and necessary social services, and the right to security in the event
of unemployment, sickness, disability, widowhood, old age or other lack of livelihood in circumstances beyond his control' (1). As the popular saying goes,
'home is where the heart is', and being homeless has a huge impact on the existence of an individual. It is estimated that the global count of the homeless
population is between 100 million to 1 billion (2). Research on the psychosocial
and health impacts on the homeless population reports a high mental morbidity in the population (3). The homeless mentally ill (HMI) often present with
a complex combination of physical, psychological, and social problems. The
HMI population can be subdivided into various groups: individuals with severe
mental illness who have been rendered homeless because of the illness; those
who have a mental illness but never approach the treatment services with the
underlying illness, contributing to drift; and those whose mental health problems are the consequence of becoming homeless. As in many other countries,
the scenario in India about HMI is grave with high vulnerabilities, disadvantaged economic support, prevalent social stigma, and also sluggish implementation of mental health policies. The vicious cycle of poverty, ill health, and
homelessness makes the context of mental health and homelessness in India an
important one. People suffering from mental illness are very often neglected,
abused, and deprived from their rights in the society, but when a mentally ill
person is homeless too, the problem of neglect, abuse, and violation of human

right increases multifold. Poverty in developing countries like India plays a major role in both homelessness and mental health.

Definition of homelessness in the Indian context

Homelessness has been defined widely over studies and between countries and this has affected the measurement of epidemiology and the creation of the required services (4). The fourfold aspects (according to the European Federation of National Organisations Working with Homeless) comprise rooflessness, houselessness, insecure accommodation, and substandard or inadequate housing (5). According to the Census of India, homeless people are those 'who do not live in census houses [a census house is referred to a structure with a roof] which is either self-owned or rented', but instead reside in a houseless household such as on the roadside, under flyovers or staircases, in places of worship, or railway platforms or spend nights at transit homes, short stay homes, or beggar homes, or reside in temporary structures without walls and roofs such as under plastic sheets, in parks and other common spaces (6). This official definition is used primarily for the entitlements and policymaking of the government. For example, pavement dwellers, Hindu sadhus (wandering ascetics), squatters whose settlement has not been recognized as a 'slum', Banjaras (Gypsies), and Loharas (nomadic blacksmiths) are not considered as houseless according to the census and are thus not entitled to any benefits. But the discussion of homelessness in the perspective of mental health and illness needs a broader dimension. Working definitions are adopted by non-governmental organizations (NGOs) in order to focus on and prioritize the most deprived population. The National Campaign for Housing Rights in India defines home as 'a place where one lives with dignity, has security and can access basic essential housing resources like water, fuel, land, building materials etc.'. The Aashray Adhikar Abhiyan defines a homeless person as 'an individual with no place which can be referred as a home in that city where home implies a shelter and also nurturance of one's cultural, social, health and economic needs' (7).

Epidemiology

There is availability of extensive research data on HMI from high-income countries and also some Asian countries. But there is a general lack of scientific data from India. This may be because this population is difficult to access and there may be physical and linguistic barriers. Humanitarian grounds take an upper hand over scientific investigations, thus studies are mostly exploratory and also sometimes compromise on their methodology (8). The lack of a standardized definition also plays a major obstacle in obtaining epidemiological data. The Census of India 2011 estimated the prevalence of the houseless population as 449,761 households/families by point in time estimation. The houseless number accounts to 1,772,889 people with a distribution of 834,541 in rural and 938,348 in urban settings. There is a 28% drop from rural setting but a 20% rise in the urban setting since the 2001 census. The point estimation has a major methodological flaw in the form of the transient nature of the population. Other epidemiological data available show that there are 78 million homeless people (Action Aid, 2003) and 11 million homeless children in India (Child Relief and You, 2006). The UN-HABITAT (2005) says that 63% of all slum dwellers from South Asia are in India which amounts to a figure of 170 million people (17% of the total slum dwellers in the world) (9).

Epidemiological data for the homeless population who are mentally ill is even more scarce. Very few epidemiological studies provide us with descriptive data as there is a dearth of published data. Table 9.1 gives a summary of the available epidemiological data about the HMI in the Indian population (8,10,11).

Another North Indian study from Haryana in inmate girls of a female shelter home included 36 runaway or 'throwaway' female participants. It was seen that more than 60% had received at least one psychiatric diagnosis; 22.2% had a diagnosis of depression, 13.88% had a diagnosis of post-traumatic stress disorder, 11.11% had conversion disorder, 5.55% had panic disorder, 2.8% had generalized anxiety disorder, and 11.11% had intellectual disability (12). Thus, the studies point to the fact that psychotic illnesses comprise a majority of the wandering mentally ill and intellectual disability is also a common entity either alone or as a comorbid condition.

The National Mental Health Survey guestimates that HMI numbers in some states are high and vary across districts and states. There is a lack of awareness of the key informant and also there is difficulty in procuring data (14).

The various factors contributing to homelessness in India

Various factors are responsible for the coexisting mental illness and homelessness. These are not dissimilar to those reported from other countries as described elsewhere in this volume. The possible reasons can be summarized as follows (15):

1. Factors related to administration and policy.
2. Factors related to delivery of service.
3. Factors related to the illness.
4. Factors related to the society.

Table 9.1 Summary of the key findings about the clinical profiles of the HMI population in the major clinical epidemiological studies of India

Variables	Gowda et al., 2017 Southern India (Bangalore) (11)	Singh et al., 2016 Western India (Gujarat) (10)	Tripathi et al., 2013 Northern India (Lucknow) (8)
Number of patients included in the study	78	82	140
Time period	January 2002–December 2015	March 2012–February 2014	February 2005–July 2011
Type of study	Retrospective chart review of inpatients	Retrospective chart review of inpatients	Retrospective chart review of inpatients
Prevalence of mental disorder in the study population	All patients were HMI	All patients recruited were wandering mentally ill	90.7% (127 patients)
Primary diagnosis			
Schizophrenia and other psychotic disorder	65.4%	54.9% schizophrenia 26.8% psychosis not otherwise specified	65% (30.7% schizophrenia, 15% other non-organic psychotic disorder, 12.85% psychosis not otherwise specified, 4.3% schizoaffective disorder, 2.1% acute psychosis)
Mood disorders	14.1%	12.2% (bipolar)	12.9% (bipolar)
Intellectual disability	30.8%	8.5%	25.7% (12.8% had low average intelligence)
Substance use disorder	29.5%	6.1%	44.3% (tobacco 25.7%, cannabis 15.7%, alcohol 8.6%, others 4.3%)
Other diagnosis			Anxiety not otherwise specified (2.1%) Personality disorder (0.71%)
Outcome	82% completely improved at discharge	23% had 70–100% improvement 24% had 30–70% improvement	24.4% very much improved 58.3% much improved (according to CGI-I scale)

Table 9.1 Continued

Variables	Gowda et al., 2017 Southern India (Bangalore) (11)	Singh et al., 2016 Western India (Gujarat) (10)	Tripathi et al., 2013 Northern India (Lucknow) (8)
Reestablishment of ties with family/caregiver	51.3%	47% (54.9% could provide address)	68.6%
Other ways of reintegration	19.2% sent to state-run homes for women 21.8% taken up by NGOs	21.8% taken up by NGOs	8.6% sent to NGOs for long-term rehabilitation 3 females sent to nearby women's welfare organization

CGI-I, Clinical Global Impression-Improvement scale.

Factors related to administration and policy

Psychosocial rehabilitation services really began after deinstitutionalization became a norm around the 1960s. The custodial type of mental hospitals had abysmal conditions but acted as a shelter to some mentally ill people. These patients faced a worse situation and became destitute; they were not taken care of by their families and the hospitals could not provide any long-time solution (15,16).

Factors related to delivery of service

◆ Lack of rehabilitation services: although there are developments in pharmacological treatment, community rehabilitation is grossly lacking. In low- and middle-income countries, there is dearth of any rehabilitative services. Many HMI people who are reached by agencies receive acute treatment but an adequate follow-up with rehabilitation back into community and family is often not possible simply because of a lack of workforce and financial resources (17).

◆ Scarcity of adequate resources for mental health: there remains a huge scarcity of mental health resources. The available services are also more urban centred, hospital based, and fragmented (18). It has been showed in a large survey conducted over multiple countries that 76–85% of the mentally ill received no treatment in less developed countries when compared to developed countries where 35–50% received no treatment (19). The Mental Health Atlas of 2017 found that there are fewer than two mental health workers per 100,000 population in India and other low-income countries. The Mental

Health Atlas 2014 depicted the ratio of mental health professionals as 0.07 clinical psychologists and psychiatric social workers and 0.12 psychiatric nurses per 100,000 population (14).

+ Lack of political will: the massive underestimation of the suffering of mentally ill people, lack of political will, negative attitudes towards mental ill-health, and lack of a strong leadership at national level have resulted in inadequacy of appropriate care in low- and middle-income countries like India (17).

Factors related to the illness

+ Untreated mental disorder: it is seen that severe mental illness has a rapidly deteriorating course if not treated effectively. Unfortunately, only about one-third of the HMI receive treatment (20).

+ Impaired ability to self-care: essential aspects of daily life are hampered in patients with severe mental illness. Self-care and household management are hampered very severely. Research has shown that most patients develop symptoms of mental illness before becoming homeless (21).

+ Disrupted interpersonal relationships: maintaining a stable relationship is sometimes prevented due to the mental illness. This also may lead to misin-terpretation of the offer of someone's help; as a result, the assistance is often rejected by the mentally ill person.

+ Deficits in cognition: cognitive problems due to illness prove to be an impeding factor in maintaining compliance with treatment and thus can pre-dispose to loss of contact with the therapist, leading to homelessness.

+ Comorbidities: comorbid physical illnesses reduce the capacity to seek treat-ment and thus further decrease any chance of obtaining treatment.

+ Substance abuse: mentally ill people have a higher propensity to abuse sub-stances. This deadly combination of substance use and mental illness, along with physical poor health, puts residential stability at risk, resulting in homelessness.

Factors related to the society

+ Social stigma: stigma attached to mental illness is a definite issue for patients with mental illness residing across the globe, including those in developing countries. Stigma can lead to treatment seeking from faith healers or from providers of alternative medicine, resulting in an increase in the time taken to reach a mental health specialist. It also leads to the mentally ill being clas-sified as social outcasts. Social isolation and thus lack of social support plays a major role in homelessness (22).

◆ Poverty and low literacy: poverty in low- and middle-income countries such as India along with low levels of literacy are important contributing factors to the inability to access mental health services, which in turn contributes to homelessness in mentally ill (23).

◆ Rapid urbanization and the change of social structure: urbanization has brought about significant socioeconomic changes in societal structure. Industrialization and a better economic situation in urban areas caused migration of the rural population to urban areas in search of job opportunities and better living conditions. This rapid urbanization has a deleterious effect on the mental health condition of an individual. Various stressors and adverse events such as poverty, pollution, overcrowding, prevailing cash economy, rising violence, and poor social support all lead to an increased vulnerability to both mental illness and homelessness.

◆ Lack of employment: people with serious mental illness have a high rate of unemployment as there may be an inability to work consistently due to active symptoms and the disability of the illness. The menial jobs they qualify for do not pay good wages and also do not include healthcare benefits, making them more vulnerable to becoming and remaining homeless. People with substance use behaviour also frequently have employment problems (24).

◆ Housing barriers: scarcity of accessible, appropriate, and affordable housing remains one of the biggest barriers for residential stability in patients with serious mental illness.

The duality and the direction

It has been seen that individuals living within poverty are highly vulnerable to develop mental health issues. These include both severe mental illness and also common mental health disorders. The social causation gives an explanation of how poverty can result in mental health problems whereas the social drift hypothesis states that the mental health problems can contribute to poverty and lower socioeconomic status (25). The homeless population with mental illnesses comprises both the HMI and the mentally ill homeless. The distinction lies in the fact of whether the mental illness is the cause or effect of homelessness. There exists a duality and there is a need for exploration of the cause–effect relationship. It has been seen that one of the most common reasons for homelessness is wandering away from home due to a mental disorder which has not been treated adequately. Thus, the direction of the mentally ill becoming homeless is established (26). The mentally ill can result being homeless by two means. They can drift away from their residence because of their illness or they can

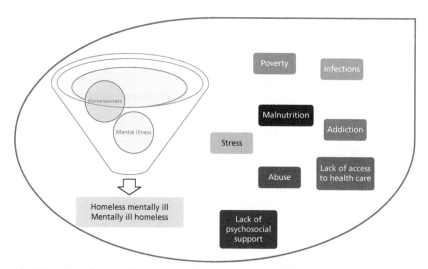

Fig. 9.1 Various factors affecting homelessness and mental illness.

be thrown out from their house due to the mental illness. Fig. 9.1 summarizes various other factors that might play a role in causing mental illness in a homeless person and vice versa.

Studies have also shown that homelessness can be a contributing factor to the development of mental illness. Thus, mental illness and homelessness form a vicious cycle and both can precipitate each other. The homeless population may well have a lack of knowledge regarding healthcare facilities and state benefits. There are also potential financial obstacles. As mentioned previously, being homeless is itself a risk factor for the development of mental illness. Poor psychosocial support, ongoing mental stressors, lack of a definitive residential place, frequent migration, increased risk of substance use behaviour, and many other reasons make the homeless population vulnerable to mental disorders. Lack of basic necessities in the homeless population such as clean water, proper sanitation, food, clothing, shelter, physical safety, education, employment, healthcare, and social security are also prominent risk factors for poor mental health in the homeless population. So, researchers and policymakers should always be aware of this duality (27,28).

Special issues in women

Women remain a particularly marginalized section of Indian society. Homelessness in mentally ill individuals is an important factor in the female population. The definition of homelessness includes lack of privacy and dispossession but for men it is more like propertylessness, while for women it involves the disruption of day-to-day routines. This confirms that homelessness is a far more serious problem for women (7). Stigma has been shown to be especially higher for the female population (2). In India, often there are less educational and occupational opportunities for women, lack of access to healthcare facilities, and a sex bias in diagnosing psychiatric disorders due to the influence of culture and gender roles. The impact of the mental disorder on women can vary. Often the male is the primary wage earner for the family thus treating him and rehabilitating back into productivity becomes a priority. On the other hand, females with mental illnesses may be seen to increase the financial burden of the family but interestingly they are also likely to be caregivers in spite of their own illnesses. It has been seen that the main onus for the care remains with elderly parents as there is always a propensity to shuttle the woman between family of origin and family of procreation (2,16). It is also not acceptable under present social norms for a female to wander around in the streets. Thus, HMI women are also not easily accepted back at home and after a psychiatric hospitalization can end up being isolated from their family (2).

A recent incident is of interest. Gitanjali Nagpal, a successful ramp model, was found in an unkempt state begging in the streets of Delhi. This led to mass media coverage and thus the special needs of this vulnerable population came to prominence. A Public Interest Litigation was undertaken by a student of Delhi University which drew the attention of the court. It was subsequently ordered by the Delhi High Court that special wards should be made for mentally ill women and specifically for the homeless population in the Nirmal Chhaya home—a state government-run shelter home (16).

The role of non-governmental organizations and other voluntary agencies

As mentioned previously, mental health rehabilitation services are scarce in many states. Voluntary agencies have taken a major role in the field of psychosocial rehabilitation in India and thus need a worthy mention. Pioneers in psychosocial rehabilitation services are the Medico-Pastoral Association and the Richmond Fellowship Society (India). These societies have opened halfway homes based on the model of 'therapeutic community' and have served as role models over the past three decades. The Richmond Fellowship Society (India) is a part of Richmond Fellowship International, UK, one of the biggest NGOs in the world working for the cause of mental health. It provides training for psychosocial rehabilitation and also has established centres at Bengaluru, New Delhi, Siddlaghata (rural Bengaluru), and Lucknow. There are also many other organizations which came into existence in the 1980s or early 1990s and have been serving for the last three decades, namely Aashray Adhikar Abhiyan in Delhi, The Banyan in Chennai, Navachetana in Guwahati, Paripurnata in West Bengal, Shraddha Foundation in Maharashtra, Ashadeep in Guwahati, Iswar Sankalpa in Kolkata, and many others (16).

The model of care followed by these organizations works in a unique way to rehabilitate the mentally ill homeless individuals. Some of these organizations work from the ground level of bringing the wandering mentally ill to the point of reintegration into their family while others provide post-clinical rehabilitation. Newer models were formulated as needed and since then tremendous work has been done to rehabilitate the wandering mentally ill. There have also been women-centric initiatives such as The Banyan. The ultimate goal has been to reconcile the HMI with their families with generation of awareness in the family and the community to remain integrated (29). Table 9.2 gives a summary of the major NGOs working in this area and their primary mode of action.

Policies and programmes

India was the first country among low-income countries to introduce a National Mental Health Programme way back in 1982. It encouraged community-based mental health services. But the actual picture was not that rosy. The National Mental Health Policy 2014 addresses the homeless population as a vulnerable group and also discusses the bidirectional nature of homelessness and mental illness. The need to reduce poverty and income disparity and thus address social exclusion is one of the strategies mentioned. It has also been recommended to encourage action to change poor living conditions like homelessness. Universal access to mental healthcare which includes rehabilitation services also remains one of the priorities. Reduction of stigma and discrimination and community participation are important areas of focus. With the health budget being so low, the out-of-pocket expenses increase manifold in India making it difficult to access for the economically deprived homeless population. The District Mental Health Programme has also focused a lot on community rehabilitation. The District Mental Health Programme addresses mental illness from a disease perspective and ignores the complex economic, emotional, and social problems. Thus, the burning problems of mental illness and homelessness are not adequately addressed. This shows that the current scenario is still severe and more active focusing is needed (25). The recently launched Ayushman Bharat campaign (2018) which targets providing healthcare to the poor and vulnerable population of India also extends to homeless people (described as households without shelter in the Socio Economic and Caste Census 2011). It provides a health cover of five lakhs rupees per family which includes primary, secondary, and tertiary treatment with cashless access.

Table 9.2 Summary of the major NGOs, their location, and their primary mode of action

Name of organization	Location	Primary work area
Richmond Fellowship Society (http://rfsindia.ngo/)	Bengaluru (1986), New Delhi, Siddlaghata (rural Bengaluru) and Lucknow	Only national-level NGO working in the area of psychosocial rehabilitation for those suffering from chronic mental illness
Aashray Adhikar Abhiyan (AAA) (https://homelesspeople. in/)	Delhi (2000)	AAA brings severely mentally ill patients from the streets to the clinic for diagnosis and treatment. Maintains record of the mentally ill homeless who come to the clinic so that their presence can be secured. Provides support mechanisms (food, clothing, hygiene items, and shelter) for the patient while in the community such as monitoring the behavioural movements of the patient and administration of prescribed medications
The Banyan (http://www.thebanyan.org)	Chennai (1993)	Care of mentally ill homeless women by providing medications and rehabilitation
Ashadeep (http://www. ashadeepindia.org)	Guwahati (1996)	Psychosocial rehabilitation for mentally disabled people. The project 'Rehabilitation of Homeless Mentally Disabled Women' provided vocational training and support for livelihood for HMI women who are being reintegrated into their families
Hope Kolkata Foundation (http://www.hopechild. org)	Kolkata (1999)	Protection and development of underprivileged children on the street and in difficult circumstances
Shraddha Rehabilitation Foundation (http://www.shraddhaReha bilitationfoundation.org)	Raigad, Mumbai (1988)	Humane and compassionate rehabilitation for mentally ill roadside destitute people
Pingla Ghar (http:// pinglaghar.com)	Jalandhar (1951)	Home for homeless, intellectually disabled, abandoned persons
Shanthivanam Trust (http:// trustshanthivanam.org)	Trichy (1994)	Provides services to underprivileged mentally ill and wandering destitute people
Marisadanam Charitable Trust (http:// mariyasadanam.org)	Kerala (1998)	Complete care to HMI which includes pharmacological management of rehabilitation
Iswar Sankalpa (http:// isankalpa.org)	Kolkata (2007)	Project 'Naya daur' for HMI

The medicolegal angle

Legal provisions for homeless people with mental illness were provided in the Mental Health Act, 1987 and also in the Mental Healthcare Act, 2017. There are legal frameworks which lay out the procedure for a mentally ill homeless person.

1. *Mental Health Act, 1987*: Section 23 empowers the police personnel to take into custody any wandering patient who is not capable of taking care of themselves. He/she should be produced before a Magistrate within the next 24 hours and then if ordered by the magistrate a reception order can be issued for admission to a mental health facility. One of the main limitations was that homeless people who were not mentally ill also ended up in mental hospitals in order to honour the judicial order and rehabilitation back to facilities for homeless persons has a limited chance of occurring.

2. *Mental Healthcare Act, 2017*:

    a. *Chapter V, Section 18*, states the 'Right to access mental healthcare' which signifies that all persons have the right to access the entire range of mental healthcare and treatment from any mental health service which is run or funded by the appropriate government. This includes sufficient provisions of rehabilitation services such as half-way homes, sheltered accommodation, and home-based, hospital-based, or community-based rehabilitation. Subclause 7 also specifies that destitute or homeless persons with mental illness are entitled to mental health treatment and services free of any charge and at no financial cost at any mental health establishment run or funded by the appropriate government and at other mental health establishments designated by it.

    b. *Chapter V, Section 19*, regards the right to community living. It states that every person with mental illness including homeless persons shall have a right to live in society, be part of and not segregated from society, and not continue to remain in a mental health establishment merely due to an absence of community facilities.

    c. *Chapter XIII, Sections 100 and 102*, mention about the duties of police officers in respect to homeless persons with mental illness found wandering in the community. Fig. 9.2 represents how the procedure is followed.

    d. *Chapter V, Section 27*: the treating mental health professional should educate the HMI about the right to free legal aid. This would help in situations when the family members are reluctant to take the patient back home even after they improve (14).

    e. *Chapter XII, Sections 89 and 90*: for admitting an HMI patient where there is no availability of advanced directive or nominated representative. A person appointed by the Mental Health Review Board/Director

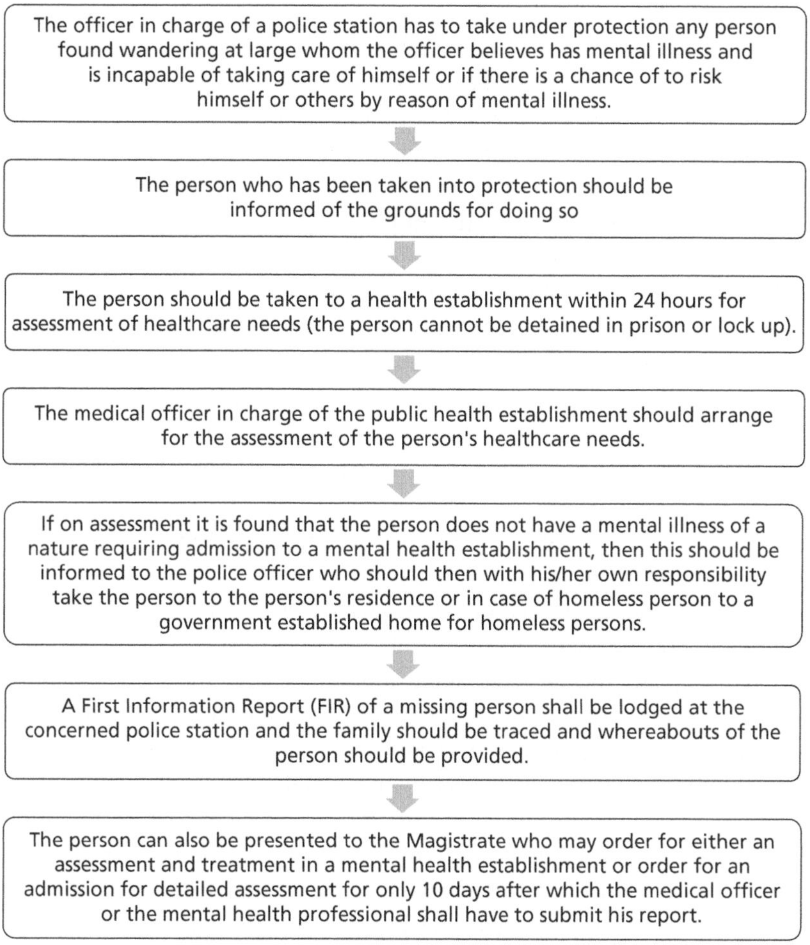

The officer in charge of a police station has to take under protection any person found wandering at large whom the officer believes has mental illness and is incapable of taking care of himself or if there is a chance of to risk himself or others by reason of mental illness.

The person who has been taken into protection should be informed of the grounds for doing so

The person should be taken to a health establishment within 24 hours for assessment of healthcare needs (the person cannot be detained in prison or lock up).

The medical officer in charge of the public health establishment should arrange for the assessment of the person's healthcare needs.

If on assessment it is found that the person does not have a mental illness of a nature requiring admission to a mental health establishment, then this should be informed to the police officer who should then with his/her own responsibility take the person to the person's residence or in case of homeless person to a government established home for homeless persons.

A First Information Report (FIR) of a missing person shall be lodged at the concerned police station and the family should be traced and whereabouts of the person should be provided.

The person can also be presented to the Magistrate who may order for either an assessment and treatment in a mental health establishment or order for an admission for detailed assessment for only 10 days after which the medical officer or the mental health professional shall have to submit his report.

Fig. 9.2 Duties of police officers with respect to homeless persons with mental illness found wandering in the community (MHCA, 2017 Sections 100 and 102).

of Department of Social Welfare/person from an organization under the Societies Registration Act (the NGOs mostly working with HMI)/a representative from Rogi Kalyan Samiti from the hospital can act as the nominated representative for the time being.

The future

There is no doubt that the actual provision of mental health services for the HMI is very limited indeed in India. Utilizing the general health services to provide mental health support, making essential psychiatric medications available free of cost in government health facilities, and integration at the government–NGO level would make things easier. The government has included taking care of the HMI in the newly drafted Mental Healthcare Act, 2017, as mental healthcare needs should be provided by the appropriate government free of cost to all HMI people. However, a lot still needs to be done. Creating awareness, reduction of stigma, and multisectoral, joined-up approaches are needed to fight the major obstacles in the way. The government–NGO–corporate partnership creates an ideal solution with the government providing security for the shelter. The NGO can provide services such as detecting illness, access to treatment, re-habilitation services, and vocational training which can be fulfilled with the help of corporate support. With the development of community psychiatric services there has been some development in rehabilitation but there is still a long way to go. There is a concept of 'critical time intervention' in preventing homelessness in mentally ill persons by ensuring continuity of care post dis-charge until harmonious community living is restored (see Chapter 21). This critical intervention needs to be planned at the point of deinstitutionalization (30). Identifying high-risk vulnerable people (such as psychotic patients living alone, comorbidity of severe mental disorder with substance use, lack of so-cial support, and intellectual disabilities with severe mental disorder) in the community can be done. Surveillance of the streets, identification of homeless persons by police officers, and taking appropriate steps thereafter should be ensured. Involvement of family by supporting them and also, if needed, the use of legal aids for prompting families who refuse to accept recovered patients can be done. Some facilities which can help in social inclusion and engagement of community are listed in Table 9.3 (2,16). It needs an active participation from all spheres—the mental health fraternity, the healthcare provider at the com-munity level, community workers, the community members, the family, and the patient. Community workers such as accredited social health activists who are engaged for medical illnesses should also be included in mental health ac-tivities to enhance the outreaching of facilities.

The recently concluded National Mental Health Survey of India (2015–2016) attempted to assess the burden and status of the HMI in India by conducting focused group discussions and key informant interviews in India. The parti-cipants of focused group discussions and key informant interviews were local stakeholders, media persons, family members of persons with mental illness, police personnel, and doctors. It was found that the exact estimate of HMI was difficult to calculate. In the urban areas, HMI people are seen more commonly than in rural areas. Most of the HMI are having longer durations of mental illness. In the community, people are mostly not aware of the facilities available for restoration and rehabilitation of homeless patients with mental illnesses.

Table 9.3 Various facilities for provision of rehabilitation services

Facility	Services to be provided
Day care centres	Vocational options along with involvement of family in the care of the patient. Reduces burden on the family and models are replicable in the family by family members. Largely located in urban areas in India and run both by governmental and NGO sectors. Low cost, family involvement, and patient participation are its key promising factors
Halfway homes	To facilitate gradual reintegration with family and community post discharge for those who are incapable of independent living or living with their family. Mostly run by NGOs but needs more initiative from government sector for establishing and running such residential rehabilitation
Community rehabilitation	Community-based programmes are done for social integration, rehabilitation, and opportunity equalization. There is a need for creation of a positive attitude along with provisions of training and education, long-term care provision, generation of income, cognitive remediation, training in social skills, etc.
Home rehabilitation	Empowerment of family members and removal of stigma and discrimination. Needs an active intervention by the mental health professional to integrate family into the treatment procedure

NGOs that work with HMI are often located in big cities. People who notice an HMI person in the street often ignore them and don't take any action. Only when such persons become violent or meet with an accident are specific actions being taken. The HMI are often abused physically or sexually in the streets. Generally, people often blame the government for failing to address this issue (31).

Conclusion

The issue of homelessness and mental health remains a vicious cycle with one contributing and worsening the situation of the other. The biggest challenge in India remains a lack of awareness and high prevalence of social stigma around mental illness. Difficulties in accessing, utilizing, and maintaining contact with mental healthcare services are common at the best of times but are probably worst for homeless individuals. Community mental health initiatives in India have started focusing on the rehabilitation services. Well-designed epidemiological studies would help to get better data on the numbers and needs of homeless individuals, which in turn would assist the policymakers in focusing attention on this vulnerable group.

References

1. **UN General Assembly.** Universal Declaration of Human Rights. Paris: UN General Assembly; 1948.

2. **Moorkath F, Vranda MN, Naveenkumar C.** Lives without roots: institutionalized homeless women with chronic mental illness. Indian J Psychol Med. 2018;**40**(5):476–481.

3. **Scott J.** Homelessness and mental illness. Br J Psychiatry. 1993;**162**(3):314–324.

4. **Patra S, Anand K.** Homelessness: a hidden public health problem. Indian J Public Health. 2008;**52**(3):164–170.

5. **Amore K, Baker M, Howden-Chapman P.** The ETHOS definition and classification of homelessness: an analysis. Eur J Homelessness. 2011;**5**(2):19–37.

6. **Office of the Registrar General and Census Commissioner, India.** Census of India 2011. Available from: https://www.censusindia.gov.in/2011-Common/CensusData2 011.html.

7. **Tipple G, Speak S.** Definitions of homelessness in developing countries. Habitat Int. 2005;**29**(2):337–352.

8. **Tripathi A, Nischal A, Dalal P,** et al. Sociodemographic and clinical profile of HMI inpatients in a north Indian medical university. Asian J Psychiatr. 2013;**6**(5):404–409.

9. **Kumar P.** Homelessness and mental health: challenging issue in an Indian context. Am Int J Res Humanit Arts Soc Sci. 2014;**7**(2):160–163.

10. **Singh G, Shah N, Mehta R.** The clinical presentation and outcome of the institutionalized wandering mentally ill in India. J Clin Diagn Res. 2016;**10**(10):VC13–VC16.

11. **Gowda GS, Gopika G, Manjunatha N,** et al. Sociodemographic and clinical profiles of HMI admitted in mental health institute of South India: 'Know the Unknown' project. Int J Soc Psychiatry. 2017;**63**(6):525–531.

12. **Gupta R, Nehra DK, Kumar V, Sharma P, Kumar P.** Psychiatric illnesses in homeless (runaway or throwaway) girl inmates: a preliminary study. Dysphrenia. 2013;**4**(1):31–35.

13. **Gowda GS, Gopika G, Kumar CN,** et al. Clinical outcome and rehabilitation of HMI patients admitted in mental health institute of South India: "Know the Unknown" project. Asian J Psychiatr. 2017;**30**:49–53.

14. **Swaminath G, Enara A, Rao R, Kumar KVK, Kumar CN.** Mental Healthcare Act, 2017 and homeless persons with mental illness in India. Indian J Psychiatry. 2019;**61**(Suppl 4):S768–S772.

15. **Kukreti P, Khanna P, Khanna A.** Chronic mental illnesses and homelessness. In: **Prasad B** (Ed), Chronic Mental Illness and the Changing Scope of Intervention Strategies, Diagnosis, and Treatment. Hershey, PA: IGI Global; 2017:1–20.

16. **Chatterjee R, Hashim U.** Rehabilitation of mentally ill women. Indian J Psychiatry. 2015;**57**(Suppl 2):S345–S353.

17. **Saraceno B, Saxena S.** Mental health resources in the world: results from Project Atlas of the WHO. World Psychiatry. 2002;**1**(1):40–44.

18. **Thirunavukarasu M.** Closing the treatment gap. Indian J Psychiatry. 2011;**53**(3):199–201.

19. **Demyttenaere K, Bruffaerts R, Posada-Villa J,** et al. Prevalence, severity, and unmet need for treatment of mental disorders in the World Health Organization World Mental Health Surveys. JAMA. 2004;**291**(21):2581–2590.

20. **Bines W.** The Health of Single Homeless People. Centre for Housing Policy. Discussion Paper 9. York: University of York; 1994.

21. **Cisneros HG.** Searching for home: mentally ill homeless people in America. Cityscape. 1996;**Dec**:155–172.

22. **Trivedi J, Jilani AQ.** Pathway of psychiatric care. Indian J Psychiatry. 2011;**53**(2):97–98.

23. **Lund C, Breen A, Flisher AJ,** et al. Poverty and common mental disorders in low and middle income countries: a systematic review. Soc Sci Med. 2010;**71**(3):517–528.

24. **Argeriou M, McCarty D.** Treating Alcoholism and Drug Abuse Among Homeless Men and Women: Nine Community Demonstration Grants. Hove: Psychology Press; 1990.

25. **Gopikumar V.** Understanding the Mental Ill Health-Poverty-Homelessness Nexus in India: Strategies that Promote Distress Alleviation and Social Inclusion. Chennai: Lokavani Southern Printers Pvt. Ltd; 2014.

26. **Dean R, Craig T.** Pressure Points: Why People with Mental Health Problems Become Homeless. London: Crisis; 1999.

27. **Speak S, Tipple G.** Perceptions, persecution and pity: the limitations of interventions for homelessness in developing countries. Int J Urban Reg Res. 2006;**30**(1):172–188.

28. **Editorial.** Health of the homeless. Lancet. 2014;**384**(9953):1478.

29. **Thara R, Patel V.** Role of non-governmental organizations in mental health in India. Indian J Psychiatry. 2010;**52**(Suppl 1):S389–S395.

30. **Susser E, Valencia E, Conover S, Felix A, Tsai WY, Wyatt RJ.** Preventing recurrent homelessness among mentally ill men: a "critical time" intervention after discharge from a shelter. Am J Public Health. 1997;**87**(2):256–262.

31. **Gururaj G, Varghese M, Benegal V,** et al. National Mental Health Survey of India, 2015–16: Summary. Bengaluru: National Institute of Mental Health and Neurosciences. 2016.

Chapter 10

Homelessness and mental illness in Hong Kong

Larina Chi-Lap Yim and
Henry Chi-Ming Leung

Introduction

Hong Kong became a British colony in the nineteenth century. By that time, the population of Hong Kong was less than 8000. Hong Kong became a Special Administrative Region of the People's Republic of China on 1 July 1997. Situated at a strategic location at the southeast coast of China, the 1106 km² fishing village turned into a cosmopolitan city with a population of 7.5 million by 2018 (1), with the highest housing cost (2) and highest cost of living in the world (3).

Increase in the homeless population

The Hong Kong government uses the notion of 'street sleeper' to conceptualize homelessness. Surveys and research in Hong Kong defined 'a homeless person' as a person who had slept in a public place, street, shelter, abandoned building, or places not intended to be dwellings.

Escalating housing costs in Hong Kong have led to an increase in the number of homeless residents over the years. According to the Social Welfare Department, the number of registered street sleepers increased from 403 in 2009 to 1075 in 2017 (4), and the percentage of female cases increased from 3% to 9% (Fig. 10.1). However, these data undoubtedly underestimate the true situation, as a significant proportion of homeless clients are not registered.

The Homeless Outreach Population Estimation survey was conducted in 2013 and 2015 (5) by social workers and volunteers affiliated with non-governmental organizations (NGOs). This survey adopted a more comprehensive and structured method, relative to the Social Welfare Department, and consequently identified a much larger number of homeless clients (Fig. 10.2). During this survey, hundreds of trained volunteers were sent out on a particular night to screen for clients in streets, temporary homes, and 24-hour restaurants that

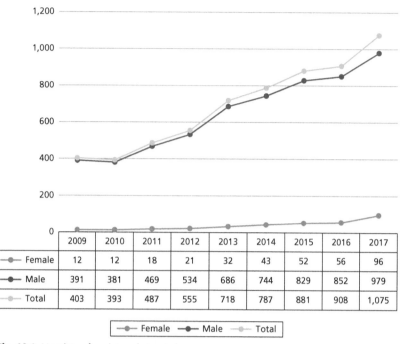

	2009	2010	2011	2012	2013	2014	2015	2016	2017
Female	12	12	18	21	32	43	52	56	96
Male	391	381	469	534	686	744	829	852	979
Total	403	393	487	555	718	787	881	908	1,075

Fig. 10.1 Number of registered street sleepers.
Source data from the Social Welfare Department.

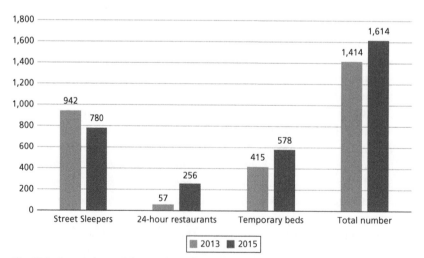

Fig. 10.2 Comparison of the number of homeless clients in 2013 and 2015.
Source data from H.O.P.E. Hong Kong.

had been pre-visited by social workers. These volunteers identified nearly twice the number of registered homeless clients as reported by the Social Welfare Department (1414 versus 718 in 2013; 1614 versus 881 in 2015) and found that the number of homeless clients who stayed in 24-hour restaurants had tripled from 2013 to 2015. Furthermore, the survey reported that almost half of the clients had been homeless for more than 10 years.

Limited housing services

For many years, locally high rental costs have been cited as the main cause of homelessness. Local studies have reported that at the time of the interview, approximately one-third of the surveyed homeless clients were employed (5–7). However, their salaries could not cover the rental costs, and the limited governmental housing subsidies precluded even the rental of a cage-like bed space or subdivided unit. Many homeless clients who had previously rented a bed space or subdivided unit, many of which were housed in very old or illegal structures, left because of the extremely poor living conditions. Although subsidized temporary hostels for homeless clients were available, these facilities did not permit active drug abusers or clients with mental illness, who comprised a significant proportion of the homeless population. Additionally, some clients refused to live in these hostels because of the limited service hours and suboptimal hygiene conditions. Other NGOs ran homeless hostels with better living conditions but set limits on the duration of stay. Taken together, these factors explain why the majority of homeless clients returned to the street even after initially finding shelter (5,8).

Available services for the homeless

Hong Kong experienced a period of economic downturn after the Asian financial crisis in 1997. The number of street sleepers increased rapidly in the following years. In 2001, the Social Welfare Department and several NGOs received funding for the development of a 3-year action plan to help the street sleepers. The evaluation report indicated that an integrated approach, that is, provision of a continuum of services including outreach, emergency and temporary accommodation, emergency funding, employment assistance, network building, and aftercare was effective in helping street sleepers leave the street and be self-reliant (9). Since 2004, the government has subsidized three NGOs (St James' Settlement, Salvation Army, and Christian Concern for Homeless Association) to provide services to homeless clients. Each NGO operates an integrated services team in a specified area, which provides counselling, night outreach, group activities, personal care, employment guidance, emergency financial assistance, emergency shelter, and temporary hostel placement. Many other parties, including public hospitals, correctional services, detoxification centres, and the Social Welfare Department, also play significant roles in addressing the various problems of this marginalized population. However, as there is no central policy for the homeless, there is a lack of coordination between the related groups.

Mentally ill homeless clients

Case studies

Case 1

Mr F had slept under a flyover near a public housing estate for more than 10 years. He looked emaciated and had the appearance of a person in his eighties. Although social workers had visited him regularly over the past 10 years, he refused to receive any welfare assistance. During his period of homelessness, residents of the nearby housing estate had provided him with food, drinks, and clothes. In recent years, his physical state had deteriorated, and he walked with a limping gait. He urinated and defaecated on the street. Although he was previously able to communicate using simple sentences, despite prominent self-muttering, he had recently remained mute most of the time. He had extremely poor hygiene, and a pungent odour could be detected from a distance.

Case 2

Mr H was a young man in his twenties who hoarded a large number of belongings next to a highway. The authorities had received complaints regarding Mr H's disturbing behaviour in public for several months. For example, he danced and shouted aloud at night and ran across the highway, regardless of potential danger. During previous interactions, he told police officers that he had recently left a mental hospital after receiving treatment for his drug abuse problem. He had no fixed abode and had been sleeping next to the highway for months.

Case 3

Mr T was previously a professor in English literature who had been sleeping outside a theatre for several years. He had worn the same shirt and trousers for years and with his filthy clothes and long, messy hair, one could hardly imagine that he had once taught in universities. His former students visited him and occasionally gave him money. Mr T was friendly and forthcoming and spoke readily about his persecutory delusions. In recent months, his lower limbs had become swollen and erythematous, and he had experienced anal bleeding of some duration. Still, he refused to undergo a medical check-up and instead believed that his condition could be healed by the power of nature.

One does not require training as a mental health professional to comment confidently on the obvious mental illnesses of Mr F, Mr H, and Mr T. It is not uncommon to observe obvious signs of mental illness or serious physical illness in homeless clients on the streets. Hong Kong provides an essentially free medical service to residents who cannot afford to pay, and even non-citizens can easily access emergency medical treatment. Theoretically, public hospitals employ designated teams of psychiatrists and nurses who provide outreach services to known and unknown mentally ill patients in the community. In Hong Kong, the mental health ordinance grants physicians and designated social workers the power to arrange compulsory medical treatment for patients with serious mental illness who may pose a risk to themselves or others. Police officers also have the power to remove individuals with suspected mental illness who are potentially at risk of harming themselves or others to the hospital for a proper assessment. Given these policies, why do severely mentally ill homeless clients remain untreated for years?

Local data

Prior to 2010, no report or study had addressed homelessness and mental illness in Hong Kong. Several NGOs collaboratively investigated mental health problems in the homeless population using a self-rated questionnaire (10). The study found that approximately 60% of homeless clients might have suffered from mental illness. However, only 10% of the suspected cases had been diagnosed in a public hospital, and only one of the suspected cases had been visited previously by the community psychiatric team.

In another study (6), psychiatrists used randomized sampling and the Structured Clinical Diagnostic Interview for the *Diagnostic and Statistical Manual of Mental Disorders*, fourth edition (SCID-IV) to determine that approximately half of the subjects were mentally ill at the time of the interview. Moreover, 70% had a lifetime history of mental illness, 30% had a mood disorder, 25% had an alcohol use disorder, 25% had a substance use disorder, 10% had a psychotic disorder, 10% had an anxiety disorder, and 6% had dementia. Although 41% of the subjects with mental illness had undergone a previous psychiatric assessment, only 13% were receiving psychiatric care at the time of interview.

Severely mentally ill clients

The above-mentioned results are unsurprising. Overseas studies reported similar figures. Exploring why these mentally ill street sleepers remain on the street is more important. The most significant finding was that nearly 20% of the subjects initially selected via random sampling were too ill to consent validly to participate in a more detailed study and were accordingly not included in the data analysis. Many of these severely ill subjects had extremely poor hygiene, florid psychotic symptoms, formal thought disorders, cognitive impairment, and malnourishment, and none had utilized services for homeless people. As none had been assessed by community psychiatric teams from the public mental health service, the rate of undertreatment was hugely underestimated. This limitation (i.e. severe illness preventing interview participation) meant that previous studies and surveys could not reflect the severity of the problems faced by the homeless people most strongly affected by mental illness. Because these mentally incapacitated clients do not possess the ability to provide valid consent to participate in any formal study, their situation often goes unnoticed. In summary, for the most severely ill clients, their underlying mental illnesses prevented them from receiving proper medical treatment for their physical and mental illnesses.

As severely ill patients clearly lack the ability to make rational treatment decisions, physicians would undoubtedly be forced to arrange compulsory treatment for members of this population who appear in clinical or hospital settings, regardless of the reason (e.g. collapse in the street). Once a mentally incapacitated patient has entered a clinical setting, physicians and social workers can initiate a guardianship order. Subsequently, the Social Welfare Department would address the patient's welfare issues and medical treatments. However, homeless clients with no contactable relatives are labelled as 'unknown', 'not violent', or 'in no imminent danger' and will remain on the street until they eventually collapse. This scenario indicates an obvious service gap in the current healthcare delivery system.

Substance abuse

Another subgroup of mentally ill homeless clients who actively abuse substances represented approximately a third of the homeless population. People in this subgroup often went unnoticed and untreated but had a longer duration of homelessness and higher frequencies of forensic records, drug-related crimes, violence-related crimes, and suicide attempts. Moreover, these clients faced increased health hazards. Several service sectors cooperate to assist this subgroup, including correctional service departments, detoxification services, and NGOs that serve the homeless population. However, public healthcare services only become involved upon the emergence of serious physical or psychiatric complications. Homeless shelters do not accept clients who are actively abusing drugs, while detoxification rehabilitation hostels initially require clients to undergo an acute detoxification programme. Currently, there is a lack of concerted effort to provide holistic care for clients in this subgroup, who are known to be difficult to engage.

Dementia

Only one local study (6) evaluated this subgroup of homeless residents and found a fifth of subjects who were able to complete the Mini-Mental State Examination scored lower than the cut-off point. Still, the true prevalence should be much higher, as approximately a fifth of the initially identified clients were deemed mentally unfit to participate in the study. Only four of 15 subjects determined to have a cognitive impairment or dementia underwent an assessment of their cognitive issues by a public healthcare service. The effects of cognitive impairment were frequently overlooked by service providers, as these clients were usually quiet and submissive and had no active complaints and no history of violence or self-harm. Moreover, clients in this subgroup were also prone to receiving abuse.

Intellectual disability

No local report or survey has specifically targeted this group of homeless clients, and little is currently known about this population. The lack of data concerning intellectually disabled homeless people reflects the inadequacy of attention given to these vulnerable clients who face a greater risk of abuse. Social workers did observe that some homeless clients found it difficult to solve problems and to understand certain conversations and concepts but did not usually manifest other symptoms of mental illness. For these clients, poor judgement and problem-solving skills, impaired occupational ability, and susceptibility to abuse often trapped them in a homeless status. In Hong Kong, the government provides residential or day care services for residents with a moderate to severe level of intellectual disability. However, those with borderline intellectual impairment and those with mild intellectual disability and a lower level of impairment tend to remain with their families or live alone, and their needs were often neglected.

Medical problems and help-seeking

A local study reported that a third of homeless interviewees had attended regular follow-up visits for the management of chronic physical illnesses (5). This figure was higher than the corresponding figure of 19% in the general population (11). The most commonly reported physical problems were skin infections and musculoskeletal disorders. Still, more than half of the interviewees with physical symptoms did not seek medical attention, and more than half perceived that they did not need to consult a physician regarding their symptoms (6). In summary, mentally ill homeless clients are more likely to receive undertreatment for medical or psychiatric illnesses.

New service models

The current local healthcare delivery model fails to reach the most underprivileged populations, particularly severely mentally ill residents whose physical problems also remain untreated for years, especially if they are homeless. The community psychiatric teams from public hospitals do not provide outreach services for street sleepers who have no immediate danger to self or to others. These severely mentally ill patients do not seek help by themselves and must be reached proactively by healthcare workers. Although public hospitals employ community psychiatric teams who provide care to mentally ill patients in the community, the limited outreach hours often present a significant barrier to use. In addition, most mentally ill clients are classified as non-urgent because they do not present an imminent danger to themselves or others. Moreover, communication between the frontline social workers and the hospital administration is a lengthy process. In recent years, social workers and volunteer healthcare workers have explored the potential development of a new service model for underprivileged groups. This effort began with a joint night-time outreach mediated by psychiatrists and social workers. The following cases demonstrate the practical difficulties encountered by frontline social workers and the attempts to overcome these issues through joint efforts made by social workers and medical staff.

Mr F's mental condition worsened over time. However, his physical condition was of greater concern. Mr F no longer ate the food provided by his neighbours but instead picked food waste from bins. Social workers contacted the community psychiatric team at a nearby hospital. However, the request for an outreach assessment was declined because Mr F was not considered imminently dangerous. He had never performed an act of self-harm and had not indicated that he would consent to an assessment by mental health professionals. Mr F's condition was only expected to worsen over time. Although social workers attempted to call an ambulance directly, Mr F refused when asked to board the ambulance. The ambulance workers were uncertain whether they had the power to transport a patient with an unknown history of mental illness (though Mr F was clearly very ill) to the hospital against the patient's will, and subsequently left the area. A volunteer psychiatrist assessed Mr F and concluded that he likely suffered from dementia and was a mentally incapacitated person requiring urgent medical attention. This assessment result was stated in a letter kept by the social worker, who again called the ambulance. That time, Mr F was sent to the accident and emergency department with the letter from the psychiatrist. He was admitted compulsorily to a mental hospital for further management.

Mr H, the young man with a drug abuse problem, was visited by the volunteer outreach team one night. He made irrelevant statements and could not hold a meaningful conversation. Two police officers performing a routine patrol arrived at the scene, and the outreach team seized the opportunity to report Mr H's condition as a psychotic man with a drug abuse problem who performed disturbing and dangerous acts in public. However, the police found Mr H to be calm and non-disruptive at the time of interview and did not actively intervene. At the time, Mr H was only presenting with disorganized speech and self-giggling. The police left. While the team debated the next step, Mr H dashed out onto a road with heavy traffic and fortunately was not struck. Two team members ran to the opposite side of the road and attempted to catch Mr H, while another team member called the police and an ambulance. The remaining volunteer physician quickly wrote a letter stating Mr H's condition. He was subsequently sent to the nearby accident and emergency department, which arranged his compulsory admission to a mental hospital.

Mr T, the professor with gastrointestinal bleeding, insisted that his problem would resolve naturally, despite the relentless attempts of his former students and social workers to persuade him to seek proper medical attention. His body was later found at a popular tourist spot.

Mr A, a man in his eighties, lived in a rented subdivided unit and earned a very small amount of money by bringing cardboard to a recycling facility. The social worker noticed that Mr A often looked for food in the rubbish bin and his pants were often stained with urine and faeces. Mr A said he was receiving a government subsidy and did not need any other welfare assistance. He was invited to take a shower at the NGO offices and received a free haircut from volunteers, as well as donated clothes to replace his stained ones. After building a rapport, the social workers were able to visit Mr A's rented unit, where they found a horrible level of hygiene. Mr A revealed that he gave his entire government subsidy, as well as the small amount of money earned from recycling, to the landlord every month. In return, the landlord brought him a meal every day. The landlord also kept Mr A's identity card. Other residents in the same flat were found to be in the same situation as Mr A, and the social worker suspected that the landlord had been taking advantage of Mr A. Following a suggestion to consider applying for a place in an old age home, Mr A visited several private homes but did not like the environment. Mr A was then assessed by a volunteer physician who identified a severe cognitive impairment which made him vulnerable to financial abuse. Although the social workers attempted to explain this problem to Mr A, he did not seem to understand. Mr A indicated verbally that he did not want to go to a hospital for assessment and had no major physical problems. The volunteer physician wrote a letter stating the results of the assessment and the need to apply for a guardianship order, as the significant cognitive impairment had rendered Mr A a victim of financial abuse. Later, Mr A experienced dizziness and sought help from a social worker, who identified that he had high blood pressure and suggested a check-up at the hospital. Mr A agreed, and the letter containing his previous assessment results was presented to the medical staff upon his arrival at the hospital. Mr A was subsequently admitted to the hospital, where he was diagnosed with dementia and deemed unfit for independent living. The medical social worker proceeded with the application of guardianship and made arrangements for Mr A to live in an old age home after discharge.

Mrs W presented with auditory hallucinations and persecutory delusions. She had a history of arson and had been admitted compulsorily to a mental hospital for treatment several years earlier. Although her psychotic symptoms recurred after stopping the depot antipsychotic, she refused to return to the psychiatric clinic for follow-up. One day, Mrs W went missing and her husband notified the police, who located Mrs W in a park. The case was closed. However, Mrs W refused to go home because she believed that her persecutors would soon kill her. Her husband rented a room in a hotel for Mrs W. However, she again went missing and her husband sought help from the police again. Mrs W was again located by the police and her case was closed. Her husband sought help from a psychiatric clinic and was told to bring his wife to the clinic for an assessment. Mrs W refused to go to the clinic. Subsequently, her husband contacted an NGO social worker.

One night, Mrs W was interviewed by the volunteer outreach team but largely remained mute. When the outreach team tried to give her some food and water, she attempted to kick one of the team members. Given the information provided by Mrs W's husband, she was experiencing a relapse of schizophrenia and was at risk of violence. The police and an ambulance were summoned, and a physician quickly sent Mrs W to the accident and emergency department with a referral letter. She was subsequently sent to a mental hospital for treatment.

The outreach team located Mr K in a park on a cold night, where he had wrapped himself in layers of black plastic bags. Mr K was a street sleeper who had moved to a private hostel some time ago. He could not explain why he had left the old age home and slept in a park. He gave brief, relevant replies to simple questions and was not willing to undergo testing of his cognitive functions. No psychotic symptoms were evident. The social worker contacted the staff at the old age home, who reported that Mr K had not returned to the hostel one day. The old age home reported his disappearance to the police, who located Mr K on the street and closed the case. During repeated visits, Mr K was found to have disorganized speech and very poor self-care abilities. He wore layers of clothes during summer, slept at the same location even in heavy rain, and exhibited a decrease in body weight. Mr K probably suffered from dementia, as evidenced by his progressively poor problem-solving skills and worsening ability to communicate. The Social Welfare Department was contacted because Mr K refused to return to the old age home again and refused to receive any welfare assistance. Although a legal guardian might have been needed to ensure his welfare, the Social Welfare Department did not actively intervene. One day, the outreach team observed that Mr K's lower limbs had swollen. The volunteer medical staff attempted to remove the plastic bags wrapped around his leg. A huge wound was revealed, from which something appeared to fly. An ambulance was summoned. Given his fragile state and the horrifying condition of his wound, Mr K was sent to the hospital for further management, and arrangements were made for him to live in another old age home after discharge.

The above-described cases demonstrate how and why the current service model fails to provide timely medical care to homeless and mentally ill clients. At a superficial level, everything needed to provide medical care to the homeless mentally ill is available. A free medical service has been developed for residents who cannot pay. The Mental Health Ordinance (12) governs the supervision and treatment of mentally incapacitated and mentally disordered persons. Registered physicians have the power to apply for a guardianship order for a mentally incapacitated person, which enables the provision of timely treatment. As mentioned previously, compulsory psychiatric treatment can be initiated by a physician or designated social worker. A mentally ill person can be detained in the interest of his own health or safety or to protect other people. The Mental Health Ordinance also states that if a police officer finds any person who reasonably appears to be suffering from a mental disorder and to have an immediate need of care or control, the officer may take that person into custody and remove him or her to a place of safety (i.e. the accident and emergency department of a general hospital). Although it is not difficult to determine whether a patient is at risk of harming themselves or others, it is more difficult to decide whether a patient should be detained for treatment in the interest of his/her own health. Similarly, police often find it very difficult to exercise good judgement, especially when lacking medical support. Furthermore, the lack of collaboration between various agencies reduces the potential efficacy of the system. The frontline social workers who know the homeless mentally ill clients fairly well have not been designated to arrange compulsory treatment or apply guardianship. In contrast, physicians at public hospitals do not have the opportunity to become well acquainted with homeless mentally ill patients. The decision not to provide an outreach assessment is often justified by the determination of no imminent danger to oneself or to the others. Without support from physicians, police officers are often hesitant or reluctant to commit a suspected mentally ill person in need to a safe place.

Volunteer medical outreach team

A regular joint outreach team designed to target the needs of mentally ill homeless clients was initiated in 2014. The team initially comprised one psychiatrist and three social workers. Over time, the number of team members increased to more than 60, including general practitioners, surgeons, family physicians, anaesthetists, psychiatrists, general nurses, intensive care unit nurses, psychiatric nurses, medical students, and nursing students. These professionals provide regular night outreach services twice weekly. The volunteer medical outreach team also addresses the physical problems of both mentally ill and non-mentally ill homeless clients. Currently, clinical psychologists are joining the team with the aim of exploring the provision of counselling to homeless clients with mood disorders and active substance abuse problems. Given the success of this new service model, funding has been provided to the NGO to enable the hiring of a full-time social worker and part-time nurse to care for homeless clients with mental or physical illnesses.

Unreached clients

Ninety per cent of the homeless clients in Hong Kong were of Chinese descent (5). The majority of non-Chinese homeless clients are Vietnamese (50%), Nepalese (20%), and Indian (10%). Currently, no regular medical outreach is provided to ethnic minorities. However, interpreters and NGOs that serve ethnic minorities have collaborated to arrange the timely assessment and treatment of this population.

Furthermore, the needs of homeless clients with intellectual disabilities have not been investigated. Hopefully, the inclusion of clinical psychologists will enable the volunteer team to assess the level of disability in these clients and arrange appropriate services.

The future

Different service providers must collaborate to solve the complicated problems related to mental illness and homelessness. However, no platform on which all parties can coordinate their work is currently available.

When a frontline social worker identifies a homeless client, who looks very ill physically or mentally, but actively refuses assessment or treatment, the social worker has no way to send the client to hospital. Even if an ambulance is summoned, the ambulance staff cannot bring someone to hospital against his or her will. Police officers, who have the power to send someone with suspected mental illness that requires immediate care to a place of safety (i.e. the accident and emergency department of public hospital), may find it difficult to exercise judgement when there is a lack of medical support. Psychiatrists, who are in the position to make a diagnosis and exercise clinical judgement, cannot be reached without the bureaucratic procedures that take a long time.

A mentally ill homeless client with active use of a substance may be repeatedly sent to mental hospital for management of substance-induced psychosis. The psychotic episode usually would not last long. Then the homeless client would be discharged back to the street, and reinstates the substance soon after discharge. The only substance-free period for the client would be the period of hospitalization, during which the client could have a rational discussion of his or her future plan. A homeless client with active use of substances may be repeatedly sent to jail as well. After leaving the jail, the client would be homeless again and reinstates the substance soon after release, if no support could be rendered to him or her at that moment.

A homeless mentally client would be admitted to a general hospital if they required management of serious skin infection. After treatment of the acute condition, the client would be discharged directly to the street, if the client does not speak out about the need for accommodation assistance. The skin infection would soon recur due to the poor hygiene condition on the street.

The homeless mentally ill clients do not only need treatment of their medical and physical illness. Coordination from multidisciplinary professionals is needed to tackle the complicated problems.

Hopefully, the success of this new service model, which involves multidisciplinary volunteers, will enable the development of such a platform in the near future.

Conclusion

The collaborations between social workers and volunteer healthcare workers have successfully connected the severely mentally ill homeless clients to the public healthcare services. However, if there is no post-admission follow-up or post-discharge arrangement, the problems would most likely recur. The new service model is an informal service supported by volunteer doctors and nurses, most of whom work in public hospitals. There is no formal channel for discussion or planning between the public sector that provides acute care, and the NGOs that provide long-term care. Assigning a designated mental hospital and a designated team of healthcare workers to receive the mentally ill homeless clients would be beneficial. Such a team could orchestrate the effort from different service providers, and facilitate the communication among them. For the less severely ill clients, the new service model may not suit them, as they do not require acute or immediate care. Long-term counselling services, together with extensions of stays in temporary hostels, would be helpful for them to be integrated back to into the community. For clients with cognitive impairment and intellectual disabilities, input from psychiatrists and psychologists to look into the extent and severity of their problems is essential, before developing new services for them. Mental healthcare workers have to take up a proactive role in providing care for this underserved group, instead of waiting for patients to seek help by themselves, as some will never do so, due to their underlying mental illnesses.

References

1. Census and Statistics Department. Population [Internet]. Hong Kong: The Government of the Hong Kong Special Administrative Region; 2018. Available from: https://www.censtatd.gov.hk/hkstat/sub/so20.jsp

2. Demographia. 14th Annual Demographia International Housing Affordability Survey:2018 [Internet]. London: London School of Economics; 2018. 51p. Available from: http://www.demographia.com/dhi2018.pdf

3. Mercer. Cost of living city ranking [Internet]. New York: Mercer; 2018. Available from: https://mobilityexchange.mercer.com/Insights/cost-of-living-rankings

4. Census and Statistics Department. Street sleepers by District Council [Internet]. Hong Kong: Census and Statistics Department; 2017. Available from: https://www.censtatd.gov.hk/FileManager/EN/Content_1149/T11_04.xls

5. H.O.P.E. Hong Kong 2015. Homeless Outreach Population Estimation Hong Kong. Hong Kong: H.O.P.E. Hong Kong 2015; 2016. 55p. Available from: http://www.cityu.edu.hk/youeprj/hopehk2015_chi.pdf

6. Yim LC, Leung HC, Chan WC, Lam MH, Lim VW. Prevalence of mental illness among homeless people in Hong Kong. Plos One [Internet]. 2015: 10(10). Available from: https://journals.plos.org/plosone/article?id=10.1371/journal.pone.0140940

7. Society for Community Organization. The homeless in Hong Kong 24-hour fast food restaurant [Internet]. Hong Kong: Society for Community Organization; 2018. 53p. Available from: https://soco.org.hk/wp-content/uploads/2014/10/research_homeless_24-hour-fast-food-shops_2019.pdf

8. Society for Community Organization. Repeat Homeless Report 2017 [Internet]. Hong Kong: Society for Community Organizations; 2017. 71p. Available from: https://soco.org.hk/wp-content/uploads/2014/10/Homeless-survey_2017_2_26.pdf

9. Legislative Council of the Hong Kong Special Administrative Region. Final Report on the "Three-year Action Plan to Help Street Sleepers" and the Way Forward [Internet]. Hong Kong: Legislative Council of the Hong Kong Special Administrative Region; 2004. 13p. Available from: https://www.legco.gov.hk/yr03-04/english/panels/ws/papers/ws0308cb2-1609-13e.pdf

10. St. James' Settlement. Richmond Fellowship of Hong Kong. Mental health of the homeless [Internet]. Hong Kong: St. James' Settlement & the Richmond Fellowship of Hong Kong.

11. Census and Statistics Department. Hong Kong Monthly Digest of Statistics January 2015 [Internet]. Hong Kong: Census and Statistics Department; 2015. Available from: https://journals.plos.org/plosone/article?id=10.1371/journal.pone.0140940

12. Mental health ordinance 1999 (Hong Kong). Available from: https://www.elegislation.gov.hk/hk/cap136?xpid=ID_1438402701917_003

Section 3

Clinical issues

Chapter 11

Clinical care and rehabilitation of homeless individuals with mental illnesses

Guru S. Gowda,
Channaveerachari Naveen Kumar,
Narayana Manjunatha, and
Suresh Bada Math

Introduction

The homeless mentally ill (HMI) issue is pivotal and an urgent challenge to the mental health field and is considered a global problem. Individuals who are homeless are prone to developing mental illnesses, and those suffering from a pre-existing mental illness are at a risk of becoming homeless. Homelessness appears in virtually all countries around the globe and reasons for this vary. In many countries, it is about access to affordable housing, whereas in others, it is about the social drift among individuals with mental illness. In this chapter, we describe specific issues related to the management of HMI individuals with a special focus on rehabilitation.

Definitions

There is no consensus definition for HMI individuals as implied by Fazel et al. (1). Although several high income countries have established various criteria to define homelessness in order to provide services to those eligible and track progress in eliminating the program, uniformly agreed-upon definitions for the same are still controversial and debatable. The US and European countries consider a mentally ill person to be an HMI on the principle of persons sleeping in designated shelters (such as a overnight shelters, emergency shelter homes, and transitional housing programmes) and undesignated shelters (such as streets, cellars, attics, lobbies and abandoned buildings, multistorey car parks, and public spaces).

A few examples can illustrate the variations in definitions. In Australia, homelessness is divided into three types. These include (a) primary homelessness (a person who is without regular accommodation), (b) secondary homelessness (a person who is living in shelters or temporarily with family or friends or boarding homes), and (c) tertiary homelessness (a person who is living in substandard housing, e.g. boarding homes) (2). The European Typology of Homelessness and Housing Exclusion (ETHOS) was developed in 2005 in liaison with the European Federation of National Organisations working with Homelessness (3). ETHOS defines a person as homeless if they have a deficit in at least two domains. These domains include physical, legal, and social domains. Any person who lives without a shelter of any kind, sleeping rough, is called a 'person with rooflessness' and a person who has a place to sleep but which is temporary, in an institution or shelter, is called a 'person with houselessness'. The US had forced the Homeless Emergency Assistance, and Rapid Transition to Housing (HEARTH) Act in 2012, which replaced the previous McKinney–Vento Act (4,5). In comparison to the old act, the HEARTH Act, 2012, broadened homelessness's definition by including the individual who is at risk of homelessness. Further, it also enables a homeless person to become eligible for permanent housing through the 'Housing First' programme. It help in accelerated shift from sheltered accommodation to permanent housing. The act also directed the US Interagency Council on Homelessness (USICH) to develop a national strategic plan to end homelessness. The UK defines and offers accommodation that is 'reasonable for him to continue to occupy'; Under this, the law considers living without shelter or living in inadequate or insecure housing, as being homeless (6,7). In contrast to other high-income countries, low- and middle-income countries including India do not have any specific legislation, acts, or programmes to define HMI. However, as per literature in the Indian context, HMI as one who doesn't have either regular accommodation or shelter homes or boarding homes. For example, a person sleeping on platforms of railway stations, bus stands, pilgrim centres, beggars' homes, urban areas, and on street corners of metro cities (8,9).

Prevalence of homeless mentally ill individuals

The prevalence of HMI individuals varies across the world and cities and, inevitably, the prevalence of psychiatric disorders in these groups also varies, as shown in Table 11.1. Depending upon where the sample is collected from, the prevalence of psychosis ranges from 3.7% to 84.1%, common mental disorder 93.2%; substance use disorders range from 6% to 82%, cognitive impairment ranges from 15% to 70%, and that of intellectual developmental disorder

Table 11.1 Studies on the prevalence of psychiatric illnesses in homeless mentally ill individuals

Study group	Year	Country	Study design	Population	Sample	Results and conclusion
Ayano et al., 2017	2015	Ethiopia	Cross-sectional	Community-based	456	Most common diagnosis was substance use disorder (93.2%) followed by psychosis (77.40%) (10)
Bassuk et al., 1984	1984	Boston and Cambridge, US	Cross-sectional	Community-based	78	Most common diagnosis was psychoses (40%) followed by alcohol use disorder (21%) and personality disorders (21%) (11)
Breakey et al., 1989	1989	Baltimore, US	Cross-sectional	Community-based	203	Most common diagnosis was severe mental illness, which was present in 42% of males and 48.7% of females (12)
Chondraki et al., 2014	2009	Greece	Cross-sectional	Hospital	254	The prevalence of psychiatric disorder was 56.7% (13)
Fekadu et al., 2014	2014	Ethiopia	Cross-sectional	Community-based	217	Most common diagnosis was alcohol use disorder (60%) followed by psychosis (41.0%) (14)
Gelberg et al., 1993	1993	Los Angeles, US	Cross-sectional	Community-based	443	The prevalence of alcohol use disorder was 24% and illegal drug use was 18% (15)
Gupta et al., 2013	2013	India	Cross-sectional	Community-based	36	Most common diagnosis was depression (22.2%) followed by post-traumatic stress disorder (13.8%). 11.1% had intellectual disability (16)
Gouveia et al., 2017	2008–2010	Mozambique	Cross-sectional	Hospital-based	71	Most common diagnosis was schizophrenia (64.8%) followed by substance abuse in 29.6% and intellectual disability in 5.6% (19)
Gowda et al., 2017	2002–2015	India	Retrospective design	Hospital-based	78	Most common diagnosis was schizophrenia and other psychotic disorders (65.4%) followed by intellectual disability (30.8%) and substance use disorder (29.5%) (17)

(continued)

Table 11.1 Continued

Study group	Year	Country	Study design	Population	Sample	Results and conclusion
Heckert et al., 1999	2003	Brazil	Cross-sectional	Community-based	479	Most common diagnosis was alcohol use disorder (82%), followed by mood disorders (32.5%), drug abuse/dependence (31.3%), and schizophreniform psychosis (9.6%) (20)
Lovisi et al., 2003	2003	Brazil	Cross-sectional	Hospital-based	330	The overall prevalence of mental disorders was 49.2%. Most common diagnoses were alcohol use disorder (31%) and severe cognitive impairment (15%) (21)
Moquillaza-Risco et al., 2014	2014	Peru	Cross-sectional	Hospital-based	302	The prevalence of cognitive impairment was 70% among elderly homeless persons (22)
Nayak et al., 2015	2015	India	Cross-sectional	Centre for homeless persons	50	70% had either psychotic or affective disorders and 44% of the above had comorbid substance dependence (24)
Nuttbrock et al., 1998	1998	New York, US	Cross-sectional	Community-based	694	Most common diagnosis was substance use disorder (63.5%) followed by psychoses (48.8%) and personality disorders (22.3%) (23)
Singh et al., 2016	2012–2014	India	Cross-sectional	Hospital-based	82	Most common diagnosis was schizophrenia (84.1%) followed by bipolar affective disorder (12.2%) and substance use disorder (6%) (8)
Susser et al., 1989	1985	New York, US	Cross-sectional	Community-based	223	Most common diagnosis was schizophrenia (33%) (25)
Tripathi et al., 2013	2005–2011	India	Cross-sectional	Hospital-based	140	The most common diagnosis was either psychosis or mood disorders which were present in 77.9%. The comorbid substance dependence was seen in 44.3% (26)

ranges from 5.6% to 30.8% in both community-based and hospital-based samples (8,10–26). HMI individuals have been shown to have high rates of severe mental illnesses such as psychosis, substance abuse/use disorder, and depression, both in high- and low-income countries (1,7,27,28). On the other hand, as mentioned previously and elsewhere in this volume, mental illness also leads to homelessness, which may be due to ongoing poor social support, lack of economic resources, poverty, personal and social deterioration, underutilization of public entitlements, inability to receive care, and deinstitutionalization. These factors converge and form a vicious cycle (27,29). The prevalence of HMI individuals in the general population will be influenced by several factors, including how the law of the land defines it. Access to care, mental health establishments, deinstitutionalization, a programme for HMI individuals, mental health policy, availability of mental health resources, societal fabric, and structure are other factors which may play a role (17,18).

Interestingly, homeless people in low- and middle-income countries are more likely to have psychosis when compared to high-income countries. HMI individuals from high-income countries are more likely to have primary alcohol and other drug dependence over low- and middle-income countries (10–26).

Clinical outcome of homeless mentally ill individuals

The clinical outcome of HMI individuals is an important issue and depends upon clinical care, policy, and programme for states. Table 11.2 shows the clinical outcome of mental illness among HMI people from low-, middle-, and high-income countries (8,13,18,26,30–32). In the HMI individuals who are elderly, with higher education levels, a longer duration of homelessness is associated with an increased likelihood of being treated in a psychiatric setting (13). The clinical improvement in psychiatric condition ranged from 56.1% to 82.7% among HMI individuals admitted into a psychiatric hospital (8,26). The HMI individuals who have psychosis, mood disorder, and comorbid substance dependence had shown improvement in their clinical condition during inpatient care (26).

Rehabilitation of homeless mentally ill individuals

Rehabilitation of the HMI individuals is important and essential in terms of the rights of the person and ensuring a high-quality healthcare service and helping them settle down and lead a productive life. Table 11.3 shows the results of studies on rehabilitation of the HMI individuals. Mental health professionals and social workers attempted reintegration of the HMI individuals back into the

Table 11.2 Studies on clinical outcome of homeless mentally ill individuals

Study group	Year	Country	Study design	Population	Sample	Results and conclusion
Chondraki et al., 2014	2009	Greece	Cross-sectional	Hospital-based	254	HMI individuals who are older with higher education and longer duration of being homeless had a higher likelihood of getting treatment in a psychiatric setting (13)
Fu et al., 2017	2017	China	Comparative study	Hospital-based	500	Impaired insight is more common in HMI inpatients when compared to those mentally ill inpatients who were not homeless (30)
Gowda et al., 2017	2002–2015	India	Retrospective design	Hospital-based	78	Clinical improvement was seen in 82% of HMI individuals following inpatient care. The mean duration of inpatient care was 15 weeks (17)
Onofa et al., 2002	2004–2008	Nigeria	Retrospective design	Hospital-based	183	HMI individuals had poorer clinical profiles and treatment outcomes compared to non-homeless mentally ill patients (31)
Ran et al., 2006	1994–2004	China	Retrospective design	Community-based	510	Having unstable shelter, being unmarried, divorced, or separated, and having a diagnosis of schizophrenia are risk factors for homelessness (32)
Singh et al., 2016	2012–2014	India	Cross-sectional	Hospital-based	82	Clinical improvement was noted in 56.1% of admitted HMI individuals (8)
Tripathi et al., 2013	2005–2011	India	Cross-sectional	Hospital-based	140	Clinical improvement was noted in 82.7% of admitted HMI individuals (26)

Table 11.3 Studies on rehabilitation of homeless mentally ill persons

Study group	Year	Country	Study design	Population	Sample	Findings from the study
Chitta Prakasha Trust	2010–2015	India	Retrospective design	Rehabilitation centre-based	62	Family reintegration was achieved in 50% of HMI individuals (35)
Gouveia et al., 2017	2008–2010	Mozambique	Cross-sectional	Hospital-based	71	Family reintegration was possible in 53.5% of HMI individuals, and it was better among those with the diagnosis of substance use disorder when compared to those with the diagnosis of intellectual disability (19)
Gowda et al., 2019	2002–2015	India	Retrospective design	Hospital-based	78	Family reintegration was achieved in 50.3% and community-based reintegration was done in 41% and the remaining 7.8% required multispecialty care in a general hospital or absconded from the hospital during inpatient care (76)
Rao, 2008	1993–2008	India	Retrospective design	Community	413	The family-based rehabilitation achieved in 61% of female patients (34)
Singh et al., 2016	2012–2014	India	Cross-sectional	Hospital-based	82	After discharge from hospital, 47.6% were reintegrated to family and 41.5% were reintegrated to community centre (8)
Tripathi et al., 2013	2005–2011	India	Cross-sectional	Hospital-based	140	After discharge from hospital, 68.6% were reintegrated to family and 8.6% were reintegrated to community centre (26)

family through police, personal contacts, postal services, e-mail, Yahoo groups, well-wishers, local practitioners, and as such, they help locate addresses after taking permission/consent from the HMI individuals (17,18,33). The family-based reintegration achieved ranged from 47.6% to 83.5%, and community-based reintegration achieved ranged from 8.6% to 41.5% (8,13,18,26,34,35). The HMI individuals with a substance use disorder and severe mental illness, with an improved clinical condition had better reintegration back into community and family. HMI individuals with poor insight continued to have active psychotic symptoms, and those with intellectual disability were less reintegrated with their family and society (17,18). Recently, an organization looked into the outcome of 7000 rehabilitated HMI individuals from their non-governmental organization (NGO) registry (36). On the other hand, a follow-up survey from the Shanthivanam Trust in Tamilnadu, India, showed that 55% of them living in a community were on regular treatment and leading a respectable life, 20% of HMI individuals made their way back on the streets as homeless individuals, and 25% did not follow up for psychiatric consultation and thus were not on any treatment (37). In another study from Columbus State Hospital in Ohio, US (38), the prevalence of homelessness among 132 patients 6 months post discharge was around 36%. Providing permanent housing through a Housing First model to HMI individuals was found effective and successful in the US and Canada. The HMI individuals perceived that they had a better quality of life and stable housing through a Housing First model. A Housing First model helped in community-based vocational training programmes and made integration back into the community easier. The Mental Health Commission of Canada recommends a Housing First model for homeless people living with mental health problems or illnesses.

Evidence-based best practice model for clinical practice and rehabilitation of homeless mentally ill individuals

The HMI individual is very often deprived of all rights. They may have to struggle for food, shelter, and healthcare needs. Access to healthcare will depend very much upon the healthcare system, for example, whether it is free at the point of contact, whether it is private, or a mixture of the two. HMI individuals may also be suffering from violation of their other rights such as confidentiality, privacy, safety, ability to practise religion, etc. (39). The rehabilitation of HMI individuals is important and essential concerning the rights of the person and ensuring high-quality healthcare services as per the World Health Organization guidance (40). To achieve these goals, there is a need to assess the needs of the HMI individuals in their locality and develop comprehensive clinical and rehabilitation services which are geographically accessible.

The following aspects include an evidence-based best practice model for clinical practice and rehabilitation. The most important unmet need for HMI individuals is getting access to a comprehensive mental health service, which is multidimensional and multidisciplinary, and that is integrated into general healthcare service and systems (41). The many studies support the need for a community centre, which is in a position to provide combined clinical services for physical and mental health rehabilitation, vocational rehabilitation, housing, and outreach mental health services (42,43). Caton and colleagues) (44) also propose discharge planning and aftercare services for HMI individuals, which look into treatment, rehabilitation, living arrangements, and finance. As many studies have confirmed, inadequate discharge planning increases the risk of homelessness and rehospitalization among HMI individuals (45). An interesting option is what Chet et al. (46) propose as transitional care for HMI individuals. Transitional care facilitates the critical transition from institutional to community settings and ensures the continuity of clinical care to HMI individuals. The effective follow-ups in aftercare programmes include (a) assertive community treatment (ACT), (b) psychosocial rehabilitation, (c) employment rehabilitation, (d) residential support in the community, and (e) economic support.

Assertive community treatment

ACT is considered as a direct service model, with a low staff–client ratio, and a focus on continuity of care. ACT components include illness management, medication management, housing, finances, and a focus on helping the individuals in transition or adjusting to the community. The components and goals of an ACT programme are more suitable for HMI individuals, as they need integrated mental health treatment, housing, and rehabilitation. ACT services include assistance in routine practical problems in living and to achieve the client's immediate needs and personal goals. So, ACT is more tailor-made for community living for an HMI person, after discharge from the hospital (47–49).

Psychosocial rehabilitation

The HMI individuals often has a deficit in self-care, social skills, coping skills, crisis management, and adaptation to the community due to their psychiatric illness and separation from the community. The psychosocial interventions such as individual counselling, handling crisis intervention, providing psychological treatment for psychological issues, self-care, and social skills training will enable the HMI individuals to adapt to the community.

Vocational rehabilitation

Employment is considered an important aspect of rehabilitation for the HMI individuals. Vocational rehabilitation is important, as it makes them independent and helps improve their self-esteem. HMI individuals can be trained in prevocational, vocational, and occupational training based on their suitability. Along with training, support has to be provided to the HMI individuals to find employment and adapt at work through supported employment. It helps them to do jobs and fulfil several needs. In turn, it helps in the integration of the HMI individuals into society through employment and enables them to create networks. The individual placement and support model showed that HMI individuals do better in competitive employment than other supported employment model (50).

Residential support in the community

Residential services are graded according to different levels of independence and follow the least restrictive alternative. This helps to improve the independence and the quality of life of HMI individuals and makes possible their progressive social reintegration. A similar concept was adapted in the US called the Housing First model. It was found effective in assisting the HMI individuals with long-term housing stability and improving their quality of life (51–53).

Financial assistance/aid

An HMI individuals also needs financial assistance/aid at different treatment and rehabilitation stages. Financial assistance is through social security disability insurance, supplemental security income, disability, and welfare benefits. This is supported by a few high-income countries and low- and middle-income countries through welfare programmes.

Including the above-mentioned components into the existing health facilities for HMI individuals can improve HMI services. The facility should be based on the prevalence of HMI individuals in the locality and their needs. The centre should be planned based on available local resources and specific legislation, acts, or programmes of each country. These centres should be planned to integrate with rehabilitation centres or be included in the rehabilitation programmes based on the needs of HMI individuals after they get better from their mental illness, substance abuse, and physical illness including infectious diseases (54).

Current status of clinical care and rehabilitation of homeless mentally ill individuals worldwide

Mental illness of the homeless is a complex public health challenge and some countries are giving special attention to the highly marginalized and vulnerable groups in society but this approach is not universal. In this regard, few high-income countries have policies, laws, and acts to fulfil the basic needs of shelter, food, clothes, and so on and managing the care of HMI individuals as a civil commitment.

Different counties propose different kinds of interventions. For example, in Australia, Mental Health Services in Australia provides the specialist homelessness services (55) to the HMI individuals. The Australian National Housing and Homelessness Agreement sees early intervention and prevention as key in reducing homelessness. The Australian National Disability Insurance Scheme also provides psychosocial support services to HMI individuals. It has also started the Housing and Accommodation Support Initiative and Victoria's Housing and Support Program that provides social and affordable housing, through which the HMI individuals can get affordable housing (56).

Canada has developed a mental health policy in the provinces. All these policies aim to provide quality mental health services to the entire population, including homeless individuals. In addition, the Mental Health Commission of Canada recommends a Housing First model for homeless people living with mental health problems or illnesses (57,58). The European Union recommends a comprehensive, integrated service to HMI individuals, which includes stable housing, personalized community-based care, stigma eradication, and rights-based care (3,59). The US passed an act in 2012 called the Homeless Emergency Assistance and Rapid Transition to Housing (HEARTH) Act which replaced the previous McKinney–Vento Act (4,5). Under the HEARTH Act, the homelessness definition was broadened and included the individual who is at risk of homelessness. Furthermore, it also enables a homeless person to be eligible for permanent housing through a Housing First programme and noted an accelerated shift from sheltered accommodation to permanent housing. The act also directed USICH to develop a national strategic plan to end homelessness. USICH (53) recommends solutions for HMI individuals by providing (a) comprehensive and seamless systems of care, (b) a strategic plan to end homelessness, (c) collaboration among law enforcement and behavioural health and social service providers, and (d) help with alternative justice system strategies. The National Health Care for the Homeless Council provides comprehensive healthcare and secure housing for everyone (60). In the UK, the Homelessness

Reduction Act, 2017 (61) was enacted in April 2018. Under this, HMI individuals receive person-centred advice and support through local housing authorities. The Mental Health Act and the Mental Capacity Act of the UK help to assess the capacity of HMI to make better decisions (62,63).

Current status of clinical care and rehabilitation of homeless mentally ill people in India

In India, the Ministry of Women and Child Development, Government of India, runs a programme called 'Swadhar Greh' (its literal meaning is self-reliant home) (64). This centre is located in the headquarters of each district. The Swadhar Greh provides shelter, food, clothing, medical treatment, care, and rehabilitation for women. The Government of Karnataka (one of the 30 states of India) in collaboration with the Social Welfare and Labour Department provides food, shelter, medical care, and rehabilitation to homeless person and beggars, irrespective of mental illness status through the Nirashrithara Parihara Kendra (Centre for Homeless Persons). This service has not yet been evaluated (65). Along with this, the Government of Karnataka provides a day-care facility for the person with severe mental disorder through the 'Maanasadhaara' programme. In India, the National Mental Health Policy, 2014 (66) and the Mental Healthcare Act (MHCA), 2017 (67) talk about the care of a HMI individuals, through universal access to mental health with care and a rights-based approach to comprehensive mental healthcare through public and state responsibility. However, it may be noted that comprehensive care and rehabilitation facilities for HMI individuals are practically non-existent at present. It remains to be seen how legislation and policies translate into facilities in real life (39,66–68).

NGOs in India are key partners as they provide care and rehabilitation to HMI individuals. These include Aashray Adhikar Abhiyan; Apnaghar; Ashadeep, Guwahati; The Banyan, Chennai; Chittadhama, Karnataka; Humana, Delhi; Hans Foundation, Delhi; Karuna Trust, Mysore; Parivartan Trust; Shantivanam, Trichy; Shraddha Rehabilitation Foundation, Mumbai; and the Uday Foundation, Delhi. These centres locally identify HMI individuals in society and provide basic shelter, care, and support. The objectives of many NGOs include identifying and admitting HMI into their centres, taking care of their mental and physical health deficits by treating them, and making efforts to rehabilitate and reintegrate them back into their communities and families through the available local resources using the concept of community-based inclusive living for HMI individuals (33,35–37). Several NGOs in India have partnered with many national and international organizations on mental health policy, education, and research. Considering the homeless population in the country, NGOs are catering to the tip of the iceberg, and it may be difficult to sustain these programmes over time and on a larger scale due to multiple factors. Effective health policies and provisions are required to address the need for homeless and wandering mentally ill individuals (18,68).

Factors influencing clinical outcome and rehabilitation of homeless mentally ill people

Many factors affect clinical outcomes during the rehabilitation of HMI individuals, both personal and societal. These are described very briefly as follows.

Age

Age is considered an important factor which influences the outcome and rehabilitation of HMI individuals. Studies show a higher prevalence of psychiatric and substance use disorder in younger age homelessness over older age homelessness. This may well be due to the fact that three-quarters of psychiatric disorders in adulthood start below the age of 24. The clinical outcome and rehabilitation were difficult with late-life first-time homeless people as they had more housing problems and social problems than psychiatric illnesses (7,69,70).

Gender

Males are over-represented among HMI individuals, and they also have higher rates of substance use disorder (8,18,26,30–32). Females have unique needs, especially as they are highly vulnerable to sexual abuse, unwanted pregnancies, and sexually transmitted diseases, and may be responsible for child care. These factors also influence the clinical outcome and rehabilitation of females. Females may require additional specialized resources in a community-based rehabilitation setting (71).

Clinical diagnosis

As noted earlier in this chapter, studies on HMI individuals across countries show substantial heterogeneity in the prevalence and distribution of severe psychiatric illness (7). HMI individuals from high-income countries have more primary substance use disorders over psychotic spectrum disorder than those from low- and middle-income countries, where primary psychotic spectrum disorders are more common than the substance use disorders and are associated with the comorbid intellectual developmental disorder. The presence of substance use disorder, psychosis, common mental disorder, and compliance with treatment had a favourable clinical outcome. HMI with intellectual disability had a poor rehabilitation outcome, and experienced delays in being placed into rehabilitation homes (18). They also required ongoing care and support after discharge from psychiatric services and being placed in a rehabilitation home (72). Not surprisingly, HMI individuals who had poor insight and less motivation for treatment had negative clinical and rehabilitation outcomes (73).

Physical health

Physical health problems are also very common in HMI individuals. Reasons for this may include (a) psychiatric illness; (b) substance use disorders; (c) poor nutrition; (d) poor living conditions; (e) higher exposure to communicable diseases such as tuberculosis, HIV, and hepatitis C; (e) victimization; (f) unintentional injuries due to wandering; and (g) poor access to the healthcare system. The presence of multiple physical health problems in HMI individuals will prolong the stay in mental health establishments and rehabilitation centres and delay the reintegration of HMI individuals back into the community. The clinical care of HMI individuals must include an integrated comprehensive medical service in mental health establishments and rehabilitation centres (7,74). Some HMI individuals with severe physical health and mental health problems may require long-term care in the establishment rather than the community due to a need for intensive medical attention and care.

Poverty

Poverty is considered an important determinant of homelessness prevalence at an individual and a societal level. Studies have shown unemployment, housing, poverty, and mental illness are interlinked, thus setting up a vicious cycle.

Integrated services and aftercare planning

An HMI individuals clinical outcome and rehabilitation depend on the type of existing services available. HMI individuals require tailor-made clinical and rehabilitation services. They would benefit from targeted multidimensional care, and multidisciplinary, integrated healthcare service and systems (41), which cater to multiple needs such as physical and mental health, rehabilitation, vocational, and housing needs (42,43,75). The multidisciplinary team is also required to provide aftercare needs such as community rehabilitation, help with living arrangements, and financial support after discharge through the outreach programmes (44). Discharge planning is the most important issue, and inadequate discharge planning may increase the risk of homelessness and rehospitalization (45).

Family reintegration

Family reintegration where possible and required, may well be more helpful for an HMI individuals. Family reintegration is more successful and feasible in India and other low- and middle-income countries due to a collectivistic and interdependent joint family system. Family reintegration can lead to stable housing, favourable treatment outcomes, and recovery from mental illness (18, 26, 36, 37).

Community reintegration

The Mental Healthcare Act, 2017 of India and many high-income countries' policies and programmes strongly advocate community-based rehabilitation for HMI individuals. The community-based reintegration of HMI individuals is a more cost-effective model over keeping HMI individuals in institutions. ACT and the equivalent model in community-based reintegration were found to be effective. The community-based reintegration of HMI individuals was associated with reduced rehospitalization. HMI individuals placed in a community-based reintegration had a better quality of life and were more satisfied with services (76–81). Some studies have shown that including motivational interviewing, cognitive behavioural therapy, and contingency management in community-based reintegration of HMI individuals improved outcomes. Also, collaboration with NGOs and communities will help clients sustain stable housing (82).

Non-governmental organizations

NGOs' work on care and rehabilitation of HMI individuals is compassion driven and NGOs have committed services in India as described previously. Linking up with government may help them provide care to large groups (18,41).

Deinstitutionalization

Deinstitutionalization is a process of replacing the beds in a mental hospital with a community-based mental healthcare system. Deinstitutionalization is a positive move from governments in both high- and low-income countries as many advances have been made in the care of a person with mental illness. Governments, however, have not build community-based care to match the extent of deinstitutionalization. Many reviews hypothesize that the high prevalence of HMI individuals in the community is due to rapid deinstitutionalization and not meeting the needs of HMI in the community due to inadequate provision of community-based living arrangements and rehabilitation services (83,84), resulting in therapeutic neglect, social disintegration, and poor quality of life of HMI individuals (85). In contrast, in a recent review, there was no increased rate of homelessness, imprisonment, or suicide after the effect of deinstitutionalization (86). Studies with robust methods are required to understand the effect of deinstitutionalization on the community and HMI individuals. ACT (soon after the discharge of HMI individuals from clinical settings) can be very helpful and shows significant advantages over standard case management models in reducing homelessness and symptom severity of illness (87).

Housing and supported accommodation

Everyone has a fundamental human right to housing, as it ensures safety, security, and freedom. Governments have a moral duty to provide decent and reasonable housing to all those who need it. It has become an obligation in many countries after they signed treaties such as the Universal Declaration of Human Rights and the International Covenant on Economic Social and Cultural Rights, which advocates the right to basic housing. Stable housing is considered to be a positive and protective factor in rehabilitation among the HMI individuals (88–90). A study showed that HMI with unemployment, chronic illness, criminal justice involvement, and victimization had difficulty accessing stable housing (91) thereby proving a vicious circle exists. Involving the HMI individuals in housing and community living-related decision-making has shown better rehabilitation outcomes (92). The community living-related decision-making was not influenced by a person's mental illness or substance use disorder, but by intellectual disability (93–97).

Supported employment

As noted previously, supported employment is considered a part of community-based rehabilitation. It provides necessary support to the HMI individuals at the workplace to help them achieve the goal. The HMI individuals with physical, cognitive, and mental health problems often has a deficit in daily life skills and safety functioning, which significantly interferes with the supported employment (95,96). As every HMI individuals has many strengths, talents, and abilities, helping them through individual placement and training with continued long-term support after successfully getting a job is necessary. Studies reported that the HMI individuals with supported employment as part of vocational rehabilitation and community-based ACT had less risk of subsequent homelessness, had less substance use and criminal behaviour, and were more satisfied with the services (97–100). The individual placement and support model showed that HMI individuals tend to do better in competitive employment than the other supported employment model (50). The supported employment model for HMI individuals especially focuses on homelessness-specific work experiences in the past and internal motivation to work, employment opportunities along with co-management with the community-based care team.

Laws, policies, and programmes

Housing, healthcare, employment, welfare, and livelihood are important issues for the HMI individuals. There is a need for comprehensive, integrated services-based, specific laws, policies, and programmes for HMI individuals. The high-income countries such as Australia, Canada, the UK, the US, and European Union countries have their laws, programmes, and policies based on local needs. In contrast to many high-income countries, India and other low-income countries do not have any specific legislation, acts, or programmes to define an HMI individuals .

Human rights policy

Respecting the human rights of the HMI individuals is essential, and this also includes the rights to housing, health, and personal autonomy. The service providers need to be cognizant of human rights. They must plan the clinical care, rehabilitation services, and research on HMI individuals in a manner that does not undermine basic human rights, as many HMI individuals are unaware of their rights.

Future directions

Care for the HMI individuals must be made the highest priority in public mental health. Each country needs to develop a comprehensive system of care to address the needs of HMI individuals and their rehabilitation. The comprehensive system of care should make provision for HMI individuals, which is individualized, tailor-made, comprehensive, community-based outreach care based on local and social resources to attain the highest possible levels of functioning. There is a need for prospective studies regarding innovation-based services which can influence the public policy. There is also scope for collaboration among all different stakeholders from the community such as the public sector, NGOs, rehabilitation centres, police, judiciary, and psychiatric facilities to enhance the quality and reach the unreached HMI individuals to provide treatment and rehabilitation services.

Conclusion

Homeless individuals with mental illnesses often suffer from complex issues. The clinical outcome and rehabilitation of the HMI individuals are determined by multiple factors such as stable housing, integrated physical and mental health services, community-based care, psychiatric symptoms, favourable treatment outcomes and recovery from mental illness, employment, social support, housing status, ACT, and national mental health policy. Based on the HMI individuals specific needs, there is a need for an optimal model of clinical, social, and rehabilitation services for homeless individuals with mental illnesses.

References

1. Fazel S, Khosla V, Doll H, Geddes J. The prevalence of mental disorders among the homeless in Western countries: systematic review and meta-regression analysis. PLoS Med. 2008;5:e225.

2. Chamberlain C. Homelessness: Re-Shaping the Policy Agenda? AHURI Final Report No. 221. Melbourne: Australian Housing and Urban Research Institute; 2014. Available from: https://www.ahuri.edu.au/__data/assets/pdf_file/0017/2249/AHURI_Final_Re port_No221_Homelessness-re-shaping-the-policy-agenda.pdf.

3. European Typology of Homelessness and Housing Exclusion (ETHOS). Homepage. Available from: https://ethos-europe.eu/.

4. US Congress. Homeless Emergency Assistance and Rapid Transition to Housing Act of 2009. Definition of homelessness. 111th Congress. Public Law 111–122, Sec. 1003. Available from: https://www.onecpd.info/resources/documents/S896_HEARTH Act.pdf.

5. National Coalition for the Homeless. McKinney–Vento Act. Available from: http://www.nationalhomeless.org/publications/facts/McKinney.pdf.

6. Minnery J, Greenhalgh E. Approaches to homelessness policy in Europe, the United States, and Australia. J Soc Issues. 2007;63(3):641–655.

7. Fazel S, Geddes JR, Kushel M. The health of homeless people in high-income countries: descriptive epidemiology, health consequences, and clinical and policy recommendations. Lancet. 2014;384(9953):1529–1540.

8. Singh G, Shah N, Mehta R. The clinical presentation and outcome of the institutionalized wandering mentally ill in India. J Clin Diagnostic Res. 2016;10:VC13–VC16.

9. Gururaj G, Varghese M, Benegal V, et al. National Mental Health Survey of India, 2015–16: Prevalence, Patterns and Outcomes. NIMHANS Publication No. 129. Bengaluru: National Institute of Mental Health and Neuro Sciences; 2016. Available from: http://indianmhs.nimhans.ac.in/Docs/Report2.pdf.

10. Ayano G, Assefa D, Haile K, et al. Mental, neurologic, and substance use (MNS) disorders among street homeless people in Ethiopia. Ann Gen Psychiatry. 2017;16:40.

11. Bassuk EL, Rubin L, Lauriat A. Is homelessness a mental health problem? Am J Psychiatry. 1984;141(12):1546–1550.

12. Breakey WR, Fischer PJ, Kramer M, et al. Health and mental health problems of homeless men and women in Baltimore. JAMA. 1989;262(10):1352–1357.

13. **Chondraki P, Madianos MG, Dragioti E, Papadimitriou GN.** Homeless mentally ill in Athens area: a cross-sectional study on unmet needs and help-seeking. Int J Soc Psychiatry. 2014;**60**(6):544–553.

14. **Fekadu A, Hanlon C, Gebre-Eyesus E, et al.** Burden of mental disorders and unmet needs among street homeless people in Addis Ababa, Ethiopia. BMC Med. 2014;**12**:138.

15. **Gelberg L, Leake BD.** Substance use among impoverished medical patients: the effect of housing status and other factors. Med Care. 1993;**31**(9):757–766.

16. **Gupta R, Nethra DK, Kumar V, Sharma P, Kumar P.** Psychiatric illnesses in homeless (runaway or throwaway) girl inmates: a preliminary study. Dysphrenia. 2013;**4**(1):31–35.

17. **Gowda GS, Gopika G, Manjunatha N, et al.** Sociodemographic and clinical profiles of homeless mentally ill admitted in mental health institute of South India: 'Know the Unknown' project. Int J Soc Psychiatry. 2017;**63**(6):525–531.

18. **Gowda GS, Gopika G, Kumar CN, et al.** Clinical outcome and rehabilitation of homeless mentally ill patients admitted in mental health institute of South India: 'Know the Unknown' project. Asian J Psychiatr. 2017;**30**:49–53.

19. **Gouveia L, Massanganhe H, Mandlate F, et al.** Family reintegration of homeless in Maputo and Matola: a descriptive study. Int J Ment Health Syst. 2017;**11**:25.

20. **Heckert U, Andrade L, Alves M, Martins C.** Lifetime prevalence of mental disorders among homeless people in a southeast city in Brazil. Eur Arch Psychiatry Clin Neurosci 1999;**249**(3):150–155.

21. **Lovisi GM, Mann AH, Coutinho E, Morgado AF.** Mental illness in an adult sample admitted to public hostels in the Rio de Janeiro metropolitan area, Brazil. Soc Psychiatry Psychiatr Epidemiol. 2003;**38**(9):493–498.

22. **Moquillaza-Risco M, León E, Dongo M, Munayco CV.** [Socio-demographics characteristics and health conditions of older homeless persons of Lima, Peru]. Rev Peru Med Exp Salud Publica. 2015;**32**(4):693–700.

23. **Nuttbrock LA, Rahav M, Rivera JJ, Ng-Mak DS, Link BG.** Outcomes of homeless mentally ill chemical abusers in community residences and a therapeutic community. Psychiatr Serv. 1998;**49**(1):68–76.

24. **Nayak RB, Patil S, Patil N, Chate SS, Koparde VA.** Psychiatric morbidity among inmates of center for destitutes: a cross sectional study. J Sci Soc. 2015;**42**(2):92–94.

25. **Susser E, Struening EL, Conover S.** Psychiatric problems in homeless men. Lifetime psychosis, substance use, and current distress in new arrivals at New York City shelters. Arch Gen Psychiatry. 1989;**46**(9):845–850.

26. **Tripathi A, Nischal A, Dalal PK, et al.** Sociodemographic and clinical profile of homeless mentally ill inpatients in a north Indian medical university. Asian J Psychiatr. 2013;**6**(5):404–409.

27. **Fischer PJ, Breakey WR.** The epidemiology of alcohol, drug, and mental disorders among homeless persons. Am Psychol. 1991;**46**(11):1115–1128.

28. **Folsom DP, Hawthorne W, Lindamer L, et al.** Prevalence and risk factors for homelessness and utilization of mental health services among 10,340 patients with serious mental illness in a large public mental health system. Am J Psychiatry. 2005;**162**(2):370–376.

29. **Nieto G, Gittelman M, Abad A.** Homeless mentally ill persons: a bibliography review. Int J Psychosoc Rehabil. 2008;**12**:2–7.

30. **Fu YN, Cao XL, Hou CL,** et al. Comparison of insight and clinical variables in homeless and non-homeless psychiatric inpatients in China. Psychiatry Res. 2017;**255**:13–16.

31. **Onofa L, Fatiregun AA, Fawole OI, Adebowale T.** Comparison of clinical profiles and treatment outcomes between vagrant and non-vagrant mentally ill patients in a specialist neuropsychiatric hospital in Nigeria. Afr J Psychiatry (Johannesbg). 2012;**15**(3):189–192.

32. **Ran MS, Chan CL, Chen EY, Xiang MZ, Caine ED, Conwell Y.** Homelessness among patients with schizophrenia in rural China: a 10-year cohort study. Acta Psychiatr Scand. 2006;**114**(2):118–123.

33. **Swaminath G.** Indian Psychiatric Society-South Zone: innovations and challenges in providing psychiatric services to disadvantaged populations: a pilgrim's progress. Indian J Psychol Med. 2015;**37**(2):122–130.

34. **Rao NP.** Rehabilitation of the wandering seriously mentally ill (WSMI) women. J Soc Work Health Care. 2005;**39**(2):49–65.

35. **Chittaprakasha Trust.** Homepage. Available from: https://www.chittaprakasha.in.

36. **Sharadha Foundation.** Homepage. Available from: https://www.shraddharehabilitationfoundation.org.

37. **Shanthivanam.** Homepage. Available from: http://www.trustshanthivanam.org/shanthivanam.php.

38. **Belcher JR.** Rights versus needs of homeless mentally ill persons. Soc Work.1988;**33**(5):398–402.

39. **Swaminath G, Enara A, Rao R, Kumar KVK, Kumar CN.** Mental Healthcare Act, 2017 and homeless persons with mental illness in India. Indian J Psychiatry. 2019;**61**(Suppl 4):S768–S772.

40. **Wright MJ, Tompkins CN.** How Can Health Care Systems Effectively Deal with the Major Health Care Needs of Homeless People? Copenhagen: WHO Regional Office for Europe's Health Evidence Network (HEN); 2005. Available from: http://www.euro.who.int/__data/assets/pdf_file/0009/74682/E85482.pdf.

41. **Smartt C, Prince M, Frissa S, Eaton J, Fekadu A, Hanlon C.** Homelessness and severe mental illness in low- and middle-income countries: scoping review. BJPsych Open. 2019;**5**(4):e57.

42. **Leda C, Rosenheck R.** Mental health status and community adjustment after treatment in a residential treatment program for homeless veterans. Am J Psychiatry. 1992;**149**(9):1219–1224.

43. **Lettner BH, Doan RJ, Miettinen AW.** Housing outcomes and predictors of success: the role of hospitalization in street outreach. J Psychiatr Ment Health Nurs. 2016;**23**(2):98–107.

44. **Caton CL.** Mental health service use among homeless and never-homeless men with schizophrenia. Psychiatr Serv. 1995;**46**(11):1139–1143.

45. **Allan J, Kemp M.** The prevalence and characteristics of homelessness in the NSW substance treatment population: implications for practice. Soc Work Health Care. 2014;**53**(2):183–198.

46. **Chen FP.** Developing community support for homeless people with mental illness in transition. Community Ment Health J. 2014;**50**(5):520–530.

47. **Bond GR, Drake RE.** The critical ingredients of assertive community treatment. World Psychiatry. 2015;**14**(2):240–242.

48. **Killaspy H.** Assertive community treatment in psychiatry. BMJ. 2007;**335**(7615):311–312.

49. **de Vet R, van Luijtelaar MJ, Brillesljper-Kater SN, Vanderplasschen W, Beijersbergen MD, Wolf JR.** Effectiveness of case management for homeless persons: a systematic review. Am J Public Health. 2013;**103**(10):e13–e26.

50. **Leddy M, Stefanovics E, Rosenheck R.** Health and well-being of homeless veterans participating in transitional and supported employment: six-month outcomes. J Rehabil Res Dev. 2014;**51**(1):161–175.

51. **Davis KE, Devitt T, Rollins A, O'Neill S, Pavick D, Harding B.** Integrated residential treatment for persons with severe and persistent mental illness: lessons in recovery. J Psychoactive Drugs. 2006;**38**(3):263–272.

52. **Donovan S, Shinseki EK.** Homelessness is a public health issue. Am J Public Health. 2013;**103**(2):S180–181.

53. **United States Interagency Council on Homelessness (USICH).** Searching out solutions: constructive alternatives to criminalization. 2012. Available from: https://www.usich.gov/resources/uploads/asset_library/RPT_SoS_March2012.pdf.

54. **Gonzalez RG, Gonzalez FJ, Fernandez-Aquirre MV.** Rehabilitation and social insertion of the homeless chronically mentally ill. Int J Psychosoc Rehabil. 2001;5:79–100.

55. **Australian Institute of Health and Family Welfare.** Mental health services in Australia; specialist homelessness services. Available from: https://www.aihw.gov.au/reports/men tal-health-services/mental-health-services-in-australia/report-contents/specialist-homelessness-services.

56. **NSW Government.** Housing and accommodation support initiative. Available from: https://www.health.nsw.gov.au/mentalhealth/Pages/services-hasi-cls.aspx.

57. **Mental Health Commission of Canada.** Homepage. Available from: https://mentalhealt hcommission.ca/English.

58. **David HJ, Philippa C, Shirley C, Stephen H, Emily P.** Mental health, mental illness, & homelessness in Canada. In: Finding Home: Policy Options for Addressing Homelessness in Canada. Cities Centre, University of Toronto; 2009. Available from: https://www.homelesshub.ca/resource/finding-home-policy-options-addressing-homel essness-canada.

59. **Mental Health Europe.** Homepage. Available from: https://www.mhe-sme.org/.

60. **National Health Care for the Homeless Council.** Homepage. Available from: https://nhchc.org/.

61. **Legislation.gov.uk.** Homelessness Reduction Act, 2017. Available from: http://www.legi slation.gov.uk/ukpga/2017/13/contents/enacted.

62. **Legislation.gov.uk.** Mental Capacity Act, 2005. 2005. Available from: http://www.legi slation.gov.uk/ukpga/2005/9/pdfs/ukpga_20050009_en.pdf.

63. **Legislation.gov.uk.** Mental Health Act, 1983. 1983. Available from: http://www.legislat ion.gov.uk/ukpga/1983/20/contents.

64. **Ministry of Women and Child Development, Government of India.** Swadhar Greh: a scheme that caters to primary needs of women in difficult circumstances. Available from: http://wcd.nic.in/sites/default/files/Guidelines7815_2.pdf.

65. **Nirashrithara Parihara Kendra.** Homepage. Available from: https://www.karnataka. gov.in/crcbng/Pages/Home.aspx.

66. **Ministry of Health and Family Welfare, Government of India.** National Mental Health Policy of India. 2014. Available from: http://nhm.gov.in/images/pdf/National_Health_ Mental_Policy.pdf.

67. **Ministry of Health and Family Welfare Department, Government of India.** The Mental Healthcare Act, 2017. Available from: http://www.prsindia.org/uploads/media/ Mental%20Health/Mental%20Healthcare%20Act,%202017.pdf.

68. **Gowda GS, Gopika G, Sanjay TN, et al.** Challenge faced by state and society in providing care to homeless mentally ill patients: "Know the Unknown" project. Indian J Soc Psychiatry. 2019;**35**:75–79.

69. **Institute of Medicine (US) Committee on Health Care for Homeless People.** Health problems of homeless people. In: Homelessness, Health, and Human Needs. Washington, DC: National Academies Press (US); 1988:39–75. Available from: https:// www.ncbi.nlm.nih.gov/books/NBK218236/.

70. **Brown RT, Goodman L, Guzman D, Tieu L, Ponath C, Kushel MB.** Pathways to homelessness among older homeless adults: results from the HOPE HOME Study. PLoS One. 2016;**11**(5):e0155065.

71. **Tsai J, Kasprow WJ, Kane V, Rosenheck RA.** National comparison of literally homeless male and female VA service users: entry characteristics, clinical needs, and service patterns. Womens Health Issues. 2014;**24**(1):e29–35.

72. **Van Straaten B, Rodenburg G, Van der Laan J, Boersma SN, Wolf JR, Van de Mheen D.** Self-reported care needs of Dutch homeless people with and without a suspected intellectual disability: a 1.5-year follow-up study. Health Soc Care Community. 2017;**25**(1):123–136.

73. **Kellinghaus C, Lowens S, Eikelmann B, Reker T.** [Homeless men in inpatient psychiatric treatment—a controlled study. 1: Health status and self assessment at intake]. Psychiatr Prax. 2000;**27**(1):19–23.

74. **Patra S, Anand K.** Homelessness: a hidden public health problem. Indian J *Public Health*. 2008;**52**(3):164–170.

75. **Lee SJ, Crowther E, Keating C, Kulkarni J.** What is needed to deliver collaborative care to address comorbidity more effectively for adults with a severe mental illness? Aust N Z J Psychiatry. 2013;**47**(4):333–346.

76. **Morse GA, Calsyn RJ, Allen G, Tempelhoff B, Smith R.** Experimental comparison of the effects of three treatment programs for homeless mentally ill people. Hosp Community Psychiatry. 1992;**43**(10):1005–1010.

77. **Morse GA, Calsyn RJ, Klikerberg WD, et al.** An experimental comparison of three types of case management for homeless mentally ill persons. Psychiatr Serv. 1997;**48**(4):487–503.

78. **Salize HJ, Horst A, Dillmann-Lange C, et al.** [How do mentally ill homeless persons evaluate their quality of life]. Psychiatr Prax. 2001;**28**(2):75–80.

79. **Starrfield JH, Avnon M, Starrfield W, Rabinowitz J, Heifetz S.** Effects of psychosocial rehabilitation for hospitalized mentally ill homeless persons. Psychiatr Serv. 1995;**46**(9):948–950.

80. **Baumgartner JN, Herman DB.** Community integration of formerly homeless men and women with severe mental illness after hospital discharge. Psychiatr Serv. 2012;**63**(5):435–437.

81. **Helfrich CA, Simpson EK, Chan DV.** Change patterns of homeless individuals with mental illness: a multiple case study. Community Ment Health J. 2014;**50**(5):531–537.

82. **Sun AP.** Helping homeless individuals with co-occurring disorders: the four components. Soc Work. 2012;**57**(1):23–37.

83. **Lamb HR.** Deinstitutionalization and the homeless mentally ill. Hosp Community Psychiatry. 1984;**35**(9):899–907.

84. **Lamb HR.** Deinstitutionalization at the crossroads. Hosp Community Psychiatry. 1988;**39**(9):941–945.

85. **Eikelmann B.** [Limits of deinstitutionalization?—perspective of the specialty clinic]. Psychiatr Prax. 2000;**27**(Suppl 2):S53–S58.

86. **Salisbury TT, Thornicroft G.** Deinstitutionalisation does not increase imprisonment or homelessness. Br J Psychiatry. 2016;**208**(5):412–413.

87. **Coldwell CM, Bender WS.** The effectiveness of assertive community treatment for homeless populations with severe mental illness: a meta-analysis. Am J Psychiatry. 2007;**164**(3):393–399.

88. **Holmes A, Carlisle T, Vale Z, Hatvani G, Heagney C, Jones S.** Housing First: permanent supported accommodation for people with psychosis who have experienced chronic homelessness. Australas Psychiatry. 2017;**25**(1):56–59.

89. **Gabrielian S, Young AS, Greenberg JM, Bromley E.** Social support and housing transitions among homeless adults with serious mental illness and substance use disorders. Psychiatr Rehabil J. 2018;**41**(3):208–215.

90. **Nelson G, Patterson M, Kirst M, et al.** Life changes among homeless persons with mental illness: a longitudinal study of housing first and usual treatment. Psychiatr Serv. 2015;**66**(6):592–597.

91. **Gray HM, Nelson SE, Shaffer HJ, Stebbins P, Farina AR.** How do homeless adults change their lives after completing an intensive job-skills program? A prospective study. J Community Psychol. 2017;**45**(7):888–905.

92. **Richter D, Hoffmann H.** Independent housing and support for people with severe mental illness: systematic review. Acta Psychiatr Scand. 2017;**136**(3):269–279.

93. **Schutt RK, Goldfinger SM.** Housing preferences and perceptions of health and functioning among homeless mentally ill persons. Psychiatr Serv. 1996;**47**(4):381–386.

94. **Larsen M, Nordentoft M.** [Evidence-based treatment of mentally ill homeless persons]. Ugeskr Laeger. 2010;**172**(22):1669–1675.

95. **Gutman SA, Raphael-Greenfield EI, Berg J, et al.** Feasibility and satisfaction of an apartment living program for homeless adults with mental illness and substance use disorder. Psychiatry. 2018;**81**(3):228–239.

96. **Gutman SA, Amarantos K, Berg J, et al.** Home safety fall and accident risk among prematurely aging, formerly homeless adults. Am J Occup Ther. 2018;**72**(4):1–9.

97. **Urbanoski K, Veldhuizen S, Krausz M,** et al. Effects of comorbid substance use disorders on outcomes in a Housing First intervention for homeless people with mental illness. Addiction. 2018;**113**(1):137–145.

98. **Poremski D, Whitley R, Latimer E.** Building trust with people receiving supported employment and housing first services. Psychiatr Rehabil J. 2016;**39**(1):20–26.

99. **Poremski D, Rabouin D, Latimer E.** A randomised controlled trial of evidence based supported employment for people who have recently been homeless and have a mental illness. Adm Policy Ment Health. 2017;**44**(2):217–224.

100. **Gray HM, Nelson SE, Shaffer HJ, Stebbins P, Farina AR.** How do homeless adults change their lives after completing an intensive job-skills program? A prospective study. J Community Psychol. 2017;**45**(7):888–905.

Chapter 12

Chronic pain in homeless persons

Marc Vogel, Christian G. Schütz, and
Stephen W. Hwang

Introduction and epidemiology

Pain, and chronic pain in particular, has adverse effects on many aspects of
health and quality of life. It has been shown to be associated with an increased
burden of mental health symptoms, substance use, and reduced ability to perform activities of daily living. Among the risk factors for the development of
chronic pain are untreated physical conditions, so it is not surprising that it is
common among homeless persons who experience multiple barriers to medical, psychiatric, and social care.

Acute pain is a normal reaction of the body to injuries, surgery, infections,
or another disease, and typically lasts for up to 3–6 months, which is assumed
to be the time required for normal tissue healing. The underlying condition
usually resolves with or without therapy and pain remits. However, sometimes
pain may persist beyond this period, and pain persisting longer than 3 months
is considered to be chronic. Chronic pain is not merely considered a symptom
of other conditions, but it is now understood to be a medical entity by itself.

Due to varying definitions of chronic pain and different assessment methods
used by the existing studies, research on the prevalence of chronic pain in the
general population has produced a range of estimates. Surveys in the general
Canadian population and in Western Europe reported a proportion of around
19% suffering from chronic pain (1,2). However, a 2016 meta-analysis from the
UK found an estimate as high as 43.5% (3).

Research on the epidemiology of chronic pain in homeless populations is
scarce but where available it shows consistently higher rates compared to the
general population. For instance, a study of 150 shelter users in the UK reported a prevalence of 59%, with a mean duration of more than 6 years (4). In
Canadian shelters, Hwang et al. (5) found a prevalence of 52%, persisting for a
mean of 10 years. In a subsample of the Canadian 'At Home' study investigating

homeless persons with mental illness, chronic pain occurred in 58% and was deemed clinically significant in 43% (6).

What are the reasons for the higher occurrence of chronic pain in homeless populations? The socioeconomic disadvantage has been shown to be a risk factor for chronic pain, potentially mediated by a variety of mechanisms such as inefficient pain coping strategies or occupational factors (7). Moreover, homeless individuals experience a much higher than average rate of intentional and unintentional injuries (8); these injuries cause acute pain and an attendant risk that the pain will become chronic. The transition of acute to chronic pain is a complex, multifactorial process highly influenced by psychological factors, for which a single risk factor is neither necessary nor sufficient. Many risk factors for the transition have been identified, many of which are over-represented in homeless individuals, such as exposure to violence, traumatic experiences in childhood or adult life, and also mental health conditions (8–10).

Homeless people may be more vulnerable to the development of chronic pain because they often do not receive adequate treatment due to a multitude of barriers to care. People experiencing homelessness frequently lack access to primary care (11), which is a cornerstone of effective pain treatment. Even when individuals who are homeless do have access to primary care, their healthcare providers may be understandably reluctant to treat pain with prescribed opioids due to the high prevalence of substance use disorder and the risk of addiction in this population (12). In addition, homeless individuals usually have limited or no access to non-medical therapies that are effective in treating pain, such as physical therapy (13). As a result of these factors, homeless individuals are at increased risk of experiencing severe and protracted pain due to highly treatable conditions.

In many countries, such as the US, the homeless population is ageing (14). With age, there comes a multitude of geriatric conditions, often also associated with pain. Homeless individuals are at higher risk of developing geriatric syndromes compared to housed individuals (15) and may suffer from these up to 15 years earlier (8). Accelerated ageing may be explained not only by poverty, stress, and highly adverse living conditions but also by delayed and insufficient care for medical illnesses, higher rates of mental health disorders, and use of substances such as tobacco, alcohol, opioids, or stimulants. Age-associated reduced mobility and cognitive functions impact the ability to seek out help and receive adequate treatment for health conditions. This is aggravated by a reduction of supportive social contacts such as family or other caregivers. Ageing may, therefore, contribute to the development of chronic pain by a higher likelihood to develop age-associated painful conditions while at the same time, limiting the ability to organize and receive adequate healthcare interventions.

Clinical issues

Chronic pain is a matter of interest in homeless populations because it can have detrimental effects on various aspects of health and quality of life. Conditions related to pain and chronic pain are among the leading causes of disease burden and disability worldwide (16). Two studies investigated the interference with activities of daily living in homeless persons with chronic pain. Up to 94% reported any interference with activities of daily living, with the strongest impact on general activities (80–86%), walking (75%), mood (74%), sleep (71–78%), and social interactions (61%) (4,6). Interference in vital activities is likely to contribute to the perpetuation of homelessness and accentuate unstable living conditions. For example, community reintegration usually requires navigating the service system and attending appointments for a range of social and health services. Reduced mobility due to pain makes this much harder to accomplish. This barrier to receiving services is aggravated by the fact that homeless persons are more likely than housed individuals to experience foot pain when walking (17), which is the primary mode of transportation for a large proportion of this population.

The most common body locations affected by chronic pain include the back, joints (mostly knees and shoulders), lower limbs (in particular feet), and the teeth and oral cavity (4–6). Improper footwear plays a significant role in the development of back, knee, and foot pain. A small study investigating a simple intervention of properly fitting footwear was able to reduce pain levels and improve walking speed in homeless individuals (18).

Chronic pain and mental health

Chronic pain is correlated with a variety of physical and mental health symptoms. While the onset often occurs in the context of physical conditions, the relation with mental health is bidirectional (19,20). Chronic pain may lead to mental health symptoms or even be the root cause of psychiatric disorders such as major depression or anxiety (21,22). Conversely, mental illness can also facilitate the occurrence of chronic pain and increase pain sensitivity (23–25). Chronic pain and mental illness share common neural mechanisms and risk factors (e.g. the experience of sexual violence) (19).

Chronic pain commonly co-occurs with psychiatric disorders and the bidirectional association is supported by preclinical and brain imaging studies (26–28). In non-homeless patients with chronic pain, major depressive disorder is prevalent in 2–61%, bipolar disorder in 1–21%, generalized anxiety disorder in 1–10%, and post-traumatic stress disorder in 1–23% (19). It is well established that depressive symptoms may enhance pain sensitivity, and antidepressants have successfully been used as an adjunctive medication for diverse forms of pain (28,29).

Similarly, the risk for substance use disorder in chronic pain patients is two to three times higher than in individuals without chronic pain, with the prevalence of alcohol use disorder ranging from 2% to 22% and any substance use disorder from 1% to 25% (19). Conversely, substance-using patients are at a 50% increased risk of developing chronic pain (30). Smoking was demonstrated to increase the risk of pain chronification via corticostriatal circuits that are active in addictive behaviour, motivation, and learning (31).

The high proportions of homeless populations suffering from chronic pain may thus, in part, be explained by the occurrence of comorbid psychiatric disorders, which are much more common than in the general population. However, research on the interaction of these conditions in homeless populations is scarce. A recent cross-sectional study in homeless persons diagnosed with bipolar disorder and schizophrenia found an association of current moderate to severe pain with female gender, antidepressant use, bipolar diagnosis, and, to a lesser extent, with age and psychotic symptoms (32). In a subsample of the Canadian 'At Home' study, we investigated chronic pain among homeless persons with mental illness. We found associations with age, major depressive episodes, and mood disorders with psychotic features (6). Furthermore, there were significant associations with a diagnosis of post-traumatic stress disorder and panic disorder, but we did not find associations with gender.

Substance use disorders may complicate the picture by being associated with pain and mental illness (33). Substance use has been described as an often-dysfunctional form of self-medication of pain as well as of mental health symptoms (34), but at the same time, it may contribute to chronic pain and mental disorders. Understanding the interplay between these factors is of great importance to improve interventions with better outcomes. Pain, psychiatric disorders, and substance use disorders all occur more often in homeless populations, as demonstrated by the limited evidence available.

A retrospective study of 219 homeless patients who died from an overdose found a high prevalence of chronic pain (45%) along with problem substance use (85%) and psychiatric illness (61%) (35). More than 80% of overdoses in this study involved opioids, which are often used as prescribed or illicit pain killers.

In the 'At Home' study subsample mentioned previously, we found that chronic pain was associated with behavioural patterns reflecting the severity of substance use rather than the use of specific substances. Participants with chronic pain as opposed to those without were more likely to use drugs daily and via the injection route (unpublished data). At the same time, participants with chronic pain were less likely to receive treatment or be prescribed pain medication when they were using substances daily.

Substance use disorders contribute to barriers to care, complicate treatment, and seem to constitute a major challenge to the treatment system, where integrated care for the level of complexity is most often not readily available (36). Aside from being an additional barrier to adequate treatment, they also impact housing and access to any form of support.

Chronic pain is also a risk factor for suicidality. In the 'At Home' study, chronic pain was significantly associated with an almost 50% increase in the risk of suicidality, controlling for psychiatric disorders, and substance use (6). This is a finding which also has been described in non-homeless populations (37). Considering the common occurrence of chronic pain, it has to be regarded as a major preventable risk factor contributing to the elevated rate of suicide and suicide attempts among homeless individuals (38). Professionals working with homeless individuals need to be aware of this association, and clinicians should routinely assess suicidality in persons experiencing chronic pain.

Treatment and barriers to care

Unstable housing and homelessness are associated with impaired access to healthcare provision. Chronic pain aggravates this problem as it is related with premature exits from supported housing, mostly back to street living (39).

Treatment of chronic pain takes place at the intersection of somatic medicine and psychiatry/psychology. It regularly involves interventions targeting the underlying physical condition. However, often this is insufficient, and therapy will need to incorporate pharmacological and psychotherapeutic treatment of associated mental disorders such as depression or bipolar disorder. Finally, it includes interventions aimed at coping, dealing, and living with chronic pain. The treatment of chronic pain usually involves continued interactions with different treatment providers. Navigating and accessing various providers for these treatments is demanding for anybody. Homeless individuals, however, will have even more difficulties. These services will rarely be available at the same clinic, let alone with one provider.

Having a regular treatment provider and/or case manager has been shown to reduce unmet needs in older homeless individuals (40). Given the complexity of chronic pain treatment and the necessity of recurring treatment contacts, a regular provider would be desirable for the treatment of chronic pain as well. However, homeless individuals often access care via acute treatment services such as emergency rooms (41), that can hardly provide a constant and lasting therapeutic relationship to build upon to treat chronic pain effectively. A recent study using qualitative interviews reported that homeless persons often felt that clinicians were biased with regard to treatment of their chronic pain (42). Specifically, interviewees thought that primary care providers were over-emphasizing the prescription of medication, while they felt stigmatized as 'drug seekers' in emergency care settings.

Other interventions and healthy behaviours that are effective in ameliorating chronic pain may be equally hard to access. A good example is physical activity, which is useful for coping with chronic pain as well as mental health disorders (43). However, a low level of physical activity is common among homeless populations, and low activity levels are also associated with lower self-rated health (44,45). Interventions aimed at improving healthy behaviour such as physical activity may be helpful in reducing chronic pain, for example, the promotion of a healthy diet along with physical activity (46) or the above-mentioned intervention aimed at the provision of proper shoes (18). There is research indicating that homeless individuals are open to and interested in such interventions (44,47).

Given the bidirectional relationship of chronic pain and mental health disorders, the underlying shared neurobiology, and existing barriers to care for homeless populations, it is clear that pharmacological and other medical interventions should ideally be aimed at treating these conditions simultaneously. In cases where regular contact with treatment providers can be established, they need to consider physical as well as mental health issues. Furthermore, providers should check for suicidality, particularly in patients suffering from comorbid conditions.

Conclusion

Chronic pain is prevalent in homeless individuals. It adversely impacts the quality of life, interferes with activities of daily living, and contributes to the perpetuation of homelessness. Because of its bidirectional association with mental health, it is also a significant risk factor for suicidal behaviour. Providers need to be aware of the fundamental role of chronic pain, which should be assessed along with underlying causes and associated consequences. It is likely that offering treatment of chronic pain in close association with a primary care provider would be helpful. However, research on chronic pain in homeless populations is still very scant. Future studies aiming at the identification of effective treatments for chronic pain in individuals experiencing homelessness are greatly needed.

References

1. Breivik H, Collett B, Ventafridda V, Cohen R, Gallacher D. Survey of chronic pain in Europe: prevalence, impact on daily life, and treatment. Eur J Pain. 2006;**10**(4):287–333.

2. Schopflocher D, Taenzer P, Jovey R. The prevalence of chronic pain in Canada. Pain Res Manag. 2011;**16**(6):445–450.

3. Fayaz A, Croft P, Langford RM, Donaldson LJ, Jones GT. Prevalence of chronic pain in the UK: a systematic review and meta-analysis of population studies. BMJ Open. 2016;**6**(6):e010364.

4. Fisher R, Ewing JJJ, Garrett A, Harrison EK, Lwin KK, Wheeler DW. The nature and prevalence of chronic pain in homeless persons: an observational study. F1000Res. 2013;**2**:164.

5. Hwang SW, Wilkins E, Chambers C, Estrabillo E, Berends J, MacDonald A. Chronic pain among homeless persons: characteristics, treatment, and barriers to management. BMC Fam Pract. 2011;**12**(1):73.

6. Vogel M, Frank A, Choi F, et al. Chronic pain among homeless persons with mental illness. Pain Med. 2017;**18**(12):2280–2288.

7. Poleshuck EL, Green CR. Socioeconomic disadvantage and pain. Pain. 2008;**136**(3):235–238.

8. Fazel S, Geddes JR, Kushel M. The health of homeless people in high-income countries: descriptive epidemiology, health consequences, and clinical and policy recommendations. Lancet. 2014;**384**(9953):1529–1540.

9. Frencher SK, Benedicto CMB, Kendig TD, Herman D, Barlow B, Pressley JC. A comparative analysis of serious injury and illness among homeless and housed low income residents of New York City. J Trauma. 2010;**69**(4 Suppl):S191–S199.

10. Larney S, Conroy E, Mills KL, Burns L, Teesson M. Factors associated with violent victimisation among homeless adults in Sydney, Australia. Aust N Z J Public Health. 2009;**33**(4):347–351.

11. Health Quality Ontario. Interventions to improve access to primary care for people who are homeless: a systematic review. Ont Health Technol Assess Ser. 2016;**16**(9):1–50.

12. Stringfellow EJ, Kim TW, Gordon AJ, et al. Substance use among persons with homeless experience in primary care. Subst Abus. 2016;**37**(4):534–541.

13. Oosman S, Weber G, Ogunson M, Bath B. Enhancing access to physical therapy services for people experiencing poverty and homelessness: the lighthouse pilot project. Physiother Can. 2019;**71**(2):176–186.

14. Culhane DP, Metraux S, Byrne T, Stino M, Bainbridge J. The age structure of contemporary homelessness: evidence and implications for public policy. Anal Soc Issues Public Policy. 2013;**13**(1):228–244.

15. Brown RT, Kiely DK, Bharel M, Mitchell SL. Geriatric syndromes in older homeless adults. J Gen Intern Med. 2012;**27**(1):16–22.

16. Vos T, Abajobir AA, Abate KH, Abbafati C, Abbas KM, Abd-Allah F et al. Global, regional, and national incidence, prevalence, and years lived with disability for 328 diseases and injuries for 195 countries, 1990–2016: a systematic analysis for the Global Burden of Disease Study 2016. Lancet. 2017;**390**(10100):1211–1259.

17. To MJ, Brothers TD, Van Zoost C. Foot conditions among homeless persons: a systematic review. PLoS One. 2016;**11**(12):e0167463.

18. **Moes J.** Proper fitting shoes: reducing pain, increasing activity, and improving foot health among adults experiencing homelessness. Public Health Nurs. 2019;**36**(3):321–329.

19. **Hooten WM.** Chronic pain and mental health disorders: shared neural mechanisms, epidemiology, and treatment. Mayo Clin Proc. 2016;**91**(7):955–970.

20. **Kroenke K, Wu J, Bair MJ, Krebs EE, Damush TM, Tu W.** Reciprocal relationship between pain and depression: a 12-month longitudinal analysis in primary care. J Pain. 2011;**12**(9):964–973.

21. **Atkinson HJ, Slater MA, Patterson TL, Grant I, Garfin SR.** Prevalence, onset, and risk of psychiatric disorders in men with chronic low back pain: a controlled study. Pain. 1991;**45**(2):111–121.

22. **Goesling J, Lin LA, Clauw DJ.** Psychiatry and pain management: at the intersection of chronic pain and mental health. Curr Psychiatry Rep. 2018;**20**(2):12.

23. **Börsbo B, Peolsson M, Gerdle B.** The complex interplay between pain intensity, depression, anxiety and catastrophising with respect to quality of life and disability. Disabil Rehabil. 2009;**31**(19):1605–1613.

24. **Gureje O, Simon GE, Von Korff M.** A cross-national study of the course of persistent pain in primary care. Pain. 2001;**92**(1–2):195–200.

25. **Magni G, Moreschi C, Rigatti-Luchini S, Merskey H.** Prospective study on the relationship between depressive symptoms and chronic musculoskeletal pain. Pain. 1994;**56**(3):289–297.

26. **Apkarian AV, Neugebauer V, Koob G,** et al. Neural mechanisms of pain and alcohol dependence. Pharmacol Biochem Behav. 2013;**112**:34–41.

27. **Joseph EK, Reichling DB, Levine JD.** Shared mechanisms for opioid tolerance and a transition to chronic pain. J Neurosci. 2010;**30**(13):4660–4666.

28. **Strigo IA, Simmons AN, Matthews SC, Craig ADB, Paulus MP.** Association of major depressive disorder with altered functional brain response during anticipation and processing of heat pain. Arch Gen Psychiatry. 2008;**65**(11):1275–1284.

29. **Micó JA, Ardid D, Berrocoso E, Eschalier A.** Antidepressants and pain. Trends Pharmacol Sci. 2006;**27**(7):348–354.

30. **Scott KM, Lim C, Al-Hamzawi A,** et al. Association of mental disorders with subsequent chronic physical conditions: World Mental Health Surveys From 17 Countries. JAMA Psychiatry. 2016;**73**(2):150–158.

31. **Petre B, Torbey S, Griffith JW,** et al. Smoking increases risk of pain chronification through shared corticostriatal circuitry. Hum Brain Mapp. 2015;**36**(2):683–694.

32. **Fond G, Tinland A, Boucekine M, Girard V, Loubière S, Boyer L.** The need to improve detection and treatment of physical pain of homeless people with schizophrenia and bipolar disorders. Results from the French Housing First Study. Prog Neuropsychopharmacol Biol Psychiatry. 2019;**88**:175–180.

33. **Sullivan MD, Edlund MJ, Zhang L, Unützer J, Wells KB.** Association between mental health disorders, problem drug use, and regular prescription opioid use. Arch Intern Med. 2006;**166**(19):2087–2093.

34. **Khantzian EJ.** Addiction as a self-regulation disorder and the role of self-medication. Addict. 2013;**108**(4):668–669.

35. **Bauer LK, Brody JK, León C, Baggett TP.** Characteristics of homeless adults who died of drug overdose: a retrospective record review. J Health Care Poor Underserved. 2016;**27**(2):846–859.

36. **Schütz CG.** Homelessness and addiction: causes, consequences and interventions. Curr Treat Options Psychiatry. 2016;**3**(3):306–313.

37. **Racine M.** Chronic pain and suicide risk: a comprehensive review. Prog Neuropsychopharmacol Biol Psychiatry. 2018;**87**(B):269–280.

38. **Feodor Nilsson S, Hjorthøj CR, Erlangsen A, Nordentoft M.** Suicide and unintentional injury mortality among homeless people: a Danish nationwide register-based cohort study. Eur J Public Health. 2014;**24**(1):50–56.

39. **Gabrielian S, Burns AV, Nanda N, Hellemann G, Kane V, Young AS.** Factors associated with premature exits from supported housing. Psychiatr Serv. 2016;**67**(1):86–93.

40. **Kaplan LM, Vella L, Cabral E, Tieu L, Ponath C, Guzman D, Kushel MB.** Unmet mental health and substance use treatment needs among older homeless adults: results from the HOPE HOME Study. J Commun Psychol. 2019;**47**(8):1893–1908.

41. **Hwang SW, Chambers C, Chiu S, Katic M, Kiss A, Redelmeier DA, Levinson W.** A comprehensive assessment of health care utilization among homeless adults under a system of universal health insurance. Am J Public Health. 2013;**103**(Suppl 2):S294–S301.

42. **Gilmer C, Buccieri K.** Homeless patients associate clinician bias with suboptimal care for mental illness, addictions, and chronic pain. J Prim Care Community Health. 2020;**11**:2150132720910289.

43. **Geneen LJ, Moore RA, Clarke C, Martin D, Colvin LA, Smith BH.** Physical activity and exercise for chronic pain in adults: an overview of Cochrane Reviews. Cochrane Database Syst Rev. 2017;**4**:CD011279.

44. **Maness SB, Reitzel LR, Hernandez DC,** et al. Modifiable risk factors and readiness to change among homeless adults. Am J Health Behav. 2019;**43**(2):373–379.

45. **Nayyar D, Hwang SW.** Cardiovascular health issues in inner city populations. Can J Cardiol. 2015;**31**(9):1130–1138.

46. **Kendzor DE, Allicock M, Businelle MS, Sandon LF, Gabriel KP, Frank SG.** Evaluation of a shelter-based diet and physical activity intervention for homeless adults. J Phys Act Health. 2017;**14**(2):88–97.

47. **Taylor EM, Kendzor DE, Reitzel LR, Businelle MS.** Health risk factors and desire to change among homeless adults. Am J Health Behav. 2016;**40**(4):455–460.

Chapter 13

Coronavirus disease 2019 (COVID-19) and homelessness: Global perspectives on the 'dual pandemic'

Debanjan Banerjee and Prama Bhattacharya

Coronavirus disease 2019 (COVID-19): the global problem statement

When the world welcomed 2020 like any other new year, it knew little of what the next few months were to bring in. COVID-19, which began in Wuhan, China, towards the end of 2019, has now emerged as a global public health threat. Within a month of its initiation, the World Health Organization (WHO) declared it as a 'Public Health Emergency of International Concern' and subsequently after 6 weeks, it was declared as a pandemic. Since then, the number of cases has kept rising worldwide, with more than 203 million affected so far (as of August 10th, 2021) and nearly 4.3 million succumbing to the infection (1). Though less fatal than its earlier congeners (severe acute respiratory syndrome and Middle East respiratory syndrome), what makes COVID-19 alarming is its rapid human-to-human transmission, being termed as the most contagious large-scale outbreak that the modern world has seen so far (2). Pandemics are far beyond just medical phenomena. They affect societies at large, having long-lasting psychosocial and economic implications.

The lockdown imposed on several countries as a measure of social distancing is the prime strategy against the virus, in the absence of any definitive biological cure so far. Ironically, certain marginalized sections of the population are vulnerable not only to the physical effects of the virus but also the social measures (like the lockdown) implemented to control it. One such section is the homeless people all over the world, for whom 'social distancing' tends to be a myth in their overcrowded and often temporary shelters (3). The poor measures of hygiene and lack of basic amenities make them susceptible to any infection whatsoever, even more during a global biological disaster like COVID-19, which does not discriminate based on socioeconomic class. Unfortunately, however, this group is largely neglected, administratively unaccounted for with least testing and precautionary measures against the virus.

Homelessness: the global scenario

Defining the 'homeless'

The Oxford dictionary defines 'home' as 'the place where one lives permanently, especially as a member of a family or household' (4). As research progressed over the years, the 'accommodation'-based definition of home has widened to include concepts of autonomy, personal space, dignity, belongingness, trust, and security. In that regard, it is important to understand homelessness as a 'social construct' rather than merely a 'locus-based' approach (5). On similar lines, homelessness has also been conceptualized on the psychosocial grounds of coldness, social indifference, chronic stress, misery, alienation, and instability (6). The ever-evolving definition of homelessness has thus been the predominant challenge in accounting and caring for this vulnerable population. The UN-Habitat report (2015) stated that there are no internationally agreed definitions of homelessness (7). Equating it with 'rooflessness' does injustice to the varied social responsibilities towards this disadvantaged group. Since the concept of 'home' is entangled with specific sociocultural contexts, a single universal definition might not do justice to the social and emotional requirements of the homeless in every country. This fact has led to wide variations in their numbers across various geographical locations.

The global burden of homelessness

The UN Centre for Human Settlements in 1996 estimated the number of global homeless to be between 100 million to 1 billion (8). During the last global survey (UN-Habitat Report 2005), the numbers rose to 1.8 billion (9). Getting an accurate estimate of the picture is difficult due to the changing definitions, varied administrative accountability, gaps in the census, temporary shelters, and high associations of mental illness and substance abuse in this population for which they might often be segregated and scattered (10). The 'hidden homeless' thus form the bulk of the missing numbers as most reside in inadequate settlements, slums, and temporary shelters and relocate frequently. Though the initial worldwide studies have mostly been done in the industrialized countries, the last few decades have marked increased studies from the developing countries. More than one-third of the global homeless are clustered within the West African and South-East Asian countries, with unique sociocultural implications altogether (11). One of the most common ways of estimating homelessness is through 'point-in-time' counts of people sleeping on streets or shelters, on any given night. This is often contrasted with the long-term prevalence of home-lessness but has proven to be similar and more accurate. This method is util-ized by the US Department of Housing and Urban Development to release the Annual Homeless Assessment Report to Congress (AHARC) every year, which estimates 1 in 1670 Americans to be homeless (12). This is in contrast with much more populous countries like India where 1.8 million are estimated to be homeless and lower-income countries like Libya or Cameroon where 3% of the population becomes homeless every year due to internal displacement and violence (13). A working definition for homelessness is thus crucial for policy intervention, especially at times of disasters as 'who we define and how we care for them, depends on how we count' (14).

Homelessness and pandemics: the dual vulnerability

During any biological disaster, homeless individuals have unique predisposi-tions and vulnerabilities (Table 13.1). They form a marginalized population, whose access to healthcare has several barriers down the line. The homeless, understandably, remain stranded on streets and temporary shelters mostly de-prived of basic living amenities, let alone the prescribed standards of hygiene and distancing necessary during an infectious disease outbreak. The groups, often large in numbers, live densely in overcrowded places with a lack of sani-tary facilities, when using the prescribed antibacterial and sanitizers are but a far-fetched dream. Vikas (15) has rightly described them as having 'camou-flaged architecture and poor layout of interiors' in their shabby shelters, which gets compounded during pandemics by poverty, infections, lack of public hy-giene, poor waste disposal, susceptibilities to extremes of weather, risk of con-tamination, and overall poorer quality of physical and mental well-being. The high prevalence of mental disorders and substance abuse among them add to the burden (discussed in later sections). They appear to be an 'invisible burden' to the society, who are not only susceptible to infection but can also be respon-sible for community spread as their physical proximity with the higher social classes are common in urban areas (16). Additionally, as their living conditions are transient, the norms of quarantine, isolation, testing, infection control, and treatment are often not implemented in them adequately during the outbreaks (17). The general compliance with quarantine or lockdown has also been de-ficient in them in the earlier epidemics, as they mandatorily need to change locations to survive.

Table 13.1 Vulnerabilities of the homeless population during pandemics/epidemics

Factors	Vulnerabilities	Consequences during a pandemic/epidemic
Structural	• Overcrowding • Lack of sanitation • Poor public hygiene • Poor air quality • Increased risk of infection • Poor waste disposal • Changing locations/shelters • Extremes of weather	• Increased susceptibility • The faster spread of the outbreak • Lack of quarantine facilities
Situational	• Lack of adequate nutrition • Vitamin and iron deficiency • Increased parasitic infections • Low immunity • Lack of healthcare access and vaccinations • Poverty	• Chronicity of infections • Decreased antibody response • Increased morbidity and mortality
Psychological	• Increased mental disorders • Lack of awareness and treatment • Substance abuse • Violence and abuse • Poor coping	• Lack of awareness • Neglect of the precautions • Exacerbation of mental illness • Increased hospitalizations • Increased fear and health anxiety
Social	• Neglect • Avoidance • Stigma and 'othering' • Blame • Healthcare competition	• Lack of support and treatment • Under-detection • Mutual' hate' • Displacement and increased social mobility • Social segregation
Administrative	• Lack of preparedness • Lack of pandemic-policy inclusion for the homeless • Inadequate testing • Lack of awareness and media penetration • Poor accountability	• Non-compliance with isolation and quarantine • Increased uncertainty and panic • Inadequate knowledge– attitude–practice about the outbreak • Increased risk of being asymptomatic carriers (under-detection) • Increased risk of community transmission • Contribution to multiple waves of infection ('hidden viral pockets')

Studies during the earlier pandemics of severe acute respiratory syndrome and influenza have reported homeless individuals to have unique problems (18). They also pose equal risks to public health, if not cared for. Their overall health is compromised both by situational factors (poor nutrition and immunity) and structural parameters (overcrowding, lack of sanitation, increased risk of infection). The pre-existing ill health is also reportedly an independent risk factor during large-scale outbreaks. However, it is not simply their characteristics and behaviour that impact their condition. The societal responses and perceptions are often blinded by apathy, unaccountability, and neglect that makes them much more vulnerable during times of crisis (19). This also leads to stigma, polarization, 'othering', and blame directed towards the homeless, that makes them further estranged from society. Lack of emergency services, public health preparedness, and policies for the homeless in many countries makes the situation difficult during an infection. During the recent Zika outbreak and Ebola infection in West Africa and India, respectively, studies show increased mortality rate, minimum test-detection, and increased displacement among the homeless (20). Similar findings in the earlier outbreak of H1N1 influenza had prompted pandemic planning guides tailored to the needs of homeless people (21). However, their implementation continues to be dismal. As pooled statistics show the number of cases, deaths, and recoveries each day during the present COVID-19 pandemic, little is known about the inclusion and proportion of the homeless. It has already been warned that as this global outbreak increases, the 'social evil' of homelessness can have a bidirectional relationship with the spread of infection (22).

The homeless at times of COVID-19: the challenges and the unmet needs

The challenges

While the world struggles against the ever-increasing viral caseload, the WHO suggested a three-pronged strategy to contain the current pandemic, namely social distancing, hand hygiene, and respiratory hygiene. Proven to be effective in community contentment in some of the worst affected areas worldwide (23), the implementation of these measures and public compliance with them, however, is fraught with challenges. With more than half the world's population under lockdown, the most common directive from stakeholders has been to 'stay at home'. However, for hundreds of millions of homeless people across the world (24) stranded on streets and temporary shelters, the preventive measures against COVID-19 appear to be a luxurious and far-fetched idea. In this section, we will briefly discuss the basic difficulties the homeless population has been facing during the pandemic, irrespective of their country of origin.

Executing social distancing

Even with the ongoing COVID vaccination programs, there are several barriers including anti-vax campaigns, misinformation, stigma, doubt about efficacy and issues with vaccine availability and accessibility in many parts of the world. Hence, prevention becomes the most critical tool against COVID-19, and so-cial/physical distancing is the first step in that. Many countries have activated a complete or partial lockdown to reduce community transmission. Ironically, the 'stay at home' directive becomes an oxymoron when it comes to the home-less population. Maintaining social distancing remains a fantasy when one is sleeping rough on the streets or is sharing a night shelter with 50 others (22). Despite staying physically integrated into society, they remain invisible to the state and the system otherwise. However, turning a blind eye towards this mar-ginalized and vulnerable population at this juncture might be costly for the countries affected by COVID-19. Their invisible integration amid society and the proximity with others can quickly spread a contagious illness once they get affected. Dharavi (Mumbai, India), for example, is Asia's largest slum (housing 150,000 individuals within 2.16 square km), where '10–12 people live in 10×10 feet tin hutments', with 369 individuals being affected and more than 3000 people being quarantined turned out to be one of the worst hotspots in India.

Increased vulnerability due to harsh living conditions

With an already compromised immunity due to adverse living conditions, the vulnerability of homeless individuals to be affected by COVID-19, or for that matter by any disease, is much higher than the general population (22,24). An array of factors such as overcrowding, lack of public hygiene, inadequate waste disposal, weather extremes, contamination, substance abuse, malnutrition, inaccessibility to drinking water, with overall poorer quality of physical and mental health jeopardizes their immunity to a large extent (25). The interim guidance prepared by the Inter-Agency Standing Committee in March 2020 to scale up the COVID-19 outbreak readiness and response operations in humani-tarian situations identified that 'people living in collective sites are vulnerable to COVID-19 in part because of the health risks associated with movement/displacement, overcrowding, increased climatic exposure due to substandard shelter, and poor nutritional and health status among affected populations. This may also be exacerbated by modalities of services/assistance provision, which can involve large crowds' (26).

Lack of information

Surviving the lockdown is a far more significant concern for the majority of homeless people than surviving the virus. Since the active symptoms of the disease represent nothing more than flu, they feel more confident in surviving it rather than hunger (27). For most homeless people, COVID-19, quarantine, and social distancing are nothing beyond some luxurious terms that they cannot afford. With the continuous efforts of most of the states across the world, while they have gathered some information about the symptoms and the preventive measures, they hardly can do anything to maintain them (28,29). At the same time, they struggle to arrange a one-time meal, let alone shelter or maintain basic hygiene.

Lack of accountability

One of the most alienated marginalized populations, the homeless have remained invisible, unaccounted for, and ignored by the stakeholders at various systemic and structural levels. Consequently, the health policy measures hardly ever pay any heed to their 'beingness'. It thus does not come as a surprise that of all the 187 countries affected by COVID-19, only a few have taken measures to contain the spread of the virus within this population.

The unmet needs

Worldwide, professionals are working at a breakneck pace to win the race against COVID-19. The spread of COVID-19 made no distinction between developed or developing nations. Even countries with the best of public health infrastructures are finding it difficult to flatten the graph. While governments, international organizations, and policymakers, besides medical professionals and other frontline workers, are doing their bit, it may still be safely argued that very little has been done for the homeless population amid this pandemic. Homeless individuals, as discussed earlier, are more vulnerable to succumb to the virus than many others. Coordinated efforts among various stakeholders, governmental as well as non-governmental, are required. Although some initiatives are already in place in terms of sheltering them, with more than 100 million homeless globally, it is not enough to contain the spread of the virus within this marginalized population. While quarantine and social distancing are challenging to be maintained among hundreds of thousands of homeless people (at present the number has increased with migrant workers rendered homeless across borders), some critical action steps are outlined as follows:

Accessibility to shelter and food

For these basic living amenities, the governments can utilize school and college buildings, community halls, and so on to arrange the temporary shelters. Some developed nations such as the US have already done this step in some states and found this measure effective (28). However, for populous countries like India and Brazil the execution of this measure would be challenging. All the existing night-shelters and hostels should be made available for 24/7 support. Farha (24) suggested that to provide adequate housing, the states might require:

> (P)rocuring hotel or motel rooms, or repurposing buildings such as army barracks, or unused hospitals. Public authorities should be empowered to make available privately-owned vacant housing or secondary homes ... Where feasible and appropriate, governments should purchase available short and long-term housing units to ensure that homeless populations are housed during and after the pandemic and as a means of increasing their public assets. (p. 2)

While the governments in many nations are trying to ensure the supply of food to the homeless, the uncertainty of the future is causing many to hoard the supplies instead. In a recent survey conducted in India, it was found that almost 44% of the nation's population have a one-time meal or no meal to save for the future. Stakeholders should be vigilant about the proper utilization of the allocated resources.

Accessibility to basic hygiene products

Though social distancing is theoretical for this population, maintaining basic hygiene becomes crucial and critical. An adequate supply of basic hygiene essentials must be provided that includes commodities like soap, masks, and disinfectants. In her guidance note on 'Protection for those Living in Homelessness', Farha (24) suggested that states might:

> Guarantee access to public toilets, showers, and handwashing facilities and products for homeless persons living on the street who do not have access to private facilities. These facilities must be properly maintained with running water and soap on-site at all times and must be regularly disinfected. (p. 2)

Testing for the virus among the vulnerable

As mentioned previously, vulnerabilities are higher among the elderly, the immunosuppressed, or those with chronic physical ailments. An increased number of testing of those who are identified in these groups is required. Those who would have a positive result on testing must invariably be quarantined for the stipulated period and appropriate healthcare initiated. Farha (24) recommended that 'those who test positive for coronavirus, [should be provided] with a safe place to stay, immediate medical attention, access to food, and any necessary medical and other support to ensure they can manage quarantine or self-isolation' (p. 2). She further suggested that all individuals living in homelessness should have 'access to non-discriminatory and cost-free healthcare and testing. There must also be a widespread distribution of accessible, up-to-date information on COVID-19, including best health practices, government health policies and where and how health services may be accessed' (p. 2) and as per the directive of WHO, it must be ensured that they have 'emergency accommodations [that] allows for physical distancing, self-isolation, quarantine and any other health recommendations ... to stop the spread of COVID-19' (p. 2).

Educating the homeless

Complex statistics do not matter for homeless people. Necessary precautionary measures need to be explained in their language and doubts clarified. Knowledge, attitude, and practices need to be improved through community programmes. The guidance note provided by the WHO, the International Federation of Red Cross and Red Crescent Societies, and the United Nations Office for the Coordination of Humanitarian Affairs on 'COVID-19: How to include marginalized and vulnerable people in risk communication and community engagement' (30) suggested that to bridge the knowledge gap the nations might consider making information available in audiovisual format in places frequented by this population. They should further keep in mind that homeless people mostly have a lack of access to health education, low literacy levels, and lack of access to information sources like newspapers, internet, or television. Actionable alternative solutions must be provided for them to deal with the challenges that they might be facing in following health guidelines. Where the governments are not well equipped to deal with such marginalized populations, it has been suggested that they partner with organizations who work with the homeless.

The global scenario for homeless individuals amid COVID-19

Globally, the WHO has identified 215 countries or territories that have reported COVID-19 positive cases (1). As identified earlier, with one-third of the homeless population living in the Asian and African countries, the situation became more skewed as COVID-19 struck, partially because of the 'numbers', and in part due to the poor infrastructural condition of public health in many of the nations.

In developing nations like India, hardly any initial measures could be undertaken to prevent the transmission of the virus within the homeless population. Amid the nationwide lockdown, in India, most of the homeless people have been displaced by the state to shelter houses where thousands have been gathered, increasing the atrocities for them as they left behind their 'homes' on the streets. While many non-governmental organizations and governments have provided food, access to basic hygiene essentials is lacking. With thousands of migrant labourers stuck in the host cities and rendered homeless, the scenario has amplified further (25).

The developed countries like the US, the UK, Italy, Spain, and Switzerland turned out to be a few of the worst-hit nations by the COVID-19 despite having better public health infrastructures. In the US, with shelters being full or closed, or too fraught with coronavirus risk to consider sleeping, states like California and Texas have been moving the most vulnerable members of the unhoused population into hotel rooms. Los Angeles is providing them with motorhomes and RVs, which allow them to maintain social distance. In Seattle, homeless people who test positive for COVID-19 are being housed together in a shelter with full-time medical staff available. Many organizations are bringing handwashing stations and portable toilets to the existing shelter-houses (28). With their guidelines in place, the Centers for Disease Control and Prevention permits the homeless shelter-houses to screen the residents for the virus. If a resident meets the criteria, local public healthcare facilities would determine the location for testing in coordination with homeless healthcare clinics and street medicine clinics. The Centers for Disease Control and Prevention rightly pointed out in their interim guideline (31) to the containment of transmission of COVID-19 virus in the homeless population a 'whole community approach' that demands the active engagement of local and state health departments, homeless service providers and continuum of care leadership, emergency management, law enforcement, healthcare providers, housing authorities, local government leadership, other support services such as outreach, case management, and behavioural health support.

Mental illness: a confounder in the 'dual pandemic'

About 20–25% of a nation's homeless population is likely to suffer from any form of mental illness and substance abuse issues (32). During the unprecedented situation that COVID-19 has posed, surviving the harsh extremities become excruciatingly difficult for those suffering both homeless and mental illness. While resources remain scarce for the homeless, it becomes even more challenging to access for those with mental illness, particularly severe mental illnesses. Holistic care from mental health service providers to support the need for homeless individuals with mental illness should not be overlooked (33). Furthermore, the pandemic itself has posed some unique challenges for mental health globally. The anxiety and stress related to the pandemic, uncertainty, loss of a job, lockdown, and so on are likely to create the need for mental health support in anyone. Supportive psychological interventions are thus vital. For a resourceless, socially alienated population like the homeless, mental health needs become magnified in such a situation and the states should not overlook the need or underplay it (34). As the mentally ill are more vulnerable in the already marginalized homeless population, they are the most neglected. This gets compounded by the fact that they are rarely diagnosed unless their symptoms cause disruption to society at large and have poor access to all forms of healthcare. Comorbid substance abuse and intellectual deficits are also common. The knowledge and awareness about mental health issues are reported to be inadequate in their relatives and families, who are already struggling with their homelessness (35). Under such circumstances, the pandemic situation can pose a 'double-hit' to them. Not only is there susceptibility to the infection and its aftermath, there are risks of exacerbation of their mental disorders, increased substance abuse, violating precautionary measures, and absconding—all of which can put the other homeless at a greater public health risk. Cases of suicide, accidental deaths, and abuse in homeless mentally ill individuals during pandemics are not unheard of, as the societal apathy becomes more prominent towards them due to the pressing health necessities and mass hysteria (36). They are also frequently deprived of their rights and self-dignity. While psychosocial health itself should be a cornerstone of public health during pandemics, vulnerable populations like the homeless mentally ill need special and urgent considerations. They need to be identified at the earliest opportunity, triaged according to the symptoms (self-harm or violence need immediate care), and rehabilitated or quarantined as needed in time.

Conclusion

Homelessness has been identified as a 'social evil' worldwide, a growing social pandemic in itself. Unfortunately, it needs a large-scale infectious outbreak like COVID-19 to alarm us about the possible health risks to the homeless, which in any case should be an administrative priority. As COVID-19 strikes the world hard, and societies appear concerned about economies and international relations, millions of homeless globally suffer from their unique vulnerabilities, either on open streets or temporary shelters. When pandemics cross paths with homelessness, a critical zone of unmet needs is created, that needs urgent attention from stakeholders at all levels. Accountability, empathy, understanding, awareness, and research can help influence policy reforms. COVID-19 will surely modify pandemic legislation all across the world. It remains to be seen whether the challenges of the homeless and their special subgroups (such as the mentally ill) get addressed or not. The societal blind eye turned towards them, enhanced by socioeconomic class difference and capitalism, can be counterproductive, to eventually boomerang the larger community as the viral spread will not respect these arbitrary human-made classes. Keeping that in context, we have summarized the global problems of homelessness and the ongoing pandemic, their special needs, the policy implications so far, and the possible way forward. Humankind has always been amazingly resilient, but the strength lies in unity and caring for the less fortunate. This can help generate positivism, hope, and self-growth. To reiterate the concept of homelessness, 'home' is not just a structure but also an identity. Appreciating and understanding that might go a long way in addressing the evil of homelessness, hopefully, earlier than the next expected outbreak.

References

1. **World Health Organization**. Coronavirus disease 2019 (COVID-19): situation report, 72. 2020. Available from: https://www.who.int/docs/default-source/coronaviruse/situation-reports/20200401-sitrep-72-covid-19.pdf.

2. **Lai CC, Shih TP, Ko WC, Tang HJ, Hsueh PR.** Severe acute respiratory syndrome coronavirus 2 (SARS-CoV-2) and coronavirus disease-2019 (COVID-19): the epidemic and the challenges. Int J Antimicrob Agents. 2020;**55**(3):105924.

3. **Lee BA, Tyler KA, Wright JD.** The new homelessness revisited. Annu Rev Sociol. 2010;**36**:501–521.

4. **Oxford University Press.** Definition of home. Lexico.com. 2021. Available from: https://www.lexico.com/definition/home.

5. **Hollander J.** The idea of home: a kind of space. Soc Res. 1991;**58**(1):31–49.

6. **Tipple AG, Speak SE.** Homelessness in Developing Countries. Newcastle upon Tyne: Global Urban Research Unit, University of Newcastle upon Tyne; 2003.

7. **UN Habitat.** International Guidelines on Urban and Territorial Planning. Nairobi: United Nations Human Settlements Programme; 2015.

8. **United Nations Centre for Human Settlements (UNCHS).** An Urbanising World: Global Report on Human Settlements, 1996. New York: Oxford University Press; 1996.

9. **UN Habitat.** Urban Governance Index: conceptual foundation and field test report. 2005. Available from: https://mirror.unhabitat.org/downloads/docs/UGI-Report-Aug04-FINALdoc.doc.

10. **Hwang SW.** Homelessness and health. CMAJ. 2001;**164**(2):229–233.

11. **Tipple G, Speak S.** The Hidden Millions: Homelessness in Developing Countries. London: Routledge; 2009.

12. **Ortiz-Ospina E, Roser M.** Homelessness. **OurWorldInData.org**; 2020. Available from: https://ourworldindata.org/homelessness.

13. **Speak S.** Degrees of destitution: a typology of homelessness in developing countries. Hous Stud. 2004;**19**(3):465–482.

14. **Peressini T, McDonald L, Hulchanski DJ.** Estimating Homelessness: Towards a Methodology for Counting the Homeless in Canada. Ottawa: Canada Mortgage and Housing Corporation.

15. **Vikas RM.** Shelter for homeless. In: **Vijay D, Varman R** (Eds), Alternative Organisations in India: Undoing Boundaries. Cambridge: Cambridge University Press; 2018:95–124.

16. **Sanchez D.** Civil society responses to homelessness. Dev South Afr. 2010;**27**(1):101–110.

17. **O'Sullivan T, Bourgoin M.** Vulnerability in an influenza pandemic: looking beyond medical risk. Behaviour. 2010;**11**:16.

18. **Leung CS, Ho MM, Kiss A, Gundlapalli AV, Hwang SW.** Homelessness and the response to emerging infectious disease outbreaks: lessons from SARS. J Urban Health. 2008;**85**(3):402–410.

19. **Todd EP.** Homelessness: Is Society Looking the Other Way? New York: Nova Publishers; 2006.

20. **Kapiriri L, Ross A.** The politics of disease epidemics: a comparative analysis of the SARS, zika, and Ebola outbreaks. Glob Soc Welf. 2020;**7**(1):33–45.

21. **Scott M.** Pandemic Influenza Guidance. Nashville, TN: National Health Care for the Homeless Council, Inc; 2009.

22. **Tsai J, Wilson M.** COVID-19: a potential public health problem for homeless populations. Lancet Public Health. 2020;**5**(4):e186–187.

23. **Wilder-Smith A, Freedman DO.** Isolation, quarantine, social distancing and community containment: pivotal role for old-style public health measures in the novel coronavirus (2019-nCoV) outbreak. J Travel Med. 2020;**27**(2):taaa020.

24. **Farha L.** COVID-19 Guidance note. Protecting those living in homelessness. 2020. Available from: https://www.ohchr.org/Documents/Issues/Housing/SR_housing_CO VID-19_guidance_homeless.pdf.

25. **Banerjee D, Bhattacharya P.** The hidden vulnerability of homelessness in the COVID-19 pandemic: perspectives from India. Int J Soc Psychiatry. 2021;**67**(1):3–6.

26. **Inter-Agency Standing Committee.** Interim Guidance on Scaling-up COVID-19 Outbreak in Readiness and Response Operations in Camps and Camp-like Settings (jointly developed by IFRC, IOM, UNHCR and WHO). 2020. Available from: https://interagencystandingcommittee.org/other/interim-guidance-scaling-covid-19-outbr eak-readiness-and-response-operations-camps-and-camp.

27. **Lewis C, Ganesan SR, Sayed N, Aditi R.** For the homeless, corona is just a cold, the worry is food. 2020. Available from: https://timesofindia.indiatimes.com/india/For-the-homeless-corona-is-just-a-cold-the-big-worry-is-food/articleshow/74789023.cms.

28. **Ellis EG.** For homeless people, Covid-19 is horror on top of horror. 2020. Available from: https://www.wired.com/story/coronavirus-covid-19-homeless/.

29. **Siddiqui Z, Kataria S.** Some of us will die': India's homeless stranded by coronavirus lockdown. 2020. Available from: https://www.reuters.com/article/us-health-coronavi rus-india-homeless/some-of-us-will-die-indias-homeless-stranded-by-coronavirus-lockdown-idUSKBN21J56D.

30. **World Health Organization.** UN agencies issue urgent call to fund the global emergency supply system to fight COVID-19. 2020. Available from: https://www.who. int/news-room/detail/20-04-2020-un-agencies-issue-urgent-call-to-fund-the-global-emergency-supply-system-to-fight-covid-19.

31. **Centers for Disease Control and Prevention.** Interim guidance for homeless service providers to plan and respond to coronavirus disease 2019 (COVID-19). 2020. Available from: https://www.cdc.gov/coronavirus/2019-ncov/community/homeless-shelters/plan-prepare-respond.html.

32. **Gopikumar V, Narasimhan L, Easwaran K, Bunders J, Parasuraman S.** Persistent, complex and unresolved issues: Indian discourse on mental ill health and homelessness. Econ Pol Wkly. 2015;**50**(11):42–51.

33. **Bhugra D** (Ed). Homelessness and Mental Health. Cambridge: Cambridge University Press; 1996 (paperback reprint 2007).

34. **Marshall EJ, Bhugra DI.** Services for the mentally ill homeless. In: **Bhugra DI** (Ed), Homelessness and Mental Health. Cambridge: Cambridge University Press; 1996:99–109.

35. **Raoult D, Foucault C, Brouqui P.** Infections in the homeless. Lancet Infect Dis. 2001;**1**(2):77–84.

36. **Bonner A, Luscombe C.** Suicide and homelessness. J Public Ment Health. 2009;**8**(3):7.

Chapter 14

Dental care when homeless

Anjali Mago, Mario A. Brondani, and
Michael I. MacEntee

Introduction

'I felt like I didn't mean anything to them.'

Homelessness is a global phenomenon with no easy solutions among rich and poor nations (1). It is fraught with health problems and concerns among which oral infection, toothache, and tooth loss can be very distressing. Recent interviews with 25 homeless people (18 men and seven women; age range: 25–64 years) in Vancouver, Canada, revealed four dominant themes on oral healthcare and dental services for homeless people: barriers to care, service use, importance of dental health, and improving dental services (2). There was considerable anxiety about the cost of dentistry, and fear of dentists because, as one participant explained, 'I felt like I didn't mean anything to them'. This sentiment was echoed by most of the participants when describing their encounters with dentists and other oral healthcare professionals. There is little doubt that homeless people feel stigmatized by their social status and their visibly unhealthy mouths (2,3).

The challenges of oral healthcare from the perspectives of the homeless people in Vancouver are similar to those in most other affluent societies (3–8). Homeless people typically have been abused, are financially poor, suffer from psychiatric illnesses, use illicit substances, and live in very unhealthy conditions (Fig. 14.1) (9,10).

Personal abuse

Homelessness significantly increases the risk of violence, including sexual and physical abuse from both within and outside the homeless community (11). Consequently, homeless people are fearful and mistrusting of the authority they perceive in healthcare professionals. Indeed, tooth extractions can seem to them as authorized abuse generated by disrespectful dentists and support staff (3).

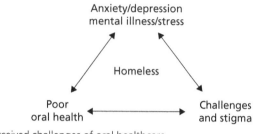

Fig. 14.1 Perceived challenges of oral healthcare.
Source data from the Social Welfare Department.

Finances

Access to dental care in industrialized societies is enabled by affluence and/ or dental insurance (12,13), and by the acceptability of available services (3). In Canada about 12% of general healthcare, but 95% of dental care, are paid directly by the recipients as out-of-pocket expenses, although some emergency dental services, typically control of pain and infection, from a physician or as in-hospital care are financed by public insurance programmes (14–16). Consequently, homeless people tend to use hospital emergency departments or even self-care for toothaches and other distressing mouth problems (17,18). Dentistry is one of the few health services in Canada financed in large part by private insurance and direct personal payments (14). Recently, public spending on healthcare services for vulnerable populations has decreased in many jurisdictions, which complicates access to dental service for homeless people even further (19). Moreover, there are many dentists who are reluctant or unwilling to accept people who cannot pay for dental treatment, and especially if complicated by mental illness or other physical or social disabilities (20–22).

Mental health and stigma

The stigma experienced by homeless people can be profoundly disturbing to their psychological well-being and ability to access and use dental services (2). More than half of the homeless population have one or more cognitive disorder (23), and homeless people compared to people with stable housing are disproportionately (3–9%) more highly infected with HIV/AIDS (24) along with the apathy, fear, lack of hygiene, and pharmacological side-effects accompanying these disorders (25). In summary, poor oral health complicates homelessness by increasing anxiety, depression, malnutrition, insomnia, and social isolation caused by toothaches from dental caries and facial disfigurement from missing teeth.

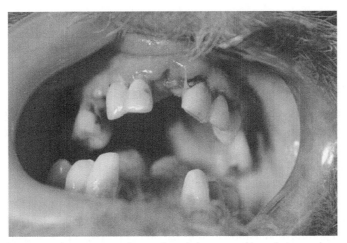

Fig. 14.2 Dry mouth, rampant caries, and tooth loss caused by substance abuse disorder.
Reproduced courtesy of Dr M Brondani.

Substance-use disorders

Substance-use is widespread among homeless people (26–28). Globally, about 1 in 20 (5.6%) of the adult population misuse drugs, and about one in nine (11%) need treatment (29). Typically this includes alcohol, tobacco, and cannabis, compounded by overprescribed or extra-medical use of opioids (30). Indeed the illicit use of steroids, hallucinogens, cocaine, amphetamines, ecstasy, heroin, and other synthetic drugs has reached epidemic status in many societies (31).

There are multiple side-effects in the mouth from most of these substances. Cannabis is associated with a dry mouth and dental caries, methamphetamines and cocaine with caries and tooth wear, and opioid-use with poor oral hygiene and frequent sugar consumption leading to rampant caries and tooth loss (Fig. 14.2) (32). Moreover, the sugar content of methadone preparations for managing heroin addiction greatly exacerbate the rampancy and rapidity of caries and tooth loss (33).

Living conditions

Homeless people with depression or other psychological illness usually struggle with personal hygiene, and oral hygiene no less so, without toothbrushes and toothpaste and easy access to clean water complicated by ready access and strong addiction to sugar-laden foods (32,34). Social relationships and health supports are usually very insecure if not completely dysfunctional within homeless communities (25), especially when missing teeth inhibit social interactions and employment (16,35–37).

Access to dental care

Difficulty accessing dental services is just one of many policy, organizational, and individual problems facing homeless people (38,39). Economic, social, and health strategies, health promotion and community campaigns, and professional and lay-person volunteers all need the attention of motivated policymakers along with a collective social sensitivity to encourage and sustain appropriate dental services. Private dental clinics can seem very unfriendly and inaccessible to homeless people who feel easily stigmatized, ostracized and misunderstood by the staff and other patients, especially when harassed about their poverty, addictions, disabilities and missed appointments(16). Dentists and their staff, on the other hand, are wary of people who they perceive as disruptive, violent, untrustworthy, dishevelled, and medically unstable (38–41). Some dentists contend that homeless people are the responsibility of government and better served by special healthcare clinics or hospital emergency departments rather than private dental clinics (18,42). Indeed, many urban communities provide dental clinics as part of a policy on homeless action (44). In British Columbia, for example, some community dental clinics provide comprehensive dental treatments from salaried dental staff in well-equipped clinics with limited government support, whereas other clinics offer only charitable services to manage acute toothaches and advanced oral infections (38).

Pathway to care

Model pathways for care help to identify the array of sociocultural, behavioural, and economic factors influencing the organization and outcome of the care (45,46). Fig. 14.3 illustrates a model pathway based on the suggestions and concerns of homeless people interviewed in Vancouver (2,47). It illustrates the organization and interaction of policies and services required to change care-seeking behaviours for better oral health through an assortment of governmental, professional, educational and motivational activities. In all, it reflects the perspectives of homeless people that are frequently excluded or overlooked in proposals on healthcare for vulnerable and socially marginalized people (48).

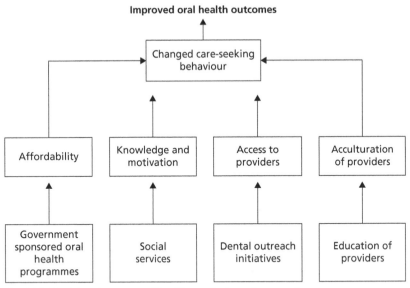

Fig. 14.3 Model pathway to oral healthcare for homeless people.
Adapted from Mago A., Brondani M., MacEntee M.I., Frankish J. (2018). A model pathway to oral health care for homeless people. Journal of the Canadian Dental Association, 84(i10).

References

1. **Ortiz-Ospina E, Roser M.** Homelessness. **OurWorldInData.org**; 2020. Available from: https://ourworldindata.org/homelessness.

2. **Mago A, MacEntee M, Brondani M, Frankish J.** Anxiety and anger of homeless people coping with dental care. Community Dent Oral Epidemiol. 2018;**46**(3):225–230.

3. **Wallace BB, MacEntee MI.** Access to dental care for low-income adults: perceptions of affordability, availability and acceptability. J Community Health. 2012;**37**(1):32–39.

4. **Parker EJ, Jamieson LM, Steffens MA, Cathro P, Logan RM.** Self-reported oral health of a metropolitan homeless population in Australia: comparisons with population-level data. Aust Dent J. 2011;**56**(3):272–277.

5. **Waplington J, Morris J, Bradnock G.** The dental needs, demands and attitudes of a group of homeless people with mental health problems. Community Dent Health. 2000;**17**(3):134–137.

6. **Nate'Bronson N.** Health Experiences of Homeless Women in LA County: Looking Beyond Individual-Level Factors. PhD Thesis, University of California Los Angeles; 2007.

7. **Daly B, Newton T, Batchelor P, Jones K.** Oral health care needs and oral health-related quality of life (OHIP-14) in homeless people. Community Dent Oral Epidemiol 2010;**38**(2):136–144.

8. **Groundswell**. Healthy Mouths: A Peer-Led Health Audit on the Oral Health of People Experiencing Homelessness. London: Groundwell; 2016. Available from: https://grou ndswell.org.uk/wp-content/uploads/2017/10/Groundswell-Healthy-Mouths-Report-Final.pdf.

9. **Nielssen OB, Stone W, Jones NM**, et al. Characteristics of people attending psychiatric clinics in inner Sydney homeless hostels. Med J Aust. 2018;4(4):169–173.

10. **Bauer LK, Brody JK, León C, Baggett TP.** Characteristics of homeless adults who died of drug overdose: a retrospective record review. J Healthc Poor Underserved. 2016;**27**(2):846–859.

11. **Quilgars D, Pleace N.** Delivering Health Care to Homeless People: An Effectiveness Review. York: Centre for Housing Policy; 2003. Available from: http://citeseerx.ist.psu. edu/viewdoc/download?doi=10.1.1.195.8567&rep=rep1&type=pdf.

12. **Schrimshaw EW, Siegel K, Wolfson NH, Mitchell DA, Kunzel C.** Insurance-related barriers to accessing dental care among African American adults with oral health symptoms in Harlem, New York City. Am J Public Health. 2011;**101**(8):1420–1428.

13. **Slack-Smith L, Hearn L, Scrine C, Durey A.** Barriers and enablers for oral health care for people affected by mental health disorders. Aust Dent J. 2017;**62**(1):6–13.

14. **Hurley J, Guindon G.** Private health insurance in Canada. In: **Thomson S, Sagan A, Mossialos E** (Eds), Private Health Insurance: History, Politics, and Performance. Cambridge: Cambridge University Press; 2020:99–141.

15. **Leake JL.** Why do we need an oral health care policy in Canada? J Can Dent Assoc. 2006;**72**(4):317.

16. **Wallace B, MacEntee MI.** Perspectives on community dental clinics in British Columbia. J Health Care Poor Underserved. 2013;**24**(2):943–953.

17. **Muirhead V, Quinonez C, Figueiredo R, Locker D.** Predictors of dental care utilization among working poor Canadians. Community Dent Oral Epidemiol. 2009;**37**(3):199–208.

18. **Brondani M, Ahmad S.** The 1% of emergency room visits for non-traumatic dental conditions in British Columbia: (mis)understanding the numbers. Can J Public Health. 2017;**108**:e279–e281.

19. **Quiñonez C, Grootendorst P.** Equity in dental care among Canadian households. Int J Equity Health. 2011;**10**:1–9.

20. **Pegon-Machat E, Tubert-Jeannin S, Loignon C, Landry A, Bedos C.** Dentists' experience with low-income patients benefiting from a public insurance program. Eur J Oral Sci. 2009;**117**(4):398–406.

21. **Quiñonez CR, Figueiredo R, Locker D.** Canadian dentists' opinions on publicly financed dental care. J Public Health Dent. 2009;**69**(2):64–73.

22. **Dharamsi S, Pratt DD, MacEntee MI.** How dentists account for social responsibility: economic imperatives and professional obligations. J Dent Educ. 2007;**71**(12):1583–1592.

23. **Funk M, Drew N, Knapp M.** Mental health, poverty and development. J Public Ment Health. 2012;**11**(4):166–185.

24. **Milloy MJ, Marshall BD, Montaner J, Wood E.** Housing status and the health of people living with HIV/AIDS. Curr HIV/AIDS Rep. 2012;**9**(4):364–374.

25. **Watt RG, Venturelli R, Daly B.** Understanding and tackling oral health inequalities in vulnerable adult populations: from the margins to the mainstream. Br Dent J. 2019;**227**(1):49–54.

26. **Fazel S, Geddes JR, Kushel M.** The health of homeless people in high-income countries: descriptive epidemiology, health consequences, and clinical and policy recommendations. Lancet. 2014;**384**:1529–1540.

27. **Hwang SW, Burns T.** Health interventions for people who are homeless. Lancet. 2014;**384**(9953):1541–1547.

28. **Brondani M, Alan R, Donnelly L.** Sigma of addiction and mental illness in health care: the case of patients' experiences in dental settings. PLoS One. 2017;**12**:e0177388.

29. **United Nations.** World drug report 2018. 2018. Available from: https://www.unodc.org/wdr2018/prelaunch/WDR18_Booklet_2_GLOBAL.pdf.

30. **Degenhardt L, Grebely J, Stone J,** et al. Global patterns of opioid use and dependence: harms to populations, interventions, and future action. Lancet. 2019;**394**(10208):1560–1579.

31. **Khalili M, Rahimi-Movaghar A, Shadloo B, Mojtabai R, Mann K, Amin-Esmaeili M.** Global scientific production on illicit drug addiction: a two-decade analysis. Eur Addict Res. 2018;**24**(2):60–70.

32. **Baghaie H, Kisely S, Forbes M, Sawyer E, Siskind DJ.** A systematic review and meta-analysis of the association between poor oral health and substance abuse. Addiction. 2017;**112**(5):765–779.

33. **Brondani M, Park PE.** Methadone and oral health–a brief review. J Am Dent Hyg Assoc. 2011;**85**(2):92–98.

34. **Moffa M, Cronk R, Fejfar D, Dancausse S, Padilla LA, Bartram J.** A systematic scoping review of environmental health conditions and hygiene behaviors in homeless shelters. Int J Hyg Environ Health. 2019;**222**(3):335–346.

35. **Halasa-Rappel YA, Tschampl CA, Foley M, Dellapenna M, Shepard DS.** Broken smiles: the impact of untreated dental caries and missing anterior teeth on employment. J Public Health Dent. 2019;**79**(3):231–237.

36. **Albright D, Gonzales A, Willits D, Broidy L, Lyons C.** Reducing Barriers to Re-Entry: Assessing the Implementation and Impact of a Pilot Dental Repair Program for Parolees. Albuquerque, NM: Institute for Social Research, The University of New Mexico; 2011. Available from: https://www.jrsa.org/pubs/sac-digest/documents/NM_DentalTreatmentReentryProgramOutcomes.pdf.

37. **Khalid A, Quiñonez C.** Straight, white teeth as a social prerogative. Sociol Health Illn. 2015;**37**(5):782–796.

38. **Wallace BB, MacEntee MI, Pauly B.** Community dental clinics in British Columbia, Canada: examining the potential as health equity interventions. Health Soc Care Community. 2015;**23**(4):371–379.

39. **El-Yousfi S, Jones K, White S, Marshman Z.** A rapid review of barriers to oral healthcare for vulnerable people. Br Dent J. 2019;**227**(2):143–151.

40. **Dharamsi S, Pratt DD, MacEntee MI.** How dentists account for social responsibility: economic imperatives and professional obligations. J Dent Educ. 2007;**71**(12):1583–1592.

41. **Wallace BB, MacEntee MI, Harrison R, Hole R, Mitton C.** Community dental clinics: providers' perspectives. Community Dent Oral Epidemiol. 2013;**41**(3):193–203.

42. **Quiñonez C, Gibson D, Jokovic A, Locker D.** Emergency department visits for dental care of nontraumatic origin. Community Dent Oral Epidemiol. 2009;37(4):331–366.

44. **Wallace B, Figueiredo R, MacEntee M, Quiñonez C.** Homelessness and oral health. In: **Guirguis-Younge M, Hwang S, McNeil R** (Eds), Homelessness & Health in Canada. Ottawa: University of Ottawa Press; 2014:189–210.

45. **Schrijvers G, van Hoorn A, Huiskes N.** The care pathway: concepts and theories: an introduction. Int J Integr Care. 2012;12(Spec Ed Integrated Care Pathways):e192.

46. **Checkland K, Hammond J, Allen P**, et al. Road to nowhere? A critical consideration of the use of the metaphor 'care pathway' in health services planning, organisation and delivery. J Soc Policy. 2019;49(2):405–424.

47. **Mago A, Brondani M, MacEntee MI, Frankish J.** A model pathway to oral health care for homeless people. J Can Dent Assoc. 2018;84:i10.

48. **Pegon-Machat E, Tubert-Jeannin S, Loignon C, Landry A, Bedos C.** Dentists' experience with low-income patients benefiting from a public insurance program. Eur J Oral Sci. 2009;117(4):398–406.

Psychiatric issues

Chapter 15

Neurocognitive impairment in homeless persons

Neha Sharma, Joshua D. Brown, and Paul Summergrad

Introduction

Mr N, a 55-year-old homeless man with schizophrenia who was discharged from an emergency room in Los Angeles because he did not meet clinical criteria for inpatient level of care, was the focus of a recent case study in social medicine (1). Mr N's homelessness, a chronic social condition, was the central issue discussed as homelessness has become seen to be more of a social rather than a medical problem. Unfortunately, such a change in policy has resulted in homelessness as 'an increasingly permanent and normalized fate' for individuals with serious mental illness in the US. Furthermore, many homeless individuals with serious mental illness, such as this patient, eventually become incarcerated which has become another tragic fate for these individuals, especially in the US. There is a need to change the culture of the medical and larger community and awake from our complacence with the current high rates of homelessness and incarceration. Practical suggestions to address these concerns including rethinking the boundaries of medical care to include programmes such as 'housing as healthcare' aimed at providing stable housing for homeless individuals with mental health conditions (1).

For many patients like Mr N, specific details remain limited; one key factor that may have influenced options for his care was his cognitive function and ability. Studies show an association between severe mental disorders, cognitive impairment, and homelessness (2–7). This chapter will highlight the important features of neurocognitive impairment and how it relates to the homeless population. The chapter is divided into three parts. The first part will define cognitive impairment. The second part will demonstrate the bidirectional cause-and-effect relationship of homelessness and cognitive dysfunction. The third part will provide guidance for potential interventions.

What is cognitive impairment?

Neurocognition is a broad term that applies to multiple different higher functions and, in some cases, areas of the brain. The *Diagnostic and Statistical Manual of Mental Disorders*, fifth edition (*DSM-5*) (8) and the International Classification of Diseases, tenth revision, Clinical Modification (ICD-10-CM) (9) specify six key areas: learning and memory, language, perceptual–motor function, executive functioning, complex attention, and social cognition (Fig. 15.1).

A deficit in any one of these areas can lead to a neurocognitive disorder. Specifically, the *DSM-5* defines this disorder as a decline from an individual's baseline in one or more cognitive domains, recognized by either the person's self-concern, by a knowledgeable informant or clinician, or by neuropsychological testing, and occurs independently of a delirious state. The severity of the cognitive impairment is based upon how significantly it interferes with an individual's independent daily activities (8). The *DSM-5* and ICD-10-CM further subtype the reasons for neurocognitive decline. This can be secondary to various types of insults. The list includes neurological conditions such as

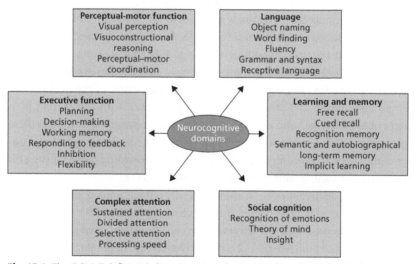

Fig. 15.1 The *DSM-5* defines six key domains of cognitive function, all with their own subdomains. Identification of the domain and subdomain relevant to an individual's neurocognitive disorder provides valuable information regarding the origin and severity of a particular impairment.

Reprinted by permission from Springer Nature: Nature Reviews Neurology 10.11, Classifying neurocognitive disorders: the DSM-5 approach, Sachdev, P. S., Blacker, D., Blazer, D. G., Ganguli, M., Jeste, D. V., Paulsen, J. S., & Petersen, R. C. (2014).

Alzheimer's disease, frontotemporal lobar degeneration, Lewy body disease, vascular dementia, prion disease, Parkinson's disease, and Huntington's disease and other medical conditions such as infections (e.g. HIV), substance/medication use, and traumatic brain injury (TBI) (8,9). Identifying these conditions is essential as they are often more prevalent in specific vulnerable populations such as the homeless (10). Generally speaking, neurocognition is referred to as a high level of information processing that includes thinking, memory, perception, attention, motivation, problem-solving, and language. Numerous psychiatric disorders have neurocognitive challenges in the above-mentioned dimensions. For example, extensive studies on schizophrenia and neurocognitive disorders indicate that impaired attention, working memory, and declarative memory are consistently associated with psychotic symptoms (11). Negative symptoms are highly correlated with greater neurocognitive deficits (12). Neurocognitive deficits have also been noted in the course of bipolar disorder (13–15) and the number of manic and depressive episodes are correlated with poor performance on verbal memory, verbal fluency, and working memory tasks (12,16). Furthermore, Kuswanto et al. (17) note that neurocognitive deficits are associated with clinical and treatment factors for psychotic spectrum conditions including schizophrenia and bipolar disorder and that deficits are primarily in executive function, working memory, verbal fluency, and motor speed.

Neurocognitive assessment

The neurobiological pathways for cognition are also complex. Studies of brain development in youth and adolescents explore this vulnerable time in the connectivity of synapses in the prefrontal cortex responsible for the executive functioning domain of cognition (18). One study in 2017 (19) explored the relationship between cortical thickening, gyrification, and neurocognitive impairment. Specifically, greater frontal and medial temporal gyrification were associated with more profound impairments similar to individuals with schizophrenia. Cortical thickening in younger patients was also correlated with more significant cognitive impairment, whereas cortical thickening in older individuals was more protective. Furthermore, when assessing cognitive function in patients who sustain a TBI, areas of abnormality found on magnetic resonance imaging (MRI) were in total grey matter volume, frontal and temporal grey matter volumes, and white matter integrity (20).

Since neurocognitive domains and thus impairment are varied, there is not a true comprehensive test to assess every domain. As such, many studies in homeless individuals have utilized the Mini-Mental State Examination (MMSE) as an indicator of cognitive function. While this test is practical for its 'inter-rater reliability' and it assesses many global areas such as orientation, immediate and short-term memory, attention and calculation, visuoconstruction skills, and praxis, its limitation is that it is not sensitive to detect focal deficits such as aphasia, higher cognitive function, or frontal lobe disorders. In addition, the test and its scoring were derived from assessing dementia in elderly hospitalized patients and so it is not necessarily a tool to assess overall cognitive impairment (21,22).

One meta-analysis underscored this point stating that 'there are more reliable and valid screening measures than the MMSE for cognitive impairment' and pointed specifically to the Montreal Cognitive Assessment (MoCA) and University of California, San Diego, Performance-based Skills Assessment (UPSA) tests (23). The MoCA is a validated assessment for dementia. Similar to the MMSE, it assesses orientation, short-term memory/delayed recall, executive function, visuospatial ability, language abilities, abstraction, animal naming, and attention. But, unlike the MMSE, it also includes the clock-drawing test. Comparatively, it has broader sensitivity and more appropriate to track changes over a period of time than the MMSE. The MoCA takes 10–12 minutes to administer and has high reliability (24). It is available in more than 35 languages and for visually impaired persons (MoCA Test Blind).

Neurocognitive impairment can alternatively be assessed by its practical effect on an individual's daily life. Termed 'functional capacity', it can be measured by such tests as the UPSA. This test explicitly includes 'five domains of everyday functioning (household chores, communication, finance, transportation, and planning recreational activities) and requires participants to use props and role play' (25). The second version of the UPSA includes the sixth domain: medication management. It takes approximately 45 minutes to administer, though an abbreviated version which only assesses two domains, financial and communication skills, takes 15 minutes. Because of its psychometric assessment of the functional capacity, it has been validated for individuals with severe and chronic mental illness in English-speaking Western countries. The UPSA has been culturally adapted to eight different languages and administered in 17 countries with moderate to strong construct validity and test–retest reliability (23).

The studies which only use the MMSE to assess neurocognitive impairments and do not use neuropsychological assessments may under-represent those with impairments[1] (26,27). On the other hand, not having a uniform diagnostic

---

[1] The study noted five categories of performance-based cognitive performance data. This includes (a) per cent below impairment criteria on cognitive screening tests on the Mini-Mental State Examination (MMSE), Abbreviated Mental Test, or Addenbrooke's Cognitive Evaluation; (b) mean performance on the MMSE; (c) mean IQ as measured by the Wechsler Adult Intelligence Scale (WAIS; various versions), Wechsler Abbreviated Scale

tool such as the MMSE makes it challenging to draw conclusions between studies. Of note, one review article in 2015 (28) investigating memory among the homeless found mixed results in the literature, with a wide variety of diagnostic tools used in studies to assess memory including the Wechsler Memory Scale Repeatable Battery for the Assessment of Neuropsychological Status, Hopkins Verbal Learning Test-Revised, Cognitive Stability Index, California Verbal Learning Test, Cognistat, and the Rey Auditory Verbal Learning Test, among others. Thus, one of the great challenges and limitations of research in this area is the lack of consistency among diagnostic tools. Despite these challenges, we hope to share available literature about the relationship between cognitive impairment and homelessness. Additionally, we recommend the MoCA for bedside diagnostic assessment due to its brevity, sensitivity, low cost, and transcultural and multilingual validation. However, the MoCA has been validated for dementia whereas the UPSA has been validated for individuals with severe mental illness and is more pragmatic to assess functionality. We recommend the UPSA to evaluate skills that can be addressed more tangibly in treatment planning.

The relationship between cognitive impairment and homelessness

Previous research has shown that homeless individuals have more profound neurocognitive impairment than the general population including lower than average full-scale intelligence quotient (IQ), attention, and memory difficulties (29). The extent of this impairment, however, is not clear as variation exists among studies in terms of populations, age, definitions of homelessness, and diagnostic tools used.[2] In a 2003 study in Brazil, using the MMSE, 36.3% of homeless individuals were found to have cognitive impairment (31). Researchers in Wisconsin utilizing the Neurobehavioral Cognitive Status Examination (Cognistat) suggested that 80% of the homeless population had cognitive impairment with specific deficits in memory (32). In Tokyo, Japan,

---

of Intelligence (WASI), Shipley, or Ravens Progressive Matrices; (d) mean premorbid IQ as measured by the Wide Range Achievement Test-3 (WRAT-3) or American National Adult Reading Test (ANART); and (e) other neuropsychological tests (e.g. Trail Making Test, Wisconsin Card Sorting Test) (26). Other studies have used neuropsychological testing such as The Hopkins Verbal Learning Test-Revised, WAIS-III, Digit Symbol and Symbol Search subtests, and Wisconsin Card Sorting Test (27).

[2] Within the MMSE, most studies (22) use 24 as a cutoff for cognitive impairment whereas one study used 26 as a cutoff (30).

one study (33) showed 44% of homeless individuals had cognitive impairment. In contrast, a different study (34) showed 78.4% of elderly homeless men met criteria for cognitive impairment.[3] In Sydney, Australia, one study (30) found 78% of older homeless individuals (45 years and older) to have cognitive impairment on the MMSE with 75% having frontal lobe dysfunction. Burra et al., in a 2009 review article (22), wrote that within 22 studies, the MMSE showed roughly 4–7% of homeless people exhibit global cognitive deficits. Depp et al., in a 2015 review article (26), cited approximately 25% of a pooled sample of 2969 homeless adults screened using various neuropsychological assessments had cognitive impairment. The results also showed that the mean full-scale IQ score was about one standard deviation below average, roughly below the 15th percentile. The authors concluded that there may be 'considerable cognitive impairment in this population that is missed by brief screening measures (e.g., the MMSE)' (26). Stergiopoulos et al. (7), utilizing a global deficit score based on a battery of neuropsychological testing, found approximately 72% of 1500 homeless individuals in Canada had neurocognitive impairment with specific deficits in processing speed (48%), verbal learning (71%), recall (67%), and executive functioning (38%).

The data are consistent that homeless individuals have more significant neurocognitive deficits than the general public. In order to derive more practical implications, research has focused on two fundamental questions that will be discussed in depth in this chapter:

1. Does cognitive impairment predispose an individual to becoming homeless or does homelessness directly impact an individual's cognition?

2. Furthermore, if the latter, does homelessness independently cause cognitive impairment or does homelessness predispose individuals to other risk factors such as TBI or substance use which, in turn, lead to neurocognitive impairment?

Cognitive impairment leading to homelessness

Cognitive impairment as a risk factor leading to homelessness is assumed by many researchers; however, there is lack of empirical evidence to discern the direct role it plays (22). Indeed, when assessing homeless youth, a review article concludes that 'because the current body of literature does not include longitudinal studies, it is unknown whether cognitive deficits precede homelessness or is a consequence of it' (18). Nevertheless, in a review in 2004, Spence et al. (21) noted that while the direct cause–effect relationship of homelessness and

---

[3] Variations in sample size and age may explain differences in these studies.

cognitive impairment has not yet been studied, the 'extent of cognitive decline is related to indices of homelessness'. Specifically, while inferring from cross-sectional data, the authors conclude that homeless individuals with significant cognitive decline are likely going to have more difficulty being able to resettle than those with less cognitive impairment. Other researchers similarly pointed out 'preserved executive function is essential to making plans, prioritizing, and completing tasks and thus may be of particular importance to homeless adults attempting to navigate complex social services' (35). In the same vein, having an address can practically help individuals obtain necessary assets such as government resources, family support, or other financial assistance. Thus, while the initial trigger for an individual's level of function is multifactorial and bidirectional, the level of executive function deficit can perpetuate a cycle of remaining homeless.

Needless to say, one can speculate that cognitive and executive function deficits predispose one to homelessness due to challenges in securing or maintaining a job. Although there is a dearth of literature on financial insecurity and homelessness, perhaps because the relationship between the two is taken for granted, there is sufficient evidence that individuals who have illnesses that affect cognitive dysfunction are more likely to be unemployed. Specifically, cognitive limitations in individuals with hepatic encephalopathy, sickle cell anaemia, attention deficit hyperactive disorder, executive function deficit, chronic substance abuse, and HIV-related encephalopathy are associated with unemployment (36–40). To no one's surprise, the sequela of unemployment when there is limited community and family support is homelessness.

Despite limited conclusive data on cognitive impairment leading to homelessness, there are some conditions that need to be reviewed to better understand the relationship between the two. As noted in the introduction, schizophrenia, bipolar disorder, intellectual disability (ID), autism spectrum disorder (ASD), and childhood trauma can impact cognitive function which, in turn, can lead to homelessness. Other conditions such as malnutrition, TBI, dementia, and substance abuse which albeit may precede homelessness are also often sequelae of it and will be reviewed in the later section of 'Homelessness leading to cognitive impairment'.

Schizophrenia

Individuals with serious mental illness have a 10–20 times higher risk of becoming homeless than those in the general population (41). More specifically, cognitive impairment has been found to affect 85% of individuals with schizophrenia, impacting their ability to maintain stable housing (5). Moreover, psychosis, which is a common symptom of schizophrenia, has been associated with living for a greater duration in unsheltered environments instead of sheltered facilities (42). This may be related to poor social cognition where individuals have difficulty managing social norms such as conflicts with other individuals that can lead to more isolating environments. However, it is also likely related to the neurocognitive impairment and decline noted in patients with schizophrenia. Individuals with schizophrenia tend to score 2.5 standard deviations below control subjects in domains of verbal memory, attention, speed of processing, and executive function (43). Challenges in memory, working memory, problem-solving, and social cognition even when not on antipsychotic medications are also noted (44,45). These deficits are present before presentation of psychotic symptoms and are independent from the symptomatic manifestation of the illness (46). Additionally, the cognitive deficits that are present at the first episode of psychosis tend to be associated with functional outcomes, such as difficulty in problem-solving, difficulty in benefitting from a psychosocial rehabilitation programmes, and inability to hold a job (47,48). Additionally, challenges in social cognition further exacerbate the ability of a person with schizophrenia to have stable housing.

One limitation is assessing cognitive function in schizophrenic individuals who are homeless is practical diagnostic assessment tools. Measurement and Treatment Research to Improve Cognition in Schizophrenia (MATRICS) and the Treatment Units of Research on Neurocognition and Schizophrenia (TURNS) were developed to assess cognition in schizophrenia for it to be better studied and for pharmacological development. MATRICS assesses seven cognitive domains including processing speed, attention, working memory, verbal learning and memory, visual learning and memory, reasoning and problem-solving, and verbal comprehension (44). These long batteries of tests are time-consuming, expensive, and require a trained administrator. To increase utility in clinical practice, the Repeatable Battery for the Assessment of Neuropsychological Status (RBANS) and the Brief Assessment of Cognition in Schizophrenia (BACS) were developed which are both reliable in showing a relationship between cognitive function and functional outcomes (49,50). However, these tools still take approximately 30 minutes to administer when an average clinical visit is much shorter. To make the tools more relevant and clinically feasible, the Brief Cognitive Assessment Tool for Schizophrenia (B-CATS) and Screen for Cognitive Impairment in Psychiatry (SCIP) were developed and compared. These tools were noted to be shorter (approximately 10–15 minutes), reliable, and valid, although the SCIP has a better predictive value of global cognitive impairment than the B-CATS (51). Another scale, the MoCA, was noted to be sensitive to detect both mild and severe cognitive impairments in schizophrenia and its score correlated with the BACS and the Brief UPSA

(52). There are thus a variety of diagnostic tools available to assess cognition in schizophrenic patients and shorter scales such as the B-CATS, SCIP, and MoCA can be useful to assess the degree of cognitive decline and need for social services for stable housing.

Bipolar disorder

Bipolar disorder is an illness with various subtypes that typically differ in their degree of mania (53). The two most common are termed bipolar I disorder and bipolar II disorder and each has been shown to cause cognitive impairment in similar domains—executive function, attention, verbal memory, non-verbal memory, and functional impairment—although individuals with bipolar I tend to have a greater severity of deficit (54). It is well established that cognitive deficits exist during acute phases of mania or depression. Many studies also show that deficits are also prevalent in individuals even after remission, with larger deficits in verbal memory and executive function with smaller deficits in visuoperception (54). One reason offered for the degree of cognitive impairment is the high levels of emotional arousal in individuals with bipolar disorder which impacts their attention and cognitive flexibility (54). It is also important to note that individuals with bipolar disorder, who had an early onset of disease, are older, or with repeated number of depressive or manic episodes have worsening cognitive function which point to a possible neurocognitive trait in the brain that worsens with cumulative insults (55). Indeed, one study assessing individuals with bipolar disorder who lived in adult congregate facilities housing (roughly defined as 'senior-based housing that is publicly supported . . . who may need support in personal care'), showed that impairment in cognitive function is found across age groups but appears to worsen in elderly individuals who typically have a greater need for services (56).

One recent study (57) investigated independent living skills in homeless veterans with serious mental illness (including bipolar disorder) and their functional adaptability to retain or lose housing. Several problems that faced these individuals included acquiring an apartment, money management, acquiring food, furniture, processing necessary paperwork such as a lease or eviction notice, and interpersonal conflict. Although not statistically significant, most 'stayers' (those who retained housing for more than 1 year) used greater anticipatory and additive problem-solving to address housing issues, suggesting a link between cognitive ability and functional adaptability within this population (57).

Not surprisingly, a study (58) that looked at cognitive function and housing in individuals with psychosis which included bipolar disorder I with psychotic features using a dimensional analytical approach, showed that greater cognitive deficits contributed to more days of unsheltered homelessness. Cognition was assessed using the MATRICS Consensus Cognitive Battery (MCCB) test and specific deficits in visual learning and social cognition were identified as critical prognostic factors. Visual learning is an important tool for functional ability and may connect with the ability to maintain employment. Poor social cognition as mentioned elsewhere in this chapter can lead to poor interpersonal relationships and impact a tenant's ability to manage conflict with a landlord.

Thus, individuals with bipolar disorder whether in acute stages of psychosis or even after remission are found to have various forms of cognitive impairment which can predispose these individuals to homelessness and often enter a vicious cycle where it also becomes challenging to obtain and sustain housing after becoming homeless.

Intellectual disability

Backer and Howard (5) pointed out that nearly one out of five individuals with developmental disabilities (which are often discovered at a young age) also have cognitive impairment. These individuals are at great risk of becoming homeless at two distinct junctures: the first is after they age out of the care system such as foster care and special education (and do not qualify for adult services) and the second time is when their lifelong caregiver passes away without making necessary arrangements. Thus, homelessness becomes an unfortunate disposition in the interplay between individuals with developmental delays, cognitive impairment, and mental health issues.

Research shows that there is a significant prevalence of homeless individuals who have ID (5). One study in the UK using the WASI found that approximately 12% of the homeless participants had ID specifically in full scale and verbal IQ. Of note, using the Adaptive Behavior Assessment Scale (ABAS) there was no significant difference among performance IQ among the same cohort (59). One recent study in the Japanese population using intellectual measures such as the WAIS-III and Japanese Adult Reading Test (JART) found up to 39% of homeless participants had ID which on further analysis was 28% when excluding decline due to ageing or mental illness (60). In a study of Dutch homeless individuals, 30% were found to have a suspected ID. In that study, the Hayes Ability Screening Index (HASI), a brief screening scale, was used instead of full-scale diagnostic tool which may have overestimated the statistic (61).

One review article (62) studying homeless individuals from Montreal with ID concluded that two key factors, substance abuse and breakdowns in social network, predisposed this population to homelessness. There were also many gender differences between males and females in regard to the relative stability of their living condition (males with less stable conditions) as well as problems with the criminal justice system (males having more problems). Oakes and Davies (59) found a similar conclusion regarding substance use which had two times greater odds of being found in individuals with suspected ID than those without ID. Thus, homeless individuals with ID are likely more susceptible to environmental issues such as substance use and are in greater need of social networks for aide and assistance. These are necessary factors to consider when working with this population.

One compelling conclusion regarding the relationship between ID and homelessness noted by Van Straaten et al. (61) is that participants with suspected ID when compared to those without ID more often preferred independent housing support available by direct appointment, instead of passively being on-call to receive it. Thus, the programme 'Housing First' which focuses on providing homeless individuals with independent stable housing without any precondition may be a more stable option for these individuals, as the cohort was noted to prefer independent housing but may not access it without more direct help and intervention (61). Moreover, Durbin et al. (63) found that there was no difference in sustaining housing stability between homeless individuals with borderline or low intellectual function compared to homeless individuals with average intellectual functioning which further supports the notion that homeless individuals with ID should be included in this programme.

Another practical conclusion by Oakes and Davies (59) showed that individuals with ID had specific challenges in understanding verbal information. Therefore, the use of more visual cues when communicating with persons with ID would likely be beneficial. In the same vein, using more straightforward screening tools by practitioners will probably be more helpful than complex assessments. Oakes and Davies (59) also conclude: 'Increased awareness of staff and the implementation of simple measures in services which include acute and primary care, substance misuse, mental health, criminal justice and housing could make a real and relevant impact on this problem.'

Autism spectrum disorder

Globally, the prevalence of autism is rising. According to the World Health Organization, one in 160 children has autism (64). However, in high-income countries, such as the US, the prevalence is as high as one in 60. Since challenges in communication and social behaviour are integral aspects of this condition, individuals with autism are particularly at danger of losing their community and family support and becoming roofless. Literature investigating the relationship between ASD and homelessness is scarce. One study (65) created a screening diagnostic tool called the '*DSM-5* Autistic Traits in the Homeless Interview' (DATHI) which is a tool that keyworkers in the UK (who are similar to social workers or case managers in the US) can use to document traits that are specific to individuals with ASD. The study found that 12.3% of homeless people had a range of autistic traits consistent with *DSM-5* diagnostic criteria, higher than the general population which is 1%. In addition, the study concluded that certain specific character traits of ASD such as lacking social emotional reciprocity and having greater sensory difficulties could be risk factors for homelessness. Indeed, each of these traits can lead to greater social isolation such as avoiding noisy public places (e.g. hostels), and inability to appropriately obtain employment, leading to poverty. It may also be challenging to help individuals transition from homeless to stable housing when they are accustomed to a routine and may have more rigidity in their thinking and behaviour.

Access to social services is one vital factor for individuals with ASD which is a problem worldwide. Indeed, even in high-income countries like the US and the UK, the linkage between healthcare services for children with autism becomes fragmented as they enter adulthood, resulting in loss of services and healthcare support (66,67). Higher functioning individuals with ASD who are either undiagnosed or do not meet the threshold for services are particularly vulnerable (68). Furthermore, in low-income countries, there is a significant unmet need for educational support, financial support, and access to trained healthcare professionals (69). These barriers are likely to impact residential stability especially as individuals with autism transition into adulthood and elderly family members are unable to provide care. Homelessness is an unfortunate result in many cases.

Childhood trauma

Stone et al. (68) cited a notable study (70) to assess a possible correlation between childhood trauma and cognitive function in homeless adults. The study utilized several different measures such as the Frontal Systems Behavior Scale (FrSBe), used to assess prefrontal cortex dysfunction, the WASI to measure IQ, and the Childhood Trauma Questionnaire, to assess childhood trauma, noting significant positive correlations between total FrSBe scores, emotional abuse, emotional neglect, and physical neglect and a negative association with IQ. While the study itself noted limitations such as mental illness as a possible confounder, the results open up a new insight into a cause of homelessness which can be attributed to earlier trauma and abuse. Childhood trauma and its impact on mental health in the homeless are discussed at greater length in another chapter in this volume.

Homelessness leading to cognitive impairment

One recent study investigated whether housing is an independent predictor of functional capacity; using multivariate regression analysis, Stergiopoulos et al. (25) concluded 'that controlling for substance abuse, symptom severity, recognition memory, and cognitive flexibility, being homeless was associated with an approximately 9-point lower score on the UPSA'. While these data are limited and as the author herself has concluded that longitudinal studies must be done, this notion of homelessness contributing independently to neurocognitive limitation is buttressed by a 2003 study by Seidman et al. (71) which looked at the reverse outcome and showed improvement in neurocognitive function after homeless individuals were provided with stable housing. Specific areas that improved on univariate analysis were delayed verbal memory, motor speed, and sequencing. The findings also showed that the type of housing given to homeless individuals led to different outcomes: individuals given independent housing had worsening performance in executive functioning from baseline; whereas, those in group homes had an increase in executive functioning performance from baseline although it did not reach statistical significance (71). Schutt et al. (72) investigating neurocognitive functioning and its relationship to community functioning came to a similar conclusion that homeless individuals with poor executive functioning tended to have more turbulent behaviour and worse self-care when given independent housing, but did better with more supportive care housing. Furthermore, one study (73) shows that chronically homeless individuals performed at a significantly poorer level than controls on the Iowa Gambling Task, Word Fluency (FAS), and the Burglar's Story, which suggest impairment in prefrontal cortex affecting judgement, inability to learn from past experiences, and emotional control. This may explain why homeless adults are unable to devise better plans to achieve greater stability on their own and require outside intervention.

The cohort who participated in the earlier-mentioned study were individuals who were initially living in stable homeless shelters (71). According to the study, during the initial and 18-month evaluation, there were no significant differences in housing compliance between those who were assigned group homes or independent apartments; however, subsequent homelessness was less prevalent in those who were assigned group homes. Thus, the difference in the latter outcomes between individuals who received independent housing versus group home housing may be attributed to a sense of social community and structure which may be limited for individuals who obtain independent housing. Thus, fully independent housing which may provide individuals with stability and safety, at the same time may also be isolating and lead to a lack of social structure which can affect executive functioning. The term housing therefore needs to be defined further.

In contrast to adults, it is not known whether homeless youth who are given stable housing have an improvement in their cognitive function. According to one study (18), homeless youth in comparison to other youth have been found to have impairments in visuomotor, problem-solving skills, judgement, logical thinking, processing speed, and verbal abilities. Homelessness, which can induce high levels of stress hormones, can disrupt the connectivity and synchrony of neural pathways during a sensitive time of brain development which may in turn have more permanent effects on areas such as the prefrontal cortex. Ultimately this may lead to a more enduring cognitive impairment which stable housing may not be able to impact. Fry et al. (74) and Saperstein et al. (75) argue that late adolescence is an opportune time to enhance cognitive development and set the stage for education and employment since it is a sensitive time for brain development. In a more recent article (76), some of these authors showed that transition-based homeless youth who received either specific cognitive remediation or more general cognitive activation (such as being taught computer skills) had a significant improvement in verbal memory, executive functioning, working memory, and processing speed. Of note, improvements in cognitive function did not improve emotional distress in the same cohort, showing independence between these two functions and the need for more specific interventions to address emotional needs.

Another way that homelessness may cause cognitive impairment is through the means of affecting an individual's perceived biological age. Chronological age indicates the period of living, whereas biological age is inclusive of one's health status (77) and is better in predicting physical frailty and mortality. Studies have shown that age independently affects cognitive impairment in healthy older adults in areas of general fluid intelligence as well as verbal declarative memory (78). Homelessness, which can impact an individual's body such that it is ageing at a faster pace, can thereby impact cognition. According to Cohen et al. (79), the relative increase in biological age in homeless individuals can be due to ailing physical health in multiple systems of the body. The two most prominent factors that appeared to affect physical health were more stressful lifetime events and individuals who had unfulfilled needs. The unfulfilled needs were assessed by a 40-item scale that comprised six major areas: 'physical health needs, mental health needs, physical self-maintenance, instrumental self-maintenance (finance, transportation), effectance (recreation, creativity), and social needs' (80). These data are further supported by assessing geriatric conditions in the homeless population. One recent study concluded that 'despite a median age of 58 years, participants had rates of geriatric conditions similar to or higher than adults in the general population with a median age of nearly 80 years' (81). These data are supported by Arranz et al. (82) who found that homeless individuals appear to have a more suppressed immune response on a cellular level when compared to housed controls. Arranz et al. (82) looked at cellular functions such as adherence, chemotaxis, phagocytosis, superoxide levels, lymphoproliferation, natural killer cell activity, interleukin-2, and plasma antioxidant levels. Thus, higher levels of stress in this population may lead to more physical and emotional ailments which in turn can impact biological age predisposing to greater cognitive impairment.

As mentioned earlier in the chapter, conditions such as malnutrition, TBI, dementia, and substance abuse are often prevalent in the homeless population. Their association with cognitive impairment, which is often bidirectional, and their relationship to homelessness will be reviewed next.

Malnutrition

Homeless individuals often have financial constraints that result in food insecurity. Thus, nutrition in the homeless population is another potential cause of cognitive dysfunction (18). In a recent systemic review (83), the authors noted that homeless individuals have poor access to food in general and especially food rich in nutrients and essential vitamins; they also lack the physical setting to store food or cook. Moreover, alcohol use, which is especially problematic in this population, can critically interfere with health in multiple ways: it is rich in calories and can provide an individual with energy (offsetting the need for consumption of healthier choices), and it impacts the absorption of nutrients in the gut and can lead to specific nutritional deficiencies such as vitamin B1 (thiamine) that can lead to cognitive impairment. Other more severe consequences such as Wernicke–Korsakoff encephalopathy and liver failure can ensue. Certain interventions were identified which although were not consistent among studies, nevertheless had some efficacy. Specifically, educational services such as workshops (allowing individuals to use cooking facilities), providing individuals with supplemental oral, or injections of, vitamins, and free or subsidized meals with nutritional value could help offset this crucial area of health and the homeless.

Traumatic brain injury

In a 2017 review article, Hurstak et al. (35) pointed out a number of studies that show an association between TBI and cognitive dysfunction in the general population. Highley and Proffitt underscored this notion by pointing out specific cognitive functions affected by TBI which include memory, ability to following instructions, read, write, or maintain appropriate boundaries among others (84).

Homeless individuals have a disproportionately high rate of TBI compared to the general population (85). Thus, a natural conclusion would be that TBI is an independent risk factor for cognitive dysfunction in the homeless population. This finding was indeed supported by one recent study (86) where individuals with TBI, assessed using the Brian Injury Screening Questionnaire, performed worse on the attention domain of the Repeatable Battery for the Assessment of Neuropsychological Status test. This diagnostic tool measures five distinct neurocognitive domains: immediate memory, delayed memory, visual-perceptual/constructional skills, attention, and language. Surprisingly, the participants with TBI only statistically performed worse on the attention domain and not on other functions like memory (which is known to be affected in patients with TBI), likely due to sample size or possible other unperceived confounders (86). Furthermore, while the consensus in the literature is that typically TBI precedes homelessness, nevertheless, those with one TBI are also susceptible to sustaining further TBI injuries which is more probable in homeless conditions and may 'have a cumulative adverse impact on cognitive functioning' (68,85,87). Indeed, homeless individuals are at increased risk for TBI due to a greater tendency towards risk-taking, higher likelihood of being a victim of assault, and a higher chance of antisocial personality disorder (5).

Other studies (7,35) have concluded, however, that TBIs do not correlate with cognitive dysfunction. One plausible explanation for this finding, as the authors of the earlier-mentioned studies have concluded, TBI may be underreported as it is generally discovered by having the population fill out a self-screening test. Because TBI affects memory, a screening tool is not a reliable means to assess impairment. Schmitt et al. (20) confirmed cognitive dysfunction by using MRI and self-reported questionnaires for assessment. The authors noted that self-reported questionnaires alone did not have clinically significant cognitive dysfunction from other individuals; however, MRI findings suggestive of TBI (decreased grey volume or white matter integrity) in addition to positive self-screening questionnaire were significant for cognitive dysfunction in the individuals with TBI (20). Thus, utilizing more diagnostic imaging tools such as MRI may influence future findings.

Dementia

Dementia is a term which is used to describe a persistent cognitive deterioration due to a medical condition such as Alzheimer's disease, Lewy body dementia, frontotemporal lobar degeneration, vascular dementia, Creutzfeldt–Jakob disease, corticobasal degeneration, and others (which include conditions such as Parkinson's disease, Huntington's disease, alcohol dementia, and AIDS-related dementia) (5,88). Dementia is also prevalent in the homeless and can result in impairments in orientation, immediate and short-term memory, attention and calculation, visuoconstruction skills, and praxis (22). Homelessness in particular is associated with early-onset dementia (33) which is significant because early-onset dementia is associated with higher mortality (88). Thus, assessing for dementia in homeless individuals as a factor of their cognitive status is vital to ensure comprehensive diagnosis and treatment. Dementia is discussed in more in detail in another chapter in this volume.

Substance use

In the general population, substance abuse is correlated with cognitive impairment and can have long-term effects on the brain (89). In a 2005 study in Glasgow, UK (90), 82% of homeless participants had a cognitive impairment (utilizing the Addenbrooke's Cognitive Examination) and approximately 21% showed a prevalence of alcohol-related brain damage. Moreover, substance use among street children was independently accounted for as causing a difference in neuropsychological function (91). Though substance abuse is correlated with cognitive impairment and homelessness independently, it is difficult to ascertain how the three factors are related to each other. The research literature is inconsistent here, especially since the choice of substance has variable effect on cognitive impairment. In addition, the severity of addiction when present can have a direct as well as an indirect impact on homelessness, potentially via cognitive impairment. The HOPE HOME study (35) established a correlation between cognitive impairment and the homeless population specifically referring to alcohol use. Another study, which was a 2-year prospective study, followed 149 individuals in the multisite Collaborative Initiative on Chronic Homelessness programme in the US, and found correlations between the type of substance abuse and the number of days of being housed in the previous 90 days. The Addiction Severity Index (ASI) was used to score the severity of substance abuse and type of substance. The results of the study indicate that active stimulant use at baseline predicts worse housing outcomes when compared to non-stimulant drug use over 2 years. Possible reasons for this may include the differences in severity of addiction among stimulant versus non-stimulant users, as demonstrated by higher ASI scores in the stimulant group (92).

In contrast, Stergiopoulos et al. (7) in a recent study concluded that substance use was not associated with cognitive performance. Rather, other factors such as age, education level, speaking a primary language other than English or French, and a history of psychosis were notable for causing variation on cognitive performance (7). Perhaps one explanation for this finding as the authors conclude is that individuals who are substance users require a certain level of cognitive ability to obtain substances.

One interesting finding by Tevendale et al. (93) showed that restraining from substance use was somewhat protective of being homeless. The study followed homeless youth aged 14–24 for 2 years to identify predictors of their housing trajectory. They assessed sheltered status, mental health impairment, substance abuse or dependence, degree of affiliation with family and home, homelessness as a way of life, and economic resources. The three trajectories that were identified were consistently sheltered (41.4%), short-term inconsistently sheltered (20.0%), and long-term inconsistently sheltered groups (38.6%). Certain factors such as being younger, female, non-white, abstaining from substances other than alcohol or cannabis, ability to go home, homelessness for less than 1 year, not receiving entitlement benefits, and lower score of psychological distress were predictive of being consistently sheltered (93). Although this study did not specifically assess cognitive impairment as it impacts the housing trajectory, it underscores the more complex socioeconomic and demographic factors involved in obtaining housing and where further resources are needed.

Future implications

One study in 2015 asked homeless participants: 'Would you like to leave your homeless life?' and those with a cognitive disability were less likely to provide a positive answer to this question which suggests that homeless individuals with cognitive impairment are less likely to accept services. The study concludes that 'one's refusal to eschew their homeless life might not be fully willful; it might be due to an awareness of difficulties related to social adaptation' (94). Thus, cognition appears to play a key role in maintaining the current disposition of homeless individuals which is often ignored in light of more pressing and acute medical issues (32). To address cognition specifically, studies have begun to investigate cognitive skills training both in youth (76) and in adults (95) with an emphasis on social skills training. In order to communicate more effectively with individuals who have a cognitive impairment, one study suggests modifying standard testing tools and adjusting word phrases to be more simplified. Instead of focusing on content, the interviewer should focus more on context and adjust the way a question is asked (96).

Depending on the relative population, more specific measures can be taken to help homeless individuals function better. In a review of geriatric patients, cognitive impairment on the MMSE in one study was significantly associated with poor adherence to medication. Thus, helping individuals utilize skills to aid with memory or interventions to directly assist with medication adherence in this population are specific areas to be targeted (97). The 'Housing First' programme as mentioned earlier in this chapter has been able to help individuals with ID sustain housing and can hopefully be implemented on larger scales. In addition, providing social services and group homes instead of independent housing by itself may provide more stability as individuals with serious mental health will likely need social structure and communal support.

Future longitudinal studies are necessary to show direct causation between cognitive impairment and homelessness. This is equally true regarding risk factors for homelessness and their relationship to a cognitive impairment such as substance use, TBI, ID, malnutrition, and childhood trauma. Future research should include universally accepted diagnostic testing to define cognitive impairment and allow for more homogeneous findings.

References

1. **Braslow JT, Messac L.** Medicalization and demedicalization—a gravely disabled homeless man with psychiatric illness. N Engl J Med. 2018;**379**(20):1885–1888.

2. **Bremner AJ, Duke PJ, Nelson HE, Pantelis C, Barnes TR.** Cognitive function and duration of rooflessness in entrants to a hostel for homeless men. Br J Psychiatry. 1996;**169**(4):434–439.

3. **Muñoz M, Vázquez C, Koegel P, Sanz J, Burnam MA.** Differential patterns of mental disorders among the homeless in Madrid (Spain) and Los Angeles (USA). Soc Psychiatry Psychiatr Epidemiol. 1998;**33**(10):514–520.

4. **Buhrich N, Hodder T, Teesson M.** Prevalence of cognitive impairment among homeless people in inner Sydney. Psychiatr Serv. 2000;**51**(4):520–521.

5. **Backer TE, Howard EA.** Cognitive impairments and the prevention of homelessness: research and practice review. J Prim Prev. 2007;**28**(3–4):375–388.

6. **Joyce DP, Limbos M.** Identification of cognitive impairment and mental illness in elderly homeless men: before and after access to primary health care. Can Fam Physician. 2009;**55**(11):1110–1111.e6.

7. **Stergiopoulos V, Cusi A, Bekele T,** et al. Neurocognitive impairment in a large sample of homeless adults with mental illness. Acta Psychiatr Scand. 2015;**131**(4):256–268.

8. **American Psychiatric Association**. Diagnostic and Statistical Manual of Mental Disorders (5th ed.). Washington, DC: American Psychiatric Association; 2013.

9. **World Health Organization**. The ICD-10 Classification of Mental and Behavioural Disorders. Geneva: World Health Organization; 1992.

10. **Fazel S, Geddes JR, Kushel MJTL.** The health of homeless people in high-income countries: descriptive epidemiology, health consequences, and clinical and policy recommendations. Lancet. 2014;**384**(9953):1529–1540.

11. **Nuechterlein KH, Dawson ME.** Information processing and attentional functioning in the developmental course of schizophrenic disorders. Schizophr Bull. 1984;**10**(2):160–203.

12. **Ancín I, Cabranes JA, Santos JL, Sánchez-Morla E, Barabash A.** Executive deficits: a continuum schizophrenia–bipolar disorder or specific to schizophrenia? J Psychiatr Res. 2013;**47**(11):1564–1571.

13. **Altshuler LL, Ventura J, van Gorp WG, Green MF, Theberge DC, Mintz J.** Neurocognitive function in clinically stable men with bipolar I disorder or schizophrenia and normal control subjects. Biol Psychiatry. 2004;**56**(8):560–569.

14. **Depp CA, Moore DJ, Sitzer D, et al.** Neurocognitive impairment in middle-aged and older adults with bipolar disorder: comparison to schizophrenia and normal comparison subjects. J Affect Disord. 2007;**101**(1–3):201–209.

15. **Ivleva EI, Morris DW, Osuji J, et al.** Cognitive endophenotypes of psychosis within dimension and diagnosis. Psychiatry Res. 2012;**196**(1):38–44.

16. **Simonsen C, Sundet K, Vaskinn A, et al.** Neurocognitive dysfunction in bipolar and schizophrenia spectrum disorders depends on history of psychosis rather than Diagnostic Group. Schizophr Bull. 2011;**37**(1):73–83.

17. **Kuswanto C, Chin R, Sum MY, et al.** Shared and divergent neurocognitive impairments in adult patients with schizophrenia and bipolar disorder: whither the evidence? Neurosci Biobehav Rev. 2016;**61**:66–89.

18. **Edidin JP, Ganim Z, Hunter SJ, Karnik NS.** The mental and physical health of homeless youth: a literature review. Child Psychiatry Hum Dev. 2012;**43**(3):354–375.

19. **Gicas KM, Giesbrecht CJ, Panenka WJ, et al.** Structural brain markers are differentially associated with neurocognitive profiles in socially marginalized people with multimorbid illness. Neuropsychology. 2017;**31**(1):28–43.

20. **Schmitt T, Thornton AE, Rawtaer I, et al.** Traumatic brain injury in a community-based cohort of homeless and vulnerably housed individuals. J Neurotrauma. 2017;**34**(23):3301–3310.

21. **Spence S, Stevens R, Parks R.** Cognitive dysfunction in homeless adults: a systematic review. J R Soc Med. 2004;**97**(8):375–379.

22. **Burra TA, Stergiopoulos V, Rourke SB.** A systematic review of cognitive deficits in homeless adults: implications for service delivery. Can J Psychiatry. 2009;**54**(2):123–133.

23. **Becattini-Oliveira AC, Dutra DF, Spenciere de Oliveira Campos B, de Araujo VC, Charchat-Fichman H.** A systematic review of a functional assessment Tool: UCSD Performance-based Skill Assessment (UPSA). Psychiatry Res. 2018;**267**:12–18.

24. **Nasreddine ZS, Phillips NA, Bédirian V, et al.** The Montreal cognitive assessment, MoCA: a brief screening tool for mild cognitive impairment. J Am Geriatr Soc. 2005;**53**(4):695–699.

25. **Stergiopoulos V, Burra T, Rourke S, Hwang S.** Housing status as an independent predictor of functional capacity in patients with schizophrenia. J Nerv Ment Dis. 2011;**199**(11):854–860.

26. **Depp CA, Vella L, Orff HJ, Twamley EW.** A quantitative review of cognitive functioning in homeless adults. J Nerv Ment Dis. 2015;**203**(2):126–131.

27. **Bousman CA, Twamley EW, Vella L, et al.** Homelessness and neuropsychological impairment: preliminary analysis of adults entering outpatient psychiatric treatment. J Nerv Ment Dis. 2010;**198**(11):790–794.

28. **Ennis N, Roy S, Topolovec-Vranic J.** Memory impairment among people who are homeless: a systematic review. Memory. 2015;**23**(5):695–713.

29. **Cotman A, Sandman.** Cognitive deficits and their remediation in the homeless. J Cogn Rehabil. 1997;**15**(1):16–23.

30. **Rogoz A, Burke D.** Older people experiencing homelessness show marked impairment on tests of frontal lobe function. Int J Geriatr Psychiatry. 2016;**31**(3):240–246.

31. **Lovisi GM, Mann AH, Coutinho E, Morgado AF.** Mental illness in an adult sample admitted to public hostels in the Rio de Janeiro metropolitan area, Brazil. Soc Psychiatry Psychiatr Epidemiol. 2003;**38**(9):493–498.

32. **Solliday-McRoy C, Campbell TC, Melchert TP, Young TJ, Cisler RA.** Neuropsychological functioning of homeless men. J Nerv Ment Dis. 2004;**192**(7):471–478.

33. **Pluck G, Nakakarumai M, Sato Y.** Homelessness and cognitive impairment: an exploratory study in Tokyo, Japan. East Asian Arch Psychiatry. 2015;**25**(3):122–127.

34. **Okamura T, Awata S, Ito K, Takiwaki K, Matoba Y, Niikawa H** et al. Elderly men in Tokyo homeless shelters who are suspected of having cognitive impairment. Psychogeriatrics. 2017;**17**(3):206–207.

35. **Hurstak E, Johnson JK, Tieu L,** et al. Factors associated with cognitive impairment in a cohort of older homeless adults: results from the HOPE HOME study. Drug Alcohol Depend. 2017;**178**:562–570.

36. **Bajaj JS, Riggio O, Allampati S,** et al. Cognitive dysfunction is associated with poor socioeconomic status in patients with cirrhosis: an international multicenter study. Clin Gastroenterol Hepatol. 2013;**11**(11):1511–1516.

37. **Sanger M, Jordan L, Pruthi S,** et al. Cognitive deficits are associated with unemployment in adults with sickle cell anemia. J Clin Exp Neuropsychol. 2016;**38**(6):661–671.

38. **Halleland HB, Sørensen L, Posserud MB, Haavik J, Lundervold AJ.** Occupational status is compromised in adults with ADHD and psychometrically defined executive function deficits. J Atten Disord. 2019;**23**(1):76–86.

39. **Cattie JE, Doyle K, Weber E,** et al. Planning deficits in HIV-associated neurocognitive disorders: component processes, cognitive correlates, and implications for everyday functioning. J Clin Exp Neuropsychol. 2012;**34**(9):906–918.

40. **Weber E, Blackstone K, Iudicello JE,** et al. Neurocognitive deficits are associated with unemployment in chronic methamphetamine users. Drug Alcohol Depend. 2012;**125**(1–2):146–153.

41. **Stergiopoulos V, Dewa C, Durbin J, Chau N, Svoboda T.** Assessing the mental health service needs of the homeless: a level-of-care approach. J Health Care Poor Underserved. 2010;**21**(3):1031–1045.

42. **Llerena K, Gabrielian S, Green MF.** Clinical and cognitive correlates of unsheltered status in homeless persons with psychotic disorders. Schizophr Res. 2018;**197**:421–427.

43. **Bratti I, Bilder R.** Neurocognitive deficits and first-episode schizophrenia; characterization and course. In: **Sharma T, Harvey P** (Ed), The Early Course of Schizophrenia. Oxford: Oxford University Press; 2006:87–110.

44. **Nuechterlein KH, Barch DM, Gold JM, Goldberg TE, Green MF, Heaton RK.** Identification of separable cognitive factors in schizophrenia. Schizophr Res. 2004;**72**(1):29–39.

45. **Saykin AJ, Shtasel DL, Gur RE,** et al. Neuropsychological deficits in neuroleptic naive patients with first-episode schizophrenia. Arch Gen Psychiatry. 1994;**51**(2):124–131.

46. **Gold JM.** Cognitive deficits as treatment targets in schizophrenia. Schizophr Res. 2004;**72**(1):21–28.

47. **Green MF, Kern RS, Braff DL, Mintz J.** Neurocognitive deficits and functional outcome in schizophrenia: are we measuring the 'right stuff'? Schizophr Bull. 2000;**26**(1):119–136.

48. Harvey et al. 1998.

49. **Gold JM, Queern C, Iannone VN, Buchanan RW.** Repeatable battery for the assessment of neuropsychological status as a screening test in schizophrenia I: sensitivity, reliability, and validity. Am J Psychiatry. 1999;**156**(12):1944–1950.

50. **Keefe RS, Poe M, Walker TM, Harvey PD.** The relationship of the brief assessment of cognition in schizophrenia (BACS) to functional capacity and real-world functional outcome. J Clin Exp Neuropsychol. 2006;**28**(2):260–269.

51. **Cuesta MJ, Pino O, Guilera G,** et al. Brief cognitive assessment instruments in schizophrenia and bipolar patients, and healthy control subjects: a comparison study between the Brief Cognitive Assessment Tool for Schizophrenia (B-CATS) and the Screen for Cognitive Impairment in Psychiatry (SCIP). Schizophr Res. 2011;**130**(1–3):137–142.

52. **Yang Z, Abdul Rashid NA, Quek YF,** et al. Montreal Cognitive Assessment as a screening instrument for cognitive impairments in schizophrenia. Schizophr Res. 2018;**199**:58–63.

53. **Culpepper L.** The diagnosis and treatment of bipolar disorder: decision-making in primary care. Prim Care Companion CNS Disord. 2014;**16**(3):PCC.13r01609.

54. **Lima IMM, Peckham AD, Johnson SL.** Cognitive deficits in bipolar disorders: implications for emotion. Clin Psychol Rev. 2018;**59**:126–136.

55. **Osuji IJ, Cullum CM.** Cognition in bipolar disorder. Psychiatr Clin North Am. 2005;**28**(2):427–441.

56. **Sheeran T, Greenberg RL, Davan LA, Dealy JA, Young RC, Bruce ML.** A descriptive study of older bipolar disorder residents living in New York City's adult congregate facilities. Bipolar Disord. 2012;**14**(7):756–763.

57. **Gabrielian S, Bromley E, Hamilton AB,** et al. Problem solving skills and deficits among homeless veterans with serious mental illness. Am J Orthopsychiatry. 2019;**89**(2):287–295.

58. **Alagna E, Santangelo OE, Raia DD, Gianfredi V, Provenzano S, Firenze A.** Health status, diseases and vaccinations of the homeless in the city of Palermo, Italy. Ann Ig. 2019;**31**(1):21–34.

59. **Oakes PM, Davies RC.** Intellectual disability in homeless adults: a prevalence study. J Intellect Disabil. 2008;**12**(4):325–334.

60. **Nishio A, Yamamoto M, Ueki H,** et al. Prevalence of mental illness, intellectual disability, and developmental disability among homeless people in Nagoya, Japan: a case series study. 2015;**69**(9):534–542.

61. **Van Straaten B, Rodenburg G, Van der Laan J, Boersma SN, Wolf JR, Van de Mheen D.** Self-reported care needs of Dutch homeless people with and without a suspected intellectual disability: a 1.5-year follow-up study. Health Soc Care Community. 2017;**25**(1):123–136.

62. **Mercier C, Picard S.** Intellectual disability and homelessness. J Intellect Disabil Res. 2011;**55**(4):441–449.

63. **Durbin A, Lunsky Y, Wang R,** et al. The effect of housing first on housing stability for people with mental illness and low intellectual functioning. Can J Psychiatry. 2018;**63**(11):07067437.

64. **World Health Organization.** Autism spectrum disorders; 2019. Available from: https://www.who.int/news-room/fact-sheets/detail/autism-spectrum-disorders.

65. **Churchard A, Ryder M, Greenhill A, Mandy WJA** 2018. The prevalence of autistic traits in a homeless population. Autism. 2019;**23**(3):665–676.

66. **Oswald DP, Gilles DL, Cannady MS,** et al. Youth with special health care needs: transition to adult health care services. **Matern Child Health J.** 2013;**17**(10):1744–1752.

67. **Watson R, Parr JR, Joyce C, May C, Le Couteur AS.** Models of transitional care for young people with complex health needs: a scoping review. Child Care Health Dev. 2011;**37**(6):780–791.

68. **Stone B, Dowling S, Cameron A.** Cognitive impairment and homelessness: a scoping review. Health Soc Care Community. 2019;**27**(4):e125–e142.

69. **Tilahun D, Hanlon C, Fekadu A, Tekola B, Baheretibeb Y, Hoekstra RA.** Stigma, explanatory models and unmet needs of caregivers of children with developmental disorders in a low-income African country: a cross-sectional facility-based survey. BMC Health Serv Res. 2016;**16**:152.

70. **Pluck G, Lee KH, David R, Macleod DC, Spence SA, Parks RW.** Neurobehavioural and cognitive function is linked to childhood trauma in homeless adults. Br J Clin Psychol. 2011;**50**(1):33–45.

71. **Seidman LJ, Schutt RK, Caplan B, Tolomiczenko GS, Turner WM, Goldfinger SM.** The effect of housing interventions on neuropsychological functioning among homeless persons with mental illness. Psychiatr Serv. 2003;**54**(6):905–908.

72. **Schutt RK, Seidman LJ, Caplan B, Martsinkiv A, Goldfinger SM.** The role of neurocognition and social context in predicting community functioning among formerly homeless seriously mentally ill persons. Schizophr Bull. 2007;**33**(6):1388–1396.

73. **Davidson D, Chrosniak LD, Wanschura P, Flinn JM.** Indications of reduced prefrontal cortical function in chronically homeless adults. Community Ment Health J. 2014;**50**(5):548–552.

74. **Fry CE, Langley K, Shelton KH.** A systematic review of cognitive functioning among young people who have experienced homelessness, foster care, or poverty. Child Neuropsychol. 2017;**23**(8):907–934.

75. **Saperstein AM, Lee S, Ronan EJ, Seeman RS, Medalia A.** Cognitive deficit and mental health in homeless transition-age youth. Pediatrics. 2014;**134**(1):e138–e145.

76. **Medalia A, Saperstein AM, Huang Y, Lee S, Ronan EJ.** Cognitive skills training for homeless transition-age youth: feasibility and pilot efficacy of a community based randomized controlled trial. J Nerv Ment Dis. 2017;**205**(11):859–866.

77. **Yoo J, Kim Y, Cho ER, Jee SH.** Biological age as a useful index to predict seventeen-year survival and mortality in Koreans. BMC Geriatr. 2017;**17**(1):7.

78. **Der G, Allerhand M, Starr JM, Hofer SM, Deary IJ.** Age-related changes in memory and fluid reasoning in a sample of healthy old people. Neuropsychol Dev Cogn B Aging Neuropsychol Cogn. 2010;**17**(1):55–70.

79. **Cohen CI, Teresi JA, Holmes D.** The physical well-being of old homeless men. J Gerontol. 1988;**43**(4):S121–S128.

80. **Cohen CI, Teresi J, Holmes D, Roth E.** Survival strategies of older homeless men. Gerontologist. 1988;**28**(1):58–65.

81. **Brown RT, Hemati K, Riley ED,** et al. Geriatric conditions in a population-based sample of older homeless adults. Gerontologist. 2017;**57**(4):757–766.

82. **Arranz L, de Vicente A, Muñoz M, De la Fuente M.** Impaired immune function in a homeless population with stress-related disorders. Neuroimmunomodulation. 2009;**16**(4):251–260.

83. **Ijaz S, Thorley H, Porter K,** et al. Interventions for preventing or treating malnutrition in homeless problem-drinkers: a systematic review. Int J Equity Health. 2018;**17**(1):8.

84. **Highley JL, Proffitt BJ.** Traumatic Brain Injury Among Homeless Persons: Etiology, Prevalence, and Severity. Nashville, TN: Health Care for the Homeless Clinicians'. Network; 2008.

85. **Topolovec-Vranic J, Ennis N, Colantonio A,** et al. Traumatic brain injury among people who are homeless: a systematic review. BMC Public Health. 2012;**12**(1):1059.

86. **Andersen J, Kot N, Ennis N,** et al. Traumatic brain injury and cognitive impairment in men who are homeless. Disabil Rehabil. 2014;**36**(26):2210–2215.

87. **Mackelprang JL, Harpin SB, Grubenhoff JA, Rivara FPJ.** Adverse outcomes among homeless adolescents and young adults who report a history of traumatic brain injury. Am J Public Health. 2014;**104**(10):1986–1992.

88. **Koedam EL, Pijnenburg YA, Deeg DJ,** et al. Early-onset dementia is associated with higher mortality. Dement Geriatr Cogn Disord. 2008;**26**(2):147–152.

89. **Wilcox CE, Dekonenko CJ, Mayer AR, Bogenschutz MP, Turner JA.** Cognitive control in alcohol use disorder: deficits and clinical relevance. Rev Neurosci. 2014;**25**(1):1–24.

90. **Gilchrist G, Morrison DS.** Prevalence of alcohol related brain damage among homeless hostel dwellers in Glasgow. Eur J Public Health. 2005;**15**(6):587–588.

91. **Pluck G, Banda-Cruz DR, Andrade-Guimaraes MV, Trueba AFJCN.** Socioeconomic deprivation and the development of neuropsychological functions: a study with 'street children' in Ecuador. Child Neuropsychol. 2018;**24**(4):510–523.

92. **Edens EL, Tsai J, Rosenheck RA.** Does stimulant use impair housing outcomes in low-demand supportive housing for chronically homeless adults? Am J Addict. 2014;**23**(3):243–248.

93. **Tevendale HD, Comulada WS, Lightfoot MA.** Finding shelter: two-year housing trajectories among homeless youth. J Adolesc Health. 2011;**49**(6):615–620.

94. **Nishio A, Yamamoto M, Horita R,** et al. Prevalence of mental illness, cognitive disability, and their overlap among the homeless in Nagoya, Japan. PLoS One. 2015;**10**(9):e0138052.

95. **Gabrielian S, Bromley E, Hellemann GS,** et al. Factors affecting exits from homelessness among persons with serious mental illness and substance use disorders. J Clin Psychiatry. 2015;**76**(4):e469–476.

96. **Adair CE, Holland AC, Patterson ML,** et al. Cognitive interviewing methods for questionnaire pre-testing in homeless persons with mental disorders. J Urban Health. 2012;**89**(1):36–52.

97. **Gellad WF, Grenard JL, Marcum ZA.** A systematic review of barriers to medication adherence in the elderly: looking beyond cost and regimen complexity. Am J Geriatr Pharmacother. 2011;**9**(1):11–23.

Chapter 16

Depression in homeless

Luiz Gustavo Maestrelli,
Anderson Sousa Martins da Silva, and
João Mauricio Castaldelli-Maia

Introduction

The definition of a homeless person is a person lacking a fixed, regular, and adequate place to sleep (1). Homeless individuals enter this state due to various conditions, such as financial difficulties due to unemployment, loss of public assistance, illnesses, health expenses, divorce, and others, which can lead these people into difficulties in finding a stable residence (1). Other factors include immigration, drug addiction, loneliness, and loss of social support. In addition, ethnic disparities and the level of formal education are also associated with living on the street. Stigmatized and excluded groups are more likely to become homeless, in particular, those representing ethnic minorities or those who have previously had a mental disorder (2). This population has a higher unemployment rate and a higher risk of being arrested (3).

Health issues

Homeless people present important social and psychological problems. Their mortality rate is much higher than those having fixed housing. In addition, they demonstrate high levels of loneliness, by not having intimate relationships and also feeling marginalized from society. Consequently, they represent a group of people who are much more susceptible to violence and victimization (4). They are, therefore considered to be a particularly vulnerable group (4,5). The health of homeless people differs significantly from those living in fixed homes. Homeless people have an increased incidence of asthma, diabetes, cardiovascular diseases such as hypertension, HIV/AIDS, tuberculosis (1,3), increased risk of hepatitis C (5) and other hepatitis diseases, sexually transmitted diseases, assaults and accidents, dental problems, and mortality than the general population (1).

Moreover, the homeless population is more likely to contract common colds and influenza, in response to the conditions of poor hygiene and housing instability that are experienced. In addition, health impairment is also directly associated with eating habits, with a lack of food prevalent in this type of population, with 45% of those declaring that their food is insufficient, or demonstrating a significant correlation between lack of food and living in the street. Approximately 73% of the homeless have at least one unmet health need, which is six to ten times higher than the general population. The most common cause is the absence of a health plan or the inability to access care (1).

Homeless individuals have more significant difficulties in accessing health systems. Despite the volume of care needed, the homeless population faces numerous factors to receive adequate attention from health services, such as little medication adherence, low links with services and continuity of care, little coordination between different health services, previous negative experiences, prejudice perceived by homeless people, difficulty in accessing prescribed medication, and availability of medication. Early intervention in this group of people has been shown to positively impact the health of homeless people and reduce hospital admissions, also resulting in an overall decrease in costs to the health system (5). The homeless population with mental disorders would benefit from more attention due to insufficient current resources. In addition, more mental services and clinics can help with this problem, as well as the proper treatment of their health (1).

Mental health issues

In addition to being more prone to the occurrence of clinical severe illnesses, homeless people are also at higher risk for the occurrence of various psychiatric illnesses, presenting, in general, with worse mental health and a higher incidence of drug and alcohol use (5). Statistical data indicate that approximately 20–25% of homeless people have psychiatric problems (3,6). High rates of substance abuse, schizophrenia, bipolar disorder, and major depression are found in the homeless group when compared to the general population, in addition to personality disorders (3). Anxiety was reported in 20.5% of the homeless population in the study by Notaro et al. (1). In the homeless population, there is substantial evidence of depression (1,4), reaching values greater than 80% (7).

Living on the street is an unwanted circumstance in life associated with adverse life events and significant stress. Homeless people generally have limited social and personal resources to cope with adverse conditions and circumstances. Consequently, depressive symptoms are prevalent among homeless people. Some depressive symptoms (problems with eating, difficulty sleeping, difficulty in relationships) may reflect the physical circumstances of the homeless people themselves. In addition, the association between depression and homeless people can be understood as evidence of psychological suffering associated with the condition of living on the street. Because of the adversities that homeless people are subjected to, the finding of depression in this population is expected (7).

Risk factors for depression in homeless people include alcoholism, biological factors, gender, experiencing trauma or stressful events, having a severe illness (e.g. cancer, heart disease, HIV/AIDS), smoking, drug addiction, and socioeconomic status (1). While suicidal ideation occurs in approximately 3% of the population annually in the US, the few studies that demonstrate suicidal ideation among homeless people indicate rates that are at least four to five times higher than in the general population (3,7).

Suicidal ideation represents a high state of emotional stress that is seen as one of the biggest indicators of poor adaptation to the precarious state in which the homeless are subjected. While depression may, in fact, be an expected response to a particularly inhuman experience, suicidal ideation is the result of feelings of discouragement and hopelessness, representing an emotional reaction highly linked to the disease. While suicidal ideation is strongly related to depressive symptoms, the chance of being depressed is much greater than having suicidal thoughts. This suggests that the finding of suicidal ideation may be a sensitive measure of the severity of the suffering experienced by the homeless. Suicidal ideation requires early detection and intervention, and an understanding of the circumstances linked to suicidal ideation can serve to improve individual intervention programmes (7). In the general population, women have higher rates of suicidal thoughts when compared to men. This finding is also consistent with the homeless population (3).

People living in shelters may also have higher rates of suicidal ideation and suicide attempts. More than 40% of these adults living in hostels had thoughts of suicide, and 27% of them had tried to kill themselves at some point in their lives. Possibly the majority of these people did not have access to suicide risk prevention therapy. Most studies report that depression is associated with suicidal thoughts in homeless people. In this group, the main predictor of suicidal ideation and suicide attempts is a previous history of suicide attempts. Thus, the literature claims that it is important to verify past attempts to predict the risk of suicide in these populations.

Depression among homeless people

Homeless people are a very vulnerable population, with a much higher rate of morbidity and mortality than the general population. In addition to being more susceptible to the occurrence of serious clinical illnesses, the homeless population is also more likely to have several psychiatric disorders, including depression. Homeless people have difficulty accessing health systems, making it challenging to understand the extent of their pathologies. The high prevalence of depression in this group of people suggests that they do not receive adequate treatment. Early diagnosis of depression in homeless people promotes a significant improvement in the health of these people. The present chapter aims to summarize data on the prevalence and treatment of depression in homeless, who can assist as tools in the recognition and early treatment of depression in this vulnerable population.

Prevalence

Great variability was found in the prevalence of depression in the homeless (10–75%). Two studies showed a prevalence of major depression in the homeless of approximately 75% (8,9), seven studies close to 50% (5,10–15), three studies close to 33% (16,17,18), two studies close to 25% (3,19), seven studies close to 15–20% (1,20–25), and one study close to 10% (26).

Among the 16 remaining studies, seven used the Center for Epidemiologic Studies–Depression (CES-D) scale (which does not provide the diagnosis of depression, but only the probability of it), there were five comparative studies, and the remaining four presented data stratified by socio-demographic variables. Among the seven studies based on the CES-D scale, the results were 77.5% with suggestive depression (27); more than 75% as 'possible depression' and 60% as 'probable depression' (28); more than 72% as 'possible depression' and more than 60% as 'probable depression' (29); more than two-thirds of the sample as 'possible depression' (7); 64% as 'possible depression' at the beginning of the study and the end of the follow-up, dropping to 49% (30); and approximately 63% as 'possible depression' (31). One study had an average scale score of 25.4 at the beginning of the study, declining to 18.91 after the therapeutic intervention (32).

Among the five comparative studies, two of them compared different populations of homeless people. Munõz et al. (33) observed that the prevalence of depression in the last 12 months was 14.9% for the sample of homeless people in Madrid, Spain, and 17.5% for the sample of homeless people in Los Angeles, US, and that the prevalence throughout life was quite similar between the two samples. O'Carrol and O'Reilly (34) identified that the prevalence of depression increased from 35% in 1997 to 51% in 2005, comparing the populations of Dublin homeless people in these years. Lee et al. (27) found that the prevalence of depression was 26.8% throughout life, compared to 2.4% in the general population. In turn, two studies compared the population of homeless people with domiciled control groups. In one of them, the homeless sample showed depression in 70% of cases against only 15% of the control group (35). In the other study, 62% of the sample of homeless people were observed presenting criteria for probable depression, against only 8% of the control group (4).

Three studies showed comparisons of the prevalence of depression between male and female homeless people. Madianos et al. (36), observed that the prevalence of the total sample for depression was 11.1%, 10.1% for men and 13.6% for women. In the study by Stuart and Arboleda-Flórez (37), a prevalence of depression of 46.3% for men and 60% for women was observed. Finally, in the 2018 study by Laporte et al. (2), it was found that 4.5% of the total sample had severe depression, with a rate of 6.2% for women and 3.6% for men. One study obtained data about the prevalence of depression in homeless individuals according to their age group. The age group that most presented depression was 30–39 years (40.68%), followed by that of 40–54 years (35.23%), and then that of 18–29 years (20.02%). The group with the least depression was older than 54 years (4.07%) (38).

Suicidal ideation

Twelve studies reported homeless suicidal ideation data. As in the case of the epidemiology of depression, high rates and great variability was found. The highest prevalence recorded was 66.2% of suicidal ideation throughout life, with 51.3% of the sample registering past suicide attempts, 26% requiring hospitalization, and 8% reporting an attempt in the last 30 days (12). It was observed that 41% of the homeless had suicidal ideation, and 21.6% had previously attempted it (27). In their study, Prigerson et al. (38) found that the prevalence of suicidal ideation and suicide attempts in the last 30 days was 37.5% and 7.9%, respectively. Keogh et al. (5) reported suicidal ideation in 18% of the total sample in the last 6 months, while 9% had attempted suicide in the same period. Fitzpatrick et al. (7) found that 31% of the sample of homeless people reported suicidal ideation, representing ten times more than the general non-homeless population. In another study, suicidal ideation was present in 24.05% for the total sample (14). Coohey et al. (3) found that 17% of the sample had suicidal ideation and that one-third of the total sample had past suicide attempts. Similar results were obtained by Kales et al. (19), who verified that almost one-third of the sample (30.3%) reported suicide attempts during lifetime. In another study, 26.9% presented a history of suicidal attempts (23). The study with the lowest prevalence found only 2% of suicidal ideation in the sample (26). Homeless people who reported a past attempt are eight times more likely to think about suicide than those who have had no previous attempts (3).

Two studies compared the last-month prevalence of suicidal ideation between men and women, reporting mixed findings. Madianos et al. (36) found a prevalence of suicidal ideation of 0.5% for the male sample and 1.5% for the female sample. However, Desai et al. (12) found almost similar rates of suicidal ideation between the sexes (8% in males and 7.8% in females).

Treatment

Some studies have investigated different therapeutic interventions in the treatment of depressive symptoms in homeless people (5,11,30,32). All of them have positive results, but with a variable effect size. Wong and Pilavin (30) investigated whether social resources and housing resources directly affected distress or mediated the impact of stress factors on depressive symptoms. Their findings, however, indicated only modest effects of social resources on psychological distress through direct effects and mediating effects of life stressors on distress (30). Lam and Rosenheck (11) investigated the effects of the famous Access to Community Care and Effective Services and Supports (ACCESS) programme. Samples of homeless people submitted to this programme showed an improvement in depressive symptoms after 12 months of follow-up. An increase in quality of life of 30% was observed in the quality-of-life scale, varying from 3.25 ± 1.7 to 4.23 ± 1.6, in 12 months (11).

An intervention nursing study was tested in homeless people who had been randomized into two groups (waiting/usual care and treatment). At first, the participants had an average on the Beck scale of 25.4. In the end, the remaining 33 had an average of 18.91 (32). The mindfulness technique was tested with a good success rate by homeless patients through weekly sessions. For 9 weeks, each group met weekly for a 2-hour session. In all, nine groups were tested, with 10–15 participants in each group. At the end of the programme, 33 of the 35 depressed patients improved from depressive symptoms. There was an average reduction of 3.45 in the PHQ-9 score for depressive symptoms. In addition to a 35.9% improvement in mental health status, the frequency of suicidal ideation also declined from 24.05% to 12.66% (14). Of the total sample of 105 patients, approximately half were depressed, and of these, nine were using some antidepressant (5).

Discussion

Despite the great variability, the prevalence of depression in adult homeless people was higher than in the general population. If the great vulnerability of this population were not enough to the myriad of clinical conditions, they are still very susceptible to the occurrence of mental disorders, such as depression

(1,3,5,8–26). Based on studies that compared homeless individuals with the general population, it was possible to find a markedly higher prevalence of depression among the former (4,35). These results serve as indicators of how not being domiciled can impact the life of the individual. Women (2,36,37) and adults aged 30–54 years (38) are the most affected.

For instance, suicidal ideation, which is the most severe symptom of depression, was also more common among the homeless. Most of the studies in this research brought general results of suicidal ideation in homeless people. One study found that the prevalence of suicidal ideation was ten times higher than in the general population of non-homeless people (7), including a 66.2% rate of suicidal ideation throughout life in the study conducted by Desai et al. (12). The prevalence of suicide attempts was also generally high, with results reaching up to or near one-third of the sample with attempts throughout life (3,19). Specifically, regarding suicidal ideation in depressive homeless people, a study showed that 10% of the sample of depressive people had suicidal ideation in the last 30 days of the interview (12). When the population of depressed, homeless people was compared with non-depressed ones, depressed people were more likely to think about suicide and also to attempt suicide (27).

All the data shown prove how vulnerable the adult homeless population is to the occurrence of depression and how much it also deserves particular attention from health professionals. Regarding treatment for depressed adult homeless people, little was found in the literature. In fact, no study has provided information regarding the effectiveness of pharmacological treatment in this sample. The therapeutic approach employing the mindfulness technique is promising. It was able to promote significant results, with improvement in depressive symptoms, in mental health status, and with decreased suicidal ideation (14).

We found some studies evaluating the ACCESS programme. This programme was administered by the Homeless Programs Branch of the Center for Mental Health Services. The long-term goal of the ACCESS programme was to foster enduring partnerships that will improve the integration of existing federal, state, local, and voluntary service systems to homeless people with serious mental illness, particularly those with co-occurring alcohol or other substance abuse disorders. The more immediate goal was to identify promising approaches to systems integration and to evaluate their effectiveness in providing services to this population. After 12 months of follow-up, there was an improvement in depressive symptoms and a 30% increase in the quality-of-life scale (11). Significant therapeutic effect in reducing depressive symptoms was also found when approximately more than one-third of the homeless managed to acquire housing after a 12-month follow-up (30), which may represent how much having their own place impacts the mental health of these individuals. Another study also found that out of 52 depressive patients, only nine were using antidepressant medication (5).

The lack of treatment research in this population further reinforces the extent to which they should receive special attention. Although little has been found in the literature, a substantial improvement in the quality of life and reduction in depressive symptoms were demonstrated through the interventions performed. Future studies, with different therapies and also including pharmacological ones, could benefit this population enormously.

Conclusion

Homeless people represent a very vulnerable segment of the population. They are subject to the most diverse clinical and also psychiatric conditions, including depression. According to our review, it is possible to establish that there is a high prevalence of depression in this subpopulation. This is a fact that is reflected in several cities around the world, identifying a global issue. In addition, the homeless also have high suicidal ideation, especially when having depression, further contributing to poor mental health in these individuals. Early diagnosis of depression in homeless people promotes a significant improvement in the health of these individuals. In view of the great vulnerability to which the homeless are subjected, the special therapeutic attention they need is evident. The high prevalence of depression also suggests that this group does not have adequate treatment for this condition. The few intervention studies (e.g. ACCESS programme, nursing interventions, mindfulness) reported positive results in reducing depressive symptoms. Therefore, it seems possible to control depression and to increase the quality of life of homeless individuals affected by depression.

References

1. Notaro, SJ, Khan M, Kim C, Nasaruddin M, Desai K. Analysis of the health status of the homeless clients utilizing a free clinic. J Community Health. 2012;38(1):172–177.

2. Laporte A, Vandentorren S, Détrez M.-A, Douay C, Le Strat Y, Le Méner E. Prevalence of mental disorders and addictions among homeless people in the Greater Paris Area, France. Int J Environ Res Public Health. 2018;15(2):241.

3. Coohey C, Easton SD, Kong J, Bockenstedt JKW. Sources of psychological pain and suicidal thoughts among homeless adults. Suicide Life Threat Behav. 2014;45(3):271–280.

4. Pluck G, Lee KH, Lauder HE, Fox JM, Spence SA, Parks, RW. Time perspective, depression, and substance misuse among the homeless. J Psychol. 2008;142(2):159–168.

5. Keogh C, O'Brien KK, Hoban A, O'Carroll A, Fahey T. Health and use of health services of people who are homeless and at risk of homelessness who receive free primary health care in Dublin. BMC Health Serv Res. 2015;**15**:58.

6. Kales JP, Barone MA, Bixler EO, Miljkovic MM, Kales JD. Mental illness and substance use among sheltered homeless persons in lower-density population areas. Psychiatr Serv. 1995;**46**(6):592–595.

7. Fitzpatrick KM, Irwin J, LaGory M, Ritchey, F. Just thinking about it. J Health Psychol. 2007;**12**(5):750–760.

8. McInnes DK, Petrakis BA, Gifford AL, et al. Retaining homeless veterans in outpatient care: a pilot study of mobile phone text message appointment reminders. Am J Public Health. 2014;**104**(4):588–594.

9. Diblasio FA, Belcher JR. Social work outreach to homeless people and the need to address issues of self-esteem. Health Soc Work. 1993;**18**(4):281–287.

10. O'Toole TP, Johnson EE, Redihan S, Borgia M, Rose J. Needing primary care but not getting it: the role of trust, stigma and organizational obstacles reported by homeless veterans. J Health Care Poor Underserved. 2015;**26**(3):1019–1031.

11. Lam JA, Rosenheck RA. Correlates of improvement in quality of life among homeless persons with serious mental illness. Psychiatr Serv. 2000;**51**(1):116–118.

12. Desai RA, Liu-Mares W, Dausey DJ, Rosenheck RA. Suicidal ideation and suicide attempts in a sample of homeless people with mental illness. J Nerv Ment Dis. 2003;**191**(6):365–371.

13. Chinman MJ, Rosenheck R, Lam JA. The case management relationship and outcomes of homeless persons with serious mental illness. Psychiatr Serv. 2000;**51**(9):1142–1147.

14. Serpa JG, Taylo SL, Tillisch, K. Mindfulness-based stress reduction (MBSR) reduces anxiety, depression, and suicidal ideation in veterans. Med Care. 2014;**52**(12 Suppl 5):19–24.

15. Swabri J, Uzor C, Laird E, O'Carroll A. Health status of the homeless in Dublin: does the mobile health clinic improve access to primary healthcare for its users? Ir J Med Sci. 2019;**188**(2):545–554.

16. Savage CL, Lindsell CJ, Gillespie GL, Dempsey A, Lee RJ, Corbin, A. Health care needs of homeless adults at a nurse-managed clinic. J Community Health Nurs. 2006;**23**(4):225–234.

17. Schanzer B, Dominguez B, Shrout PE, Caton CLM. Homelessness, health status, and health care Use. Am J Public Health. 2007;**97**(3):464–469.

18. Heckert U, Andrade L, Alves MJM, Martins C. Lifetime prevalence of mental disorders among homeless people in a southeast city in Brazil. Eur Arch Psychiatry Clin Neurosci. 1999;**249**(3):150–155.

19. Kales J, Barone M, Bixler E, Miljkovic M. Mental illness and substance use among sheltered homeless persons in lower-density population areas. Psychiatr Serv. 1995;**46**(6):592–595.

20. Kermode M, Crofts N, Miller P, Speed B, Streeton J. Health indicators and risks among people experiencing homelessness in Melbourne, 1995–1996. Aust N Z J Public Health. 1998;**22**(4):464–470.

21. Prinsloo B, Parr C, Fenton J. Mental illness among the homeless: prevalence study in a Dublin homeless hostel. Ir J Psychol Med. 2012;**29**(1):22–26.

22. Goldstein G, Luther JF, Haas GL. Medical, psychiatric and demographic factors associated with suicidal behavior in homeless veterans. Psychiatry Res. 2012;**199**(1):37–43.

23. Sarajlija M, Jugović, A, Zivaljević D, Merdović B, Sarajlija A. An assessment of health status and quality of life of homeless persons in Belgrade, Serbia. Vojnosanit Pregl. 2014;**7**(2):167–174.

24. Rhoades H, Wenzel SL, Golinelli D, Tucker JS, Kennedy DP, Ewing B. Predisposing, enabling and need correlates of mental health treatment utilization among homeless men. Community Ment Health J.2014;**50**(8):943–952.

25. Greenwood RM, Schaefer-McDaniel NJ, Winkel G, Tsemberis SJ. Decreasing psychiatric symptoms by increasing choice in services for adults with histories of homelessness. Am J Community Psychol. 2005;**36**(3–4):223–238.

26. Hamid WA, Wykes T, Stansfeld S. The social disablement of men in hostels for homeless people. Br J Psychiatry. 1995;**166**(6):806–808.

27. Lee KH, Jun JS, Kim YJ, et al. Mental health, substance abuse, and suicide among homeless adults. J Evid Inf Soc Work. 2017;**14**(4):229–242.

28. Fitzpatrick KM. How positive is their future? Assessing the role of optimism and social support in understanding mental health symptomatology among homeless adults. Stress Health. 2016;**33**(2):92–101.

29. Irwin J, LaGory M, Ritchey F, Fitzpatrick K. Social assets and mental distress among the homeless: exploring the roles of social support and other forms of social capital on depression. Soc Sci Med. 2008;**67**(12):1935–1943.

30. Wong YLI, Piliavin I. Stressors, resources, and distress among homeless persons. Soc Sci Med. 2001;**52**(7):1029–1042.

31. Wong YLI. Measurement properties of the Center for Epidemiologic Studies—Depression scale in a homeless population. Psychol Asses. 2000;**12**(1):69–76.

32. Tollett JH, Thomas, SP. A theory-based nursing intervention to instill hope in homeless veterans. Adv Nurs Sc. 1995;**18**(2):76–90.

33. Muñoz M, Vázquez C, Koegel P, Sanz J, Burnam MA. Differential patterns of mental disorders among the homeless in Madrid (Spain) and Los Angeles (USA). Soc Psychiatry Psychiatr Epidemiol. 1998;**33**(10):514–520.

34. O'Carroll A, O'Reilly, F. Health of the homeless in Dublin: has anything changed in the context of Ireland's economic boom? Eur J Public Health. 2008;**18**(5):448–453.

35. D'Amore J, Hung O, Chiang W, Goldfrank L. The epidemiology of the homeless population and its impact on an urban emergency department. Acad Emerg Med. 2001;**8**(11):1051–1055.

36. Madianos MG, Chondraki P, Papadimitriou GN. Prevalence of psychiatric disorders among homeless people in Athens area: a cross-sectional study. Soc Psychiatry Psychiatr Epidemiol. 2013;**48**(8):1225–1234.

37. Stuart H, Arboleda-Flórez J. Homeless shelter users in the postdeinstitutionalization era. Can J Psychiatry. 2000;**45**(1):55–62.

38. Prigerson H, Desai R, Liu-Mares W, Rosenheck R. Suicidal ideation and suicide attempts in homeless mentally ill persons—age-specific risks of substance abuse. Soc Psychiatry Psychiatr Epidemiol. 2003;**38**(4):213–219.

Chapter 17

Mental health and post-traumatic stress disorder in homeless migrants

Erhabor Sunday Idemudia

Introduction

Recently, there has been an upsurge in the number of migrants worldwide and this has become a top priority for development partners and governments (1). Statistics (2) show that the number of international migrants has risen from 173 million in the year 2000 to 258 million in 2017 with Asia and Europe having the largest burden. Similarly, the number of refugees or those forcedly displaced because of violations of human rights, war, violence, and persecution have remained steadily on the increase from an estimate of 40 million in 2007 to almost 70 million in 2017 (3). Although a significant number of refugees move towards developed nations, data have shown that 84% of the world's refugee population are hosted by developing countries (1,3). In Asia, Jordan and Turkey rank high in the list of countries hosting refugees (4,5) because of the war in Syria while Ethiopia, Kenya, and Uganda host the largest refugee population in Africa (5,6). Germany, Sweden, and Serbia are considered to have the largest refugee intakes in Europe (7). The continual Syrian war coupled with political unrests in Iraq, Afghanistan, Libya, Sudan, and Somalia and general economic instability in Africa have resulted in serious refugee and migrant crises for Europe (3,8,9). The statistic of migrants and refugees in both developing and developed nations is predicted to continue to rise in subsequent decades (4,10,11).

While a considerable body of scholarly and policy research exists on homelessness in general, unfortunately, homelessness among migrants and among refugees have been low areas of concern for social science researchers.

Homelessness in general is an evasive concept to define and a topical social problem among social science researchers (12). Homelessness is fluid in nature and so are the factors causing it. For example, Hartshorn (13) identified four types of homelessness: economic (homeless new arrivals of people seeking greener pastures), situational (homelessness due to domestic violence abuse, family conflicts, etc.), chronic (homelessness due to mental illness or substance abuse), and near homelessness (homelessness due to risk of vulnerabilities such as people in psychiatric or correctional facilities). By the nature of vulnerabilities associated with migrations (whether local or international), homelessness is a huge problem for migrants and refugees (14). Homeless migrants fall within the four types of homeless groups previously listed. In the main, many refugees/migrants become homeless as a result of either economic, situational, chronic, or near-homelessness factors.

Many migrants who arrive at their destinations after a perilous journey within or outside Africa using unsafe means, find that the land that was supposed to flow with 'milk and honey' actually flow with hardships, police harassment, racism, imprisonment, daily apprehension of deportation, and other hostile life situations thereby compromising their mental health (15–17). Many of them sleep on the streets irrespective of weather conditions and, in general, are stigmatized by government institutions with no hope of a job and invariably end up living on the streets as homeless. Homelessness has serious implications for mental health and post-traumatic stress disorder (PTSD).

Forceful migration and homelessness are factors that causes PTSD in people. Forceful migration can be as a result of many factors including (but not limited to) civil war, political turmoil, economic hardship, and globalization. Frequently, the reason for migration might be for exploration or for survival (18). Meanwhile, the end result of migration might be different from what was expected or planned for, as people may end up regretting their choice to migrate. Studies have established links between migration and mental health. There are sufficient works in the literature in this area (19).

Aim of chapter

Given that refugees and migrants experience significant amounts of stressors in the migration process and are often vulnerable to many negative conditions, this chapter is aimed at critically reviewing extant literature by exploring how migration processes put refugees and migrants at risk of becoming homeless, traumatized, and developing mental health problems. The outcome of the literature review will inform policymakers in national and international communities of the urgent need to recognize and address the homelessness conditions of migrants and refugees and the impact on their mental health. Refugees should not only be perceived as a source of burdens by host countries and communities but as humans with needs who can also contribute positively to the society. In view of the fact that the migration crisis has become inevitable, focusing attention on the mental well-being of refugees and migrants in the destination country will be beneficial at reducing the perceived burden constituted by this population and making them useful to the social, economic, and political lives of hosting communities.

Methodology

Databases including PubMed, ISI Web, and SCOPUS were searched to obtain articles for this chapter. Articles included were those published in English and indexed mainly from 2014 to 2018. A few notable older references were also included. The search strategy included the use of the following keywords: migrants, refugees, migrants and refugees, homelessness and refugees, stress and trauma among migrants and refugees, PTSD in refuges and migrants, and mental well-being of refugees and migrants. Hand-searching of the referenced list of selected articles from these databases was also done in order to increase the pool of articles of interest. Categories of studies included were original articles, meta-analyses, monographs, reviews, newspaper articles, and conference presentations.

Refugees versus migrants

In this chapter, the terms 'refugees' and 'migrants' are used interchangeably. It is, however, important to distinguish between the two terms. According to the United Nations (20) and FitzGerald and Arar (21), a migrant is usually considered as someone who has left his or her habitual place of residence to move to another area within a state or across an international border irrespective of the (a) legal status of the person, (b) whether the relocation is involuntary or not, (c) length of stay in the hosting country or community, and (d) the causes of the relocation. On the other hand, refugees are individuals who have been forced to 'vote with their feet' from their home country as a result of war, conflict, violence, and fear of persecution or other condition(s) which seriously threaten public order and are associated with potential loss of lives (22).

These definitions imply that while refugees are forced to move out of their countries of origin because of life-threatening dangers due to disturbances in public order, the movement of migrants may result from other factors not associated with such public disorderliness and may be voluntary. Another point of note is that migrants have different categories: international tourists, visitors, students, diplomats, economic migrants, and so on. Sometimes, students, visitors, and tourists may choose not to return to their home countries and consequently become refugees, economic migrants, or even undocumented or 'stateless' persons (17,23).

Refugees and migrants are considered highly vulnerable populations (24). Both of them are faced with many hardships and stressors in their pre-migration and post-migration experiences (25,26). Pre-migration experiences may stem from stressors in their home country such as poverty, political instability, and armed conflicts which initiated the drive for migration (27).

During post-migration experiences in the host country, migrants and refugees are exposed to humiliations and excessive force from agencies and law enforcement (28,29); lack access to support networks; have problems with obtaining legal status marked by non-issuance of work permits, non-acceptance of refugee documentation, unexpected mandatory displacement, and restriction to refugee camps; and are often faced with xenophobia, stigmatization, and discrimination (1,30). In addition, they may experience quickened return to their home countries without adequate safety or protection from host communities (11) as reflected in the deal made by the European Union (EU) with Turkey in early 2016, aimed at restricting the huge influx of migrants and refugees into the borders of the EU. In the deal, it was agreed that all new refugees and migrants transiting from Turkey to the Greek Islands later than March 2016 would be repatriated to Turkey if they did not gain entrance through asylum or if their asylum applications were not admissible in the EU (28,31). In April 2016, an agreement was made for the resettlement and deportation of migrants and refugees within the EU (32).

In recognition of the enormities of these problems, the United Nations General Assembly in 2016 at its 'Summit for Refugees and Migrants' adopted the 'New York Declaration for Refugees and Migrants' which was aimed at strengthening and facilitating an urgent response to the movement of refugees and providing sustaining support to increase the resilience of refugees and their host communities through provision of humanitarian funding and setting up a comprehensive refugee response framework (33).

Homelessness and migration

Going by the dictates of both the Universal Declaration of Human Rights and the International Covenant of Economic, Social and Cultural Rights, it is clearly recognized that the right to housing is a fundamental human right which is applicable to individuals irrespective of legal status or nationality (34). According to Bassuk and Olivet (35), homelessness is a demanding public health issue without a definite solution.

In every society, there is always intense competition for scarce housing resources for many vulnerable groups such as elderly people, young people, homeless individuals, physically and mentally impaired individuals, migrants, and refugees (31). In best international migration practices, housing ranks as one of the best indicators of a successful immigration and resettlement programme. The function of housing goes beyond meeting migrants' physical needs, helping them to re-establish connections with family, friends, and communities, which in general has a significant bearing on securing employment and having access to healthcare and education (35–37). However, considerable evidence suggests that housing and accommodation problems are major concerns among migrants, refugees, and asylum seekers (36,37).

The homelessness problem of migrants does not begin in host communities but in transit from the country of origin. For example, it is noted that Zimbabwean migrants transiting to South Africa are forced to live in precarious circumstances such as uncompleted or abandoned buildings, fields, bushes, and open spaces with limited or no access to hygienic meals and drinks, and sanitary facilities (38). The same observations are made concerning sub-Saharan migrants transiting to Europe through Morocco (17,39).

Among EU countries, accommodation systems for refugees and asylum seekers vary noticeably. Though some countries have developed efficient accommodation systems, others have poor and inadequate housing arrangements which often put refugees at potential risk of becoming homeless (31). The inadequate provision of housing is attributed to the upsurge in the number of refugees who migrated to Europe in the years 2015 and 2016 and the delay in processing of applications of asylum seekers (31). The strain on available housing facilities has contributed to the shortage and substandard accommodation systems. For example, in some areas in Italy, it was reported that the level of accommodation for refugees was below that required for good living conditions thereby exposing residents to insect infestation, poor hygiene, overcrowding, and dampness (40). Out of the 13,197 refugees who lodged applications in Greece in 2015, only 3786 were accommodated in its reception facilities (41).

Almost the same conditions have been reported in Hungary where about 10,000 refugees were transported by open trains to other locations outside the country accompanied with aid (such as food, clothing, and sanitary products) from charitable organizations and volunteers (42). In other places like Germany and Denmark, refugees take shelter in concert halls, tents, factory spaces, and sport halls at reception when existing facilities are overcrowded. This is often viewed as a deliberate attempt to dissuade migrants from entry, rather than resulting from actual overwhelming of existing systems (31).

Where asylum or refugee status is granted, refugees in countries such as Finland, Sweden, and Hungary are expected to seek social or private accommodation facilities by themselves with little assistance from authorities. In a study (37) carried out to understand the current housing situation of refugees and migrants who have lived in Australia on average for more than 2 years, it was found that 90% of respondents lived in non-stable accommodation out of which 83% live in transitional facilities made available by support services while one respondent was reported to be sleeping rough. In other countries like Greece and Italy, it is almost the sole responsibility of refugees and migrants to source their own accommodation (31). Apart from competing for scarce housing resources with citizens, refugees who have gained legal status further experience housing affordability problems compounded with poor job status. For example, in Francis and Hiebert's study (43), almost 85% of refugee households pay more than 30% of their monthly income on rent. The inability to get affordable housing constrains refugees to overcrowded accommodations thereby predisposing them to a form of secondary homelessness (37).

However, in situations where asylum applications are denied, refugees are temporally accommodated until they are repatriated. Those whose applications have been turned down (depending on the functioning of the system) vanish from temporary abodes and make it into the general population as undocumented migrants. Given that they lack legal status, undocumented migrants are economically and socially disadvantaged as they find it difficult to secure employment, housing, healthcare, and welfare benefits (15,31). It is on record that some countries within the EU prevent undocumented immigrants from gaining access to even emergency housing and publicly funded homeless services (34). Since residency status is linked to legal status, undocumented migrants including women and children are vulnerable to an increased danger of street homelessness (34). The homelessness problem may not be limited to undocumented migrants but also to non-European migrants who have legal status in Europe. As noted by Juul (44), homelessness is reportedly experienced by migrants of West African origin who have resided in southern Europe for many years but decided to move northwards due to economic recessions; despite being legal Schengen residents, they are denied work permits and live in homeless shelters.

Stress, trauma, and migration

In general, human migration is attributed to chronic stressors people experience in their homelands and host communities (26). For refugees, these stressors often become so unbearable and life-threatening that they 'vote with their feet' and are forced to transit from their abode to safe lands. Stress and trauma experienced by refugees are usually categorized into three stages of the migration process, namely pre-migration, mid-migration, and post-migration stress (8,25,26). Similarly, in Hollifield et al.'s study (45), stress among refugees was categorized as non-war and non-migration stress, war-related stress, and post-migration stress.

Wars and violence in countries of origin remain the primary pre-migration experiences that drive refugee migration (45,46). Unending wars and violence produce other stressors such as witnessing violent deaths of family and friends, state persecution, imprisonment, sexual assault, rape, torture, economic recession, poverty, hunger, food and water shortages, and other social menaces which usually are hallmarks of post-traumatic stress symptoms which plausibly can lead to PTSD (47).

Recently, studies have been carried out to understand the prevalence of stressors and traumas experienced by refugees and migrants before leaving their home country. For example, Castaneda et al. (48) established the prevalence of potentially traumatic experiences (PTEs) among Kurdish, Somali, and Russian migrants. They found that the experience of war and being eye-witnesses to violent deaths were common among Kurdish (61% and 56%, respectively) and Somali migrants (40% and 41%, respectively). For Russian migrants, the most prevalent categories of PTEs were being victims of physical assaults (10%) and witnessing pugnacious injuries or deaths (10%). These prevalence figures suggest that PTEs are common in Kurds and Somali migrants.

In another study, Mhlongo et al. (49) established the prevalence of traumatic life events among mixed female refugees and migrants who were nationals of Rwanda, DR Congo, Zimbabwe, Burundi, Mozambique, Malawi, Uganda, and Ghana. With migrants from Zimbabwe (44.59%) and DR Congo (38.85%) constituting the majority of the study sample, they found that about 72.26% had witnessed the sudden death of loved ones, 77.07% had experienced physical and sexual assault, while 49.68% had undergone combat trauma. However, no specific data were provided for specific subgroups.

Sigvardsdotter et al. (50) in a systematic review of 42 articles examined the prevalence of torture- and war-associated PTEs among refugees. Some prevalences of war-related stressors found in the study include close to being killed (90%), sudden death of loved ones (80%), experienced events associated with residing in a war-prone region (74%), experienced shooting and bombing (90%), loss of property (50%), death threats (45%), being forced to separate from family members (44%), and imprisonment (15%). The study further established that experience of torture reached a maximum of 76% with a median of 27% and was common among men and older age categories. About 70–80% of cases reported lack of food, water, shelter, sanitary facilities, and residing in refugee camps.

Tinghög et al. (51) in a cross-sectional survey reported similar prevalence for Syrian refugees resettled in Sweden since 2011. The experience of war at a close range was the most common (85%) followed by being exposed to other life-threatening circumstances (79%). Also, many had witnessed physical assaults (63%), torture (31%), forced to separate from family and friends (67.9%) while 7% had experienced sexual assaults. Reports of PTEs among Syrian Kurdish refugees in Iraq detailed rates of 41.76% for experiencing torture, 86.8% for being forced to run away from home land, 64.8% had witnessed burning, shelling, or destruction of residential buildings, while 61.5% were restricted to their homes because of violence and chaos outside.

For Zimbabwean migrants in South Africa, prevalences of pre-migration stressors include physical assaults and harassments (58.4%), near-death experiences (57.6%), personal death threat (61.6%), death threat to family members (48%), hunger (72.8%), lack of employment (80.8%), and so on (25).

Refugees; experiences of PTEs do not end at the pre-migration period but may persist through the mid-migration process to the post-migration phase. In transit, refugees face ordeals in the routes taken in transiting or crossing to the country of refuge which include travelling through multiple countries, being molested and abused by armed bandits and smugglers/traffickers, deprived of food, water, and shelter, and exposed to trauma, disease, and harsh weather conditions (52). In addition, some of these routes are very dangerous and perilous leading to death of migrants as it is commonly recorded at the Balkans and the central Mediterranean routes (3).

There is also substantial evidence for post-migration stressors among refugees and migrants. Among resettled Kurdish and Vietnamese refugees in the US, Hollifield et al. (45) reported prevalence rates for an array of post-migration stressors. The stressors with alarming prevalence include fears and worries about family members left in the home country (67%), the inability to return home during an emergency (60%), social isolation (48%), communication problems (43%), poor access to medical care (34%), delay in the application process (31%), and bad job conditions (30%). Analogously in Tinghög et al.'s study in Sweden (51), missing the social life in their home country (64.1%), feeling separated from family members (49.8%), and communicating in Swedish accounted for the highest prevalence rates for post-migration stress. Apart from the report of being forced to separate from family members (76.8%), Zimbabwean migrants in South Africa further indicated unemployment (83.2%), homelessness (80%), poverty (72.5%), and refugee documentation problems as part of post-migration stress (25). The most common types of post-migration stressors among migrants in Australia were adverse social adaptation (64%), problems with finances (59%), concern for family back home (49%), and feeling lonely (18%) (53).

Spillera et al. (54) further reported substantially higher prevalence rates for pre-migration and post-migration stressors as compared to other studies among mixed refugees from Turkey, Iran, Sri Lanka, Iraq, and Bosnia seeking outpatient treatment in two psychiatric settings in Switzerland: torture (85%), imprisonment (76.9%), assault by strangers (75.4%), experience of combat situation (75.4%), being close to death (73.1%), and killing of a family member or friend (64.9%) ranked very high among the other pre-migration trauma types examined. Post-migration stressors include loneliness and boredom (84.3%), concern about families back home (80.6%), difficulty in learning the language of the host country (73.1%), fear of being sent back home (61.2%), difficulty with accommodation (56%), financial problems (56%), and discrimination (47%).

In Völkl-Kernstock et al.'s report (55), community violence (78%), interpersonal violence (73%), war and political violence (71%), and witnessing homicides (46%) were the most prevalent trauma exposures among unaccompanied African refugee children. In a review by Li et al. (56), housing, financial, unemployment, and underemployment problems were identified as post-migration socioeconomic stressors experienced by refugees in the host countries. Other problems included discrimination and stigmatization, delays in processing asylums, temporary visa status, and cumbersome and unfriendly immigration laws of the receiving country. As a result of unfavourable immigration policies, migrants continue to be in constant fear of being either deported or detained and getting separated from their children. During the period of immigration enforcements, immigrants are always afraid of visiting public places, taking children for medical visits, and even driving a car (57).

Migration and post-traumatic stress disorder

PTSD is a deep emotional wound caused to an individual as a result of exposure to threatening or traumatic events which are perceived to be severe or extraordinary. These events pose threats when they become overwhelming and the individual resources can no longer cope. PTSD can be seen as a normal response to situations that are contrary to normal when the symptoms (physical, mental, and emotional) also move beyond the realm of normalcy with clear evidence of needs for assistance. These people may complain of being brushed aside, torn apart, devastated, used, worn out, and dead inside among others (58).

PTSD was introduced to the *Diagnostic and Statistical Manual of Mental Disorders* as an anxiety disorder in 1980 (58). The causes of this anxiety disorder are multifarious and Schiraldi (58) categorized them as intentional human, unintentional human, and natural disasters. Intentional human acts include combats, civil war, sexual abuse, emotional abuse, physical abuse, terrorist acts, criminal assault, cult abuse, kidnapping, being held hostage, exposure to homicide, death threats, forceful migration, and so on. Unintentional human acts include industrial accidents, motor vehicle accidents, plane crash, explosion, nuclear disaster, surgical damage to the body, building collapse, and so on. Natural disasters include earthquake, hurricane, flood, draught, fire, life-threatening illness, among others (58).

PTSD is therefore, a disorder of trauma and stress in which the affected individual continually experiences fear and other associated symptoms after being exposed to psychologically traumatizing events such as combat, a disaster, victimization, and abuse (59). According to the *Diagnostic and Statistical Manual of Mental Disorders* (60), the fear associated with PTSD could be so intensely debilitating as to make the individual re-experience the traumatic event through persistent nightmares, thoughts, and memory; reoccurring avoidance of stimuli connected to the trauma; numbness or psychological detachment from stimuli that once evoked pleasurable feelings; and increased level of arousal causing hyper-alertness to both internal and external stimuli. Some may feel extreme anger, guilt, anxiety, and depression because they survived the traumatic event while others with the same experience did not (61).

PTSD is not age bound and distresses associated with it significantly impair both personal and social functions (62,63). However, PTSD tends to vary according to sex where females are at least twice as likely to develop PTSD compared to males (14,64,65). Untreated PTSD has been shown to have debilitating consequence characterized by higher comorbidity rates. Individuals with PTSD have greater levels of major depressive disorder, substance use disorder, psychiatric hospitalizations, suicidal ideation, and lower mental health functioning (66). PTSD is also largely associated with anxiety and moderately related with somatic symptoms (67).

Research has consistently shown that one of the most common forms of mental disorder diagnosed among refugees is PTSD when compared to the general population (51,56,68). Along with other mental disorders, the prevalence of PTSD was about 29.9% in Syrian refugees (51). A higher rate (43.7%) was obtained for another sample of Syrian refugees taking shelter in North Lebanon (69). Using two versions of the Harvard Trauma Questionnaire (HTQ-Arab Version), Ibrahim and Hassan (70) obtained 35.16% and 38.46% prevalence rates for PTSD among Syrian Kurdish in Iraq. Almost the same prevalence figure (31%) was also reported for a mixed population of Asian and African migrants in Australia (53). In a systematic review of 29 studies, Bogic et al. (68) found prevalence rates ranging from 4.4% to 86% for PTSD among war refugees with women and older adults as the most vulnerable group. Among Yazidi refugee children and adolescents resettled in Turkey, Nasıroğlu and Çeri (71) detected a prevalence of 36% for PTSD, ranking high above depression (32.7%), nocturnal enuresis (10.9%), and anxiety (7.3%). Other works on unaccompanied refugee minors in Austria majorly from Gambia, Somalia, and Nigeria reported 17% and 29.3% respectively for full and partial criteria for PTSD (55). In a scoping review of PTSD among refugee women in Mali, Burkina Faso, Somalia, and Rwanda, Workney (72) reported prevalence rates ranging between 27.3% and 61.8% for both men and women with men having seemingly higher rates.

PTSD is shown to be strongly predicted by PTEs before, during, and after the migration process as compared to other mental disorders (68). Hollifield et al. (45) likewise demonstrated that non-war and non-migration trauma, war-related trauma, and post-migration stress were more associated with PTSD than depression and anxiety disorders in Kurdish and Vietnamese refugees. In a study carried out only with a Kurdish sample, traumatic events and torture had moderate bivariate correlations with PTSD symptoms (70). Both PTEs and post-migration stressors were moderately and positively correlated among mixed refugees in psychiatric settings in Switzerland (54). Findings from Chen et al. (53) also suggested that a number of pre-migration PTEs were positively related with PTSD. Other post-migration stressors (such as loneliness, financial stressors, being discriminated against, and feeling disturbed about loved ones in the home country) with the exception of stressors associated with the asylum process all predicted PTSD. In a longitudinal study by Bryant et al. (73), evidence was also obtained for the effect of traumas and post-migration problems on subsequent diagnoses of PTSD among refugee parents and their children in Australia. However, findings from Idemudia et al.'s study (38) revealed that only post-migration stressors such as poverty, sex abuse, and total stress were the actual predictors of PTSD among Zimbabwean refugees in South Africa and not pre-migration stressors.

Migration and general mental health of refugees

Aside from the array of studies establishing the effects of pre- and post-migration stressors on PTSD, findings also inform us of the same pattern in other mental illnesses (53). In a qualitative study among West African immigrants in the US, Akinsulure-Smith (74) indicated that participants reported higher levels of mental distress which were mainly related with immigration status problem and cultural/racial discrimination. In a systematic review comparing the mental status of immigrants and the indigenous population, Bas-Sarmiento et al. (75) found higher prevalence rates of mental disorder (especially for anxiety, depression, and somatic problems) among immigrant population in 13 out of 21 studies reviewed. Similarly, in a literature review limited to immigrants in Sweden, increased risks of depression, anxiety, suicide, paranoia, and other psychotic symptoms were reported among immigrants compared to native Swedes (76). Likewise, in other reviews, migration has also been linked with mental health problems such as psychosis, addictive disorders, affective disorders, and suicide attempts especially among young migrant women (77). Some other studies and reviews have established prevalence rates for these disorders, and the rates seem to be quite high. For instance, in a review of 29 studies with an aggregate sample size of 16,010 war-traumatized refugees, Bogic et al. (68) found high prevalence rates of 80% for depression and 88% for uncategorized anxiety disorders. According to these authors, these disorders were consistently predicted by both pre-migration trauma and post-migration stressors.

In a study using the first wave of data from a survey of migrants in Australia, Chen et al. (53) reported a 16% prevalence rate for severe mental illness which was found to be associated with pre-migration PTEs and post-migration stressors. In addition, it was reported that both loneliness and social integration stressors moderated the relationship between pre-migration PTEs and mental illness.

In a systematic and narrative review, Close et al. (78) compared first-generation migrants and refugees and asylum seekers with the general population and asylum seekers/refugees were found to have higher PTSD prevalence rates (9–36%) as compared to the general population (1–2%). The study (78) also demonstrated prevalence rates of mental health problems ranging between 5% and 44% for the migrant/refugee group and 8–12% for the general population.

Pannetiera (79) found a 24% prevalence rate of anxiety and depression in women while 18% was reported for men in a study conducted among migrants of sub-Saharan African origin resettled in Paris. Fleeing the home country because of a threat to life and problems with legal status were strongly associated with mental health problems for women and men respectively.

African migrants and refugees in Durban, South Africa, also showed elevated mental distress onset due to separation from family since migration and feeling discriminated against in the host country (80). In the study, the prevalence of mental burden was high, reported as 54.6% for depression, 49.4% for anxiety, and 24.9% for post-traumatic stress symptoms. Adolescents and children of refugees and migrants have also been shown to suffer from ill mental health. Honkanen (81) reported in a review that child and adolescent refugees suffer from three major mental health problems, namely depressive symptoms (15–45%), PTSD (31–66%), and anxiety disorders (16–50%). Gilliver et al.'s review

(76) reported that diagnosis of other disorders such as autism spectrum disorders, attention deficit hyperactivity disorder, and oppositional defiant disorder in children born to foreign parents were higher compared with natives. Another study showed that the trauma history of the caregiver and post-migration stressors indirectly predict increased hyperactivity, emotional symptoms, peer problems, and conduct problems of children through caregiver PTSD and insensitive parenting (73).

Discussion

This chapter was aimed at documenting and reviewing current literature on homelessness, mental health problems, and PTSD in refugees and migrants. The findings obtained from the studies reviewed overwhelmingly demonstrate that the migration experience constitutes a serious burden to refugee and migrant individuals. It is clearly demonstrated that refugees are a high-risk and vulnerable group considering the stressors they are exposed to during the migration process (24). Principally, the sources of these stressors are classified into three stages which include the pre-migration, mid-migration, and the post-migration periods (26,38). Each of these stages presents a significant amount of distress to refugees which overwhelm their resources to cope. In the pre-migration period, violence and wars account for the main reason why refugees flee from their home country (8,45). In many instances, refugees were exposed to bombing, shooting, physical assaults, near-death experiences, and witnessed the death of family members and loved ones (48,50). During border crossings, refugees also face the risks of abuse from smugglers and bandits, and experience hunger, disease, adverse weather conditions, and even deaths (16,52). The most common post-migration stressors were fears and worries about family members left in the home country, loneliness, accommodation problems, low job status, and legal status difficulties (38,45).

It was further demonstrated that there was a high prevalence (27.3–86%) of PTSD among refugees and migrants. Both pre-migration and post-migration stressors were shown to predict PTSD (53,73). Other mental disorders common among migrants are depression and anxiety and these are associated with both pre-migration and post-migration stressors (53,68). Studies also suggested that homelessness is a major problem faced by migrants at both reception and post-migration periods in host countries. As a result of a huge influx of refugees, accommodating refugees constitutes a major burden to host countries at reception. In some countries, refugees are left to take shelter in unsafe places and are often placed in crowded accommodation which poses risks for their physical and mental well-being. Studies further showed that the homelessness problem does not end for refugees even after being granted asylum status. Refugees source for their own accommodation with little or no assistance from the authority of the host country (31). Unfortunately, they settle for substandard housing because of the problem of affordability, thus forcing them to experience secondary homelessness (37).

Conclusion

By reviewing recent studies, this chapter has demonstrated that homelessness and mental health problems are common in refugees and migrants and are majorly precipitated by pre-migration, mid-migration, and post-migration stressors. The implication is that there is an urgent need for host countries to provide comprehensive mental health services for this vulnerable group in order to mitigate the exacerbation of psychological disorders. This will help host countries to benefit from positive aspects of migration and avert the looming burdens that untreated mental illness among refugees and migrants may cause to future social, political, and economic lives. Prospective studies in this area may expand knowledge about the mental health of refugees in Africa as recent studies carried out within the continent are few and scanty.

References

1. **United Nations Conference on Trade and Development**. Policy guide on entrepreneurship for migrants and refugees. 2018. Available from: https://unctad.org/en/PublicationsLibrary/diae2018d2_en.pdf.
2. **United Nations.** International migration report: 2017 highlights. 2017. Available from: http://www.un.org/en/development/desa/population/migration/publications/migrationreport/docs/MigrationReport2017_Highlights.pdf.
3. **United Nations High Commission for Refugees**. Global trends: forced displacement in 2017. 2018. Available from: https://www.unhcr.org/5b27be547.pdf.
4. **United Nations High Commission for Refugees**. The global compact on refugees. 2018. Available from: https://www.unhcr.org/5b3295167.pdf.
5. **Aljazeera News.** Ten countries host half of world's refugees: report. 2016. Available from: https://www.aljazeera.com/news/2016/10/4/ten-countries-host-half-of-worlds-refugees-report.
6. **WordAtlas.** Countries with the largest refugee populations: 2015 report. Available from: https://www.worldatlas.com/articles/countries-hosting-the-largest-number-of-refugees-in-the-world.html.
7. **Vox.** The European countries that take in the most refugees, in one interactive map. 2015. Available from: https://www.vox.com/world/2015/11/22/9772160/europe-syrian-refugees.
8. **Abbott A.** The mental-health crisis among migrants. Nature. 2016;**538**(7624):158.

9. **Lemmens P, Dupont H, Roosen I.** Migrants, asylum seekers and refugees: an overview of the literature relating to drug use and access to services. 2017. Available from: https://www.emcdda.europa.eu/system/files/attachments/6341/EuropeanResponsesGuide2017_BackgroundPaper-Migrants-Asylum-seekers-Refugees-Drug-use.pdf.

10. **International Organization of Migration.** World migration report 2018. 2018. Available from: https://publications.iom.int/system/files/pdf/wmr_2018_en.pdf.

11. **United Nations High Commissioner for Refugees.** Global trends: forced displacement in 2016. 2016. Available from: http://www.unhcr.org/statistics/unhcrstats/5943e8a34/globaltrends-forceddisplacement-2016.html.

12. **Idemudia ES.** Personality and criminal outcomes of homeless youth in a Nigerian jail population: results of PDS and MAACL-H assessments. J Child Adolesc Ment Health. 2007;**19**(2):137–145.

13. **Hartshorn TA.** Interpreting the City: An Urban Geography (2nd ed). New York: John Wiley; 1992.

14. **Idemudia ES, William JK, Boehnke K, Wyatt G.** Gender differences in trauma and posttraumatic stress symptoms among displaced Zimbabweans in South Africa. J Trauma Stress Disord Treat. 2013;**2**(3):1340.

15. **Idemudia ES.** Associations between demographic factors and perceived acculturative stress among African migrants in Germany. Afr Popul Stud. 2014;**28**(1):449–462.

16. **Idemudia ES.** Displaced, homeless and abused: the dynamics of gender-based sexual and physical abuses of homeless Zimbabweans in South Africa. Gender Behav. 2014;**12**(2):6312–6316.

17. **Idemudia ES, Boehnke K.** I'm an Alien in Deutschland: A Quantitative Mental Health Case Study of African Immigrants in Germany. Frankfurt: Peter Lang Publishers; 2010.

18. **Bhugra D, Gupta S** (Eds). Migration and Mental Health. Cambridge: Cambridge University Press; 2011.

19. **Giacco D, Laxhman N, Priebe S.** Prevalence of and risk factors for mental disorders in refugees. Semin Cell Dev Biol. 2018;**77**:144–152.

20. **United Nations.** Global compact for safe, orderly and regular migration (zero draft). 2018. Available from: https://refugeesmigrants.un.org/sites/default/files/180205_gcm_zero_draft_final.pdf.

21. **FitzGerald DS, Arar R.** The sociology of refugee migration. Annu Rev Sociol. 2018;**44**:387–406.

22. **United Nations High Commission for Refugees.** What is a refugee? Available from: https://www.unhcr.org/what-is-a-refugee.html.

23. **Idemudiai ES.** Perceived living conditions and reported feelings of wellbeing among Africans in Germany. Gender Behav. 2009;**7**(2):2541–2556.

24. **Meyer-Weitz A, Asante KO, Lukobeka BJ.** Healthcare service delivery to refugee children from the Democratic Republic of Congo living in Durban, South Africa: a caregivers' perspective. BMC Med. 2018;**16**(1):163.

25. **Idemudia ES, Williams JK, Madu SN, Wyatt GE.** Trauma exposures and posttraumatic stress among Zimbabwean refugees in South Africa. Life Sci J. 2013;**10**(3):349.

26. **Bustamante LH, Cerqueira RO, Leclerc E, Brietzke E.** Stress, trauma, and posttraumatic stress disorder in migrants: a comprehensive review. Braz J Psychiat. 2018;**40**(2):220–225.

27. **Schouler-Ocak M, Wintrob R, Moussaoui D, Villasenor Bayardo SJ, Zhao X-D, Kastrup MC.** Background paper on the needs of migrant, refugee and asylum seeker patients around the globe. Int J Cult Ment Health. 2016;9(3):216–232.

28. **The European Union Agency for Fundamental Rights.** Monthly data collection on the current migration situation in the EU, February 2016 monthly report. 2016. Available from: http://fra.europa.eu/sites/default/files/fra_uploads/fra-2016-monthly-compilat ion-com-update-3_en.pdf.

29. **Amnesty International.** Hotspot Italy: how EU's flagship approach leads to violations of refugee and migrant rights. 2016. Available from: https://www.amnesty.org/en/docume nts/eur30/5004/2016/en/.

30. **Idemudia ES.** Perceived racism and mental health of African male and female migrants in Germany. Gender Behav. 2008;6(2):1702–1719.

31. **Baptista I, Benjaminsen L, Geertsema V, Pleace N, Striano M.** Asylum seekers, refugees and homelessness: the humanitarian crisis and the homelessness sector in Europe. Research report. FEANTSA; 2016. Available from: http://eprints.whiterose. ac.uk/111072/.

32. **Konstantinidis A.** EU resettled some 15,000 refugees out of a planned 160,000. 2017. Available from: https://www.rt.com/news/376753-eu-refugee-resettlement-plan/.

33. **United Nations High Commission for Refugees.** New York Declaration for Refugees and Migrants. Answers to Frequently Asked Questions 2018. Available from: https:// www.unhcr.org/new-york-declaration-for-refugees-and-migrants.html.

34. **Geddie E, Schmidt-Hieber E, Keith L, LeVoy M.** Housing and homelessness of undocumented migrants in Europe: developing strategies and good practices to ensure access to housing and shelter. Platform for International Cooperation on Undocumented Migrants; 2016. Available from: http://picum.org/Documents/Publi/ 2014/Annual_Conference_2013_report_HOUSING_EN.pdf.

35. **Bassuk EL, Olivet J.** The trauma of homelessness. Center for Social Innovation; 2016. Available from: https://www.masspartnership.com/pdf/TraumaofHomelessne ss6-22-16.pdf.

36. **Allsopp J, Sigona N, Phillimore J.** Poverty among refugees and asylum seekers in the UK: an evidence and policy review. IRIS Working Paper Series, NO. 1/2014. University of Birmingham; 2014. Available from: https://www.birmingham.ac.uk/Documents/coll ege-social-sciences/social-policy/iris/2014/working-paper-series/IRiS-WP-1-2014.pdf.

37. **Flatau P, Smith J, Carson G, Miller J, Burvill A, Brand R.** The housing and homelessness journeys of refugees in Australia. Final report no. 256. Australian Housing and Urban Research Institute; 2015. Available from: https://www.ahuri.edu. au/__data/assets/pdf_file/0026/5759/AHURI_Final_Report_No256_The-housing-and-homelessness-journeys-of-refugees-in-Australia.pdf.

38. **Idemudia ES.** Trauma and PTSS of Zimbabwean refugees in South Africa: a summary of published studies. Psychol Trauma. 2017;9(3):252–257.

39. **United Nations High Commissioner for Refugees.** Global trends: forced displacement in 2016. 2016. Available from: http://www.unhcr.org/statistics/unhcrstats/5943e8a34/ globaltrends-forceddisplacement-2016.html.

40. **Medecins Sans Frontieres.** Pozzallo report: unacceptable conditions need urgent and structured responses. 2016. Available from: https://www.medicisenzafrontiere.it/

news-e-storie/news/rapporto-pozzallo-condizioni-inaccettabili-servono-risposte-urge nti-e-strutturate/.

41. **European Council on Refugees and Exiles.** Asylum Information Database (AIDA). Greece: country report. 2016. Available from: https://www.asylumineurope.org/reports/ country/greece.

42. **Hartocollis A.** Traveling in Europe's river of migrants. The New York Times. 2015. Available from: https://www.nytimes.com/interactive/projects/cp/reporters-notebook/ migrants/budapest-s-keleti-train-station-has-become-a-de-facto-refugee-camp.

43. **Francis J, Hiebert D.** Shaky foundations: refugees in Vancouver's housing market. Can Geogr. 2014;**58**(1):63–78.

44. **Juul K.** Migration, transit and the informal: homeless West-African migrants in Copenhagen. Eur J Homelessness. 2017;**11**(1):131–151.

45. **Hollifield M, Warner TD, Krakow B, Westermeyer J.** Mental health effects of stress over the life span of refugees. J Clin Med. 2018;**7**(2):25.

46. **Underwood E.** Surviving genocide: storytelling and ritual help communities heal. Science. 16 May 2017. Available from: http://www.sciencemag.org/news/2017/05/surviv ing-genocide-storytelling-and-ritual-help-communities-heal.

47. **Idemudia ES.** Value orientations, acculturative stress and mental health among African German immigrants. J Psychol Afr. 2011;**21**(3):439–445.

48. **Castaneda A, Junna L, Lilja E, Skogberg N, Kuusio H.** The prevalence of potentially traumatic pre-migration experiences: a population-based study of Russian, Somali and Kurdish origin migrants in Finland. J Trauma Stress Disord Treat. 2017;**6**:2–7.

49. **Mhlongo MD, Tomita A, Thela L, Maharaj V, Burns JK.** Sexual trauma and post-traumatic stress among African female refugees and migrants in South Africa. S Afr J Psychiatr. 2018;**24**:1208.

50. **Sigvardsdotter E, Vaez M, Rydholm Hedman A-M, Saboonchi F.** Prevalence of torture and other war-related traumatic events in forced migrants: a systematic review. Torture. 2016;**26**(2):41–73.

51. **Tinghög P, Malm A, Arwidson C, Sigvardsdotter E, Lundin A, Saboonchi F.** Prevalence of mental ill health, traumas and postmigration stress among refugees from Syria resettled in Sweden after 2011: a population-based survey. BMJ Open. 2017;**7**(12):e018899.

52. **Happe K, Steinicke H, Westermann S.** Traumatized Refugees—Immediate Response Required. Halle (Saale): German National Academy of Science; 2018. Available from: https://www.leopoldina.org/uploads/tx_leopublication/2018_Stellungnahme_traumat isierte_Fluechtlinge_EN.pdf.

53. **Chen W, Hall BJ, Ling L, Renzaho AM.** Pre-migration and post-migration factors associated with mental health in humanitarian migrants in Australia and the moderation effect of post-migration stressors: findings from the first wave data of the BNLA cohort study. Lancet Psychiatry. 2017;**4**(3):218–229.

54. **Spiller TR, Schick M, Schnyder U, Bryant RA, Nickerson A, Morina N.** Somatization and Anger are Associated with Symptom Severity of Posttraumatic Stress Disorder in Severely Traumatized Refugees and Asylum Seekers. Zurich: University of Zurich; 2016.

55. **Völkl-Kernstock S, Karnik N, Mitterer-Asadi M, et al.** Responses to conflict, family loss and flight: posttraumatic stress disorder among unaccompanied refugee minors from Africa. Neuropsychiatrie. 2014;**28**(1):6–11.

56. **Li SS, Liddell BJ, Nickerson A.** The relationship between post-migration stress and psychological disorders in refugees and asylum seekers. Curr Psychiatry Rep. 2016;**18**(9):82.

57. **The Children's Partnership.** The effect of hostile immigration policies on children's mental health. 2017. Available from: http://www.childrenspartnership.org/wp content/uploads/2017/03/The-Effect-of-Hostile-Immigration-Policies-on-Childrens-Mental-Health.pdf.

58. **Schiraldi GR.** The Post-Traumatic Stress Disorder Sourcebook: A Guide to Healing, Recovery, and Growth (2nd ed). New York: McGrawHill; 2009.

59. **Comer RJ.** Abnormal Psychology (6th ed). New York: Wadsworth; 2008.

60. **American Psychiatric Association.** Diagnostic and Statistical Manual of Mental Disorders (5th ed). Washington, DC: American Psychiatric Association; 2013.

61. **Worthen M, Rathod SD, Cohen G,** et al. Anger problems and posttraumatic stress disorder in male and female National Guard and Reserve Service members. J Psychiatr Res. 2014;**55**:52–58.

62. **Alisic E, Zalta AK, Van Wesel F,** et al. Rates of post-traumatic stress disorder in trauma-exposed children and adolescents: meta-analysis. Br J Psychiatry. 2014;**204**(5):335–340.

63. **Monson CM, Resick PA, Rizvi SL.** Posttraumatic stress disorder. In: **Barlow DH** (Ed), Clinical Handbook of Psychological Disorders (5th ed). New York: Guildford Press; 2014:80–113.

64. **Yohannes K, Gebeyehu A, Adera T, Ayano G, Fekadu W.** Prevalence and correlates of post-traumatic stress disorder among survivors of road traffic accidents in Ethiopia. Int J Ment Health Syst. 2018;**12**(1):50.

65. **Perrin M, Vandeleur CL, Castelao E,** et al. Determinants of the development of post-traumatic stress disorder, in the general population. Soc Psychiatry Psychiatr Epidemiol. 2014;**49**(3):447–457.

66. **Benítez CIP, Sibrava NJ, Kohn-Wood L,** et al. Posttraumatic stress disorder in African Americans: a two year follow-up study. Psychiatry Res. 2014;**220**(1–2):376–383.

67. **Swain KD, Pillay BJ, Kliewer W.** Traumatic stress and psychological functioning in a South African adolescent community sample. South Afr J Psychiatry. 2017;**23**(1):1008.

68. **Bogic M, Njoku A, Priebe S.** Long-term mental health of war-refugees: a systematic literature review. BMC Int Health Hum Rights. 2015;**15**(1):29.

69. **Aoun A, Joundi J, El Gerges N.** Post-traumatic stress disorder symptoms and associated risk factors: a cross-sectional study among Syrian refugees. Br J Med Pract. 2018;**11**(1):a1106.

70. **Ibrahim H, Hassan CQ.** Post-traumatic stress disorder symptoms resulting from torture and other traumatic events among Syrian Kurdish refugees in Kurdistan Region, Iraq. Front Psychol. 2017;**8**:241.

71. **Nasıroğlu S, Çeri V.** Posttraumatic stress and depression in Yazidi refugees. Neuropsychiatr Dis Treat. 2016;**12**:2941.

72. **Workneh AF.** The State of Knowledge on Posttraumatic Stress Disorder, Depression and Anxiety Among Refugee Women in Africa: A Scoping Review. MSc thesis. Ottawa: University of Ottawa; 2017.

73. **Bryant RA, Edwards B, Creamer M,** et al. The effect of post-traumatic stress disorder on refugees' parenting and their children's mental health: a cohort study. Lancet Public Health. 2018;**3**(5):e249–e58.

74. **Akinsulure-Smith AM.** Resilience in the face of adversity: African immigrants' mental health needs and the American transition. J Immigr Refug Stud. 2017;15(4):428–448.

75. **Bas-Sarmiento P, Saucedo-Moreno MJ, Fernández-Gutiérrez M, Poza-Méndez M.** Mental health in immigrants versus native population: a systematic review of the literature. Arch Psychiatr Nurs. 2017;31(1):111–121.

76. **Gilliver SC, Sundquist J, Li X, Sundquist K.** Recent research on the mental health of immigrants to Sweden: a literature review. Eur J Public Health. 2014;24(Suppl 1):72–79.

77. **Bhugra D, Gupta S, Schouler-Ocak M, et al.** EPA guidance mental health care of migrants. Eur Psychiatry. 2014;29(2):107–115.

78. **Close C, Kouvonen A, Bosqui T, Patel K, O'Reilly D, Donnelly M.** The mental health and wellbeing of first generation migrants: a systematic-narrative review of reviews. Global Health. 2016;12(1):47.

79. **Pannetier J, Lert F, Roustide MJ, du Loû AD.** Mental health of sub-Saharan African migrants: the gendered role of migration paths and transnational ties. SSM Popul Health. 2017;3:549–557.

80. **Thela L, Tomita A, Maharaj V, Mhlongo M, Burns JK.** Counting the cost of Afrophobia: post-migration adaptation and mental health challenges of African refugees in South Africa. Transcult Psychiatry. 2017;54(5–6):715–732.

81. **Honkanen M.** Mental Health Problems of Child and Adolescent Refugees and Asylum Seekers: A Literature Review. Bachelor's thesis. Turku: Turku University of Applied Sciences; 2016.

Chapter 18

Tobacco smoking and homelessness

Lucas C. Davanso and
João Mauricio Castaldelli-Maia

Introduction

The numbers regarding smoking have quite impressive values. More than
1 billion smokers consume around 6 trillion cigarettes annually (1). There is
an increasing tendency in developing countries and a decreasing tendency in
developed ones. Still, smoking prevalence tends to be higher in more developed areas, especially in Europe. This continent had the highest percentage
of smokers in its population, 29%, according to the survey performed by the
World Health Organization in 2010. The continent with the lowest prevalence
was Africa, with 12% of its population being smokers; smoking was more
common among men (22%) than among women (3%), especially in less developed areas. In Europe, 39% of men and 20% of women were smokers. This
discrepancy between the sexes is even more impressive in the Western Pacific
region, with 49% of men and 4% of women being smokers (1).

Approximately 7 million deaths per year directly connect to tobacco use, and
more than 1 million result from indirect exposure to it (2). Considering the absolute number of smokers, around 80% of them live in less developed countries.
These countries have fewer resources to treat the various complications directly caused by tobacco such as bladder cancer, liver cancer, kidney and ureteral
cancer, laryngeal cancer, cancer in the oral cavity, acute myeloid leukaemia,
lung cancer, stomach cancer, colon cancer, chronic obstructive pulmonary
disease, cardiovascular events, sexual impotence, and infertility, among many
others (2).

The prevalence of smoking among the homeless is high. It is three or four
times higher than in the general population (3–5). A combination of factors
makes smoking among the population experiencing homelessness particularly
dangerous with a higher possibility of health complications. Habits like tobacco
scavenging (6) and the high amount of money they have to spend (7), when

considering the cost of cigarettes in a context of an extremely low income, to maintain the addiction and avoid the craving symptoms resulting from nicotine abstinence places this particular group in a vulnerable situation.

The lack of support and more tangible ways to quit smoking is another complicating factor. In the general population, the quitting process demands motivation and usually the need for programmes or medical interventions. Among the homeless, their social environment makes it even harder, even though their desire to quit is considerably high (8–12).

This review chapter seeks a better understanding of what is known about tobacco use in its various forms within the homeless population. It summarizes the medical literature surrounding the topic and tries to understand if there are prevention or treatment strategies to approach smoking in this population.

Methods

Data sources

A search was conducted in PubMed and PsycINFO databases using the keywords "cigarettes", "smok*", "homeless*", "dependency", and "tobacco"; the last search was conducted in June of 2020.

Eligibility

We included in the present review studies evaluating either tobacco use or dependence among the homeless population, its clinical correlation with the use of other substances, the way of obtaining tobacco, and the quitting attempts among the homeless population. Studies in the English language, with or without intervention were considered for the present review.

Study appraisal and synthesis method

The initial search identified a total of 225 articles and 178 were excluded based on an evaluation of their titles. Then, based on the evaluation of their abstracts, 23 other studies were excluded. The remaining 24 were fully assessed—see Table 18.1.

Results

Going through the surveys assessing tobacco use among people experiencing homelessness, the social abandonment theme is the most critical issue. The role of social abandonment in their lives makes their addiction harder to manage, especially during their quitting attempts. This accumulation of factors results in a widely harmful situation for this population.

Table 18.1

Author and year	Sample	Study type	Methods	Results	Limitations
Melo APS et. al, 2018.	**N** = 2.475; **Age:** ≥40 years old: 54.6% 18-39 years old: 45.4%; **Gender:** Women: 51.6% Men: 48.4%; **Setting:** 26 mental health services in Brazil.	Cross sectional.	**Measures:** A semi-structured person-to-person interview was conducted to obtain sociodemographic, clinical and behavioral data, and psychiatric diagnoses were obtained from medical records. **Interventions:** none.	71.5% of the surveyed patients experienced cigarette smoking.	Not all of the surveyed patients have experienced homelessness; Only incarcerated persons were surveyed;
Tucker JS et. al., 2020.	**N** = 449; **Age:** mean age = 21.8 years old (SD = 2.3); **Gender:** 71.7% male, 28.3% female; **Setting:** 12 service sites and 13 street sites in Los Angeles County.	Cross sectional.	**Measures:** Semi structured questionnaire, the analysis of covariance tests and follow-up Tukey post hoc tests were conducted to compare the three mutually exclusive groups: tobacco use only; co-use, but no co-administration; or co-administration. **Interventions:** none.	Over 90% of young homeless tobacco users reported past month marijuana and tobacco co-use: 65% reported any co-administration (mixing both substances in a cigarette, joint, blunt, bong, hookah, pipe or bowl) and 27% reported only using them separately.	Focused only on co-use of tobacco and marijuana.

(continued)

Table 18.1 Continued

Author and year	Sample	Study type	Methods	Results	Limitations
Tucker JS et. al., 2019. (a)	**N** = 433 (total), 234 (didn't smoke RYO cigarettes), 199 (smokes RYO cigarettes); **Age:** Non-smokers of RYO cigarettes = mean age of 21.7 years old (SD = 2.3), Smokers of RYO cigarettes = mean age of 22.2 (SD =2.1); **Gender:** 69.8% male, 30.2% female; **Setting:** 25 street and service sites in Los Angeles County.	Cross sectional.	**Measures:** Semi structured questionnaire, T-tests and chi-square tests were used to compare past month cigarette smokers who did and did not report using RYOs on background characteristics, RYO-related social factors and cognitions, and nicotine withdrawal symptoms, nicotine dependence, and intentions to continue smoking cigarettes in the future. **Interventions:** none.	RYO use was reported by 43% of cigarette smokers. Among those who filled RYOs with tobacco, 87% rolled them with used tobacco (typically mixed with new tobacco). Most RYO smokers reported engaging in high-risk smoking practices, such as smoking discarded cigarettes.	The only analysis in this article refers to RYO (roll your own) cigarettes.
Baggett PT et. al, 2019.	**N** = 50; **Age:** mean age 45.6; **Gender:** 58% female, 42% male; **Setting:** Boston.	Clinical trial.	**Measures:** 8-week pilot randomized controlled trial (RCT) of nicotine patch therapy and weekly in-person counseling with (n=25) or without (n=25) SmokefreeTXT. **Interventions:** All participants were provided with a mobile phone and a 2-month prepaid voice and text plan at no cost. SmokefreeTXT enrollees were sent 1 to 5 automated SMS text messages daily for up to 8 weeks and could receive on-demand tips for managing cravings, mood symptoms, and smoking lapses.	Across all time points, smoking abstinence did not differ significantly between SmokefreeTXT and control arm participants (odds ratio 0.92, 95% CI 0.30-2.84). Of SmokefreeTXT enrollees who completed exit surveys (n=15), two-thirds were very or extremely satisfied with the program.	SmokefreeTXT was added to a relatively robust evidence-based tobacco treatment regimen of nicotine patch therapy and in-person counseling as well as frequent in-person abstinence monitoring; Small n; Only applicable in the Boston healthcare for the homeless program, which is much more controlled than the average homelessness scenario.

Prett R et. al., 2013.	**N** = 40 **Age:** mean age = 50.2 years old (SD = 9.2); **Gender:** 72.5% male, 27.5% female; **Setting:** 2 urban homeless shelters in upper Midwest (USA).	Clinical trial.	**Measures:** one-on-one semi-structured interviews from December 2016 to April 2017. A convenience sample of 40 participants was recruited to take part in the interviews. Interviews were conducted with both control arm and intervention arm participants; **Interventions:** Changing of their social environment and trying to find in them motivation to quit smoking.	Participants described feeling pressure to smoke and drink in and around shelters, and that this pressure had led some to start smoking or resume smoking, along with making it very challenging to quit.	*"This study has several limitations. Participants are smokers experiencing homelessness who volunteered to participate in smoking cessation study, and therefore may have some self-selecting views in favor of smoking cessation. Results may not generalize to those who lack some desire to stop smoking. Additionally, this sample reflects a group of individuals located in the Upper Midwest of the United States, and may not be representative of the view and concerns in other communities."*
Harris T et. al., 2019.	**N** = 421; **Age:** mean age = 54.44 years old (SD = 7.34); **Gender:** 71.5% Male, 28.5% female; **Setting:** permanent supportive housing programs in Los Angeles, California.	Cross sectional.	**Measures:** Independent variables examined as correlates of tobacco use and cessation attempts corresponded with demographic characteristics (i.e., age, gender, race, sexual orientation, education) and clinical characteristics (i.e., psychological disability, physical disability, lifetime mental health conditions, cannabis use, illicit substance use, binge drinking). **Interventions:** None	Any tobacco use: 60.33%; daily tobacco use: 49.64%; Lifetime diagnoses of schizophrenia, posttraumatic stress disorder, depression, bipolar disorder, and illicit substance use were associated with increased odds of daily tobacco use. A lifetime diagnosis of depression was associated with an increased likelihood of a past 3-month tobacco cessation attempt.	Study focused not on smoking itself but in psychiatric and epidemiological outcomes of substance use and quitting attempts in the mental health among patients in homeless condition.

(continued)

Table 18.1 Continued

Author and year	Sample	Study type	Methods	Results	Limitations
Tucker JS et al., 2019. (b)	**N** = 469; **Age**: mean age = 21.8 years old (SD = 2.3); **Gender**: 71% male, 29% female; **Setting**: Street spots; City/State: Los Angeles California.	Cross sectional.	**Measures**: Semi structured questionnaire, a self-administered paper survey. **Interventions**: None.	Nearly all (90%) participants reported smoking regular cigarettes, and 78% reported using at least one tobacco product other than regular cigarettes.	
Dawkings L et al., 2019.	**N** = 283; **Age**: mean age = 42.7 years old(SD = 14.02); **Gender**: 84.1% males, 15.9% females; **Setting**: homeless support services in Kent, the Midlands, London and Edinburgh.	Cross sectional.	**Measures**: 4 section questionnaire, including demographic, fagerstrom teste of cigarette dependence; data on previous quitting behavior; related to any previous e-cigarette use. **Interventions**: None.	High levels of cigarette dependence were observed (FTCD: M=7.78, sd ± 0.98). Although desire to quit was high, most had made fewer than 5 quit attempts and 90% of these lasted less than 24 h. 91.5% reported that others around them also smoked. Previous quit methods used included cold turkey (29.7%), NRT (24.7%), varenicline (22.3%) and bupropion (14.5%).	

Collins SE, 2018.	**N** = 25; **Age:** mean age = 47.88 years old (SD = 10.82); **Gender:** 80% male, 20% female; **Setting:** An emergency shelter in a large city in the Pacific Northwest.	Cross sectional.	**Measures:** One-on-one, semi-structured interviews included prompts assessing sociodemographic characteristics, smoking histories, participants' perceptions of smoking and the role of smoking in their lives, past experiences with smoking treatment, and suggestions about alternative intervention strategies or means of reducing smoking-related harm. **Interventions:** the researchers tried to motivate the surveyed to try new quitting attempts as they listened to the types of cessation attempt that the interviewed had experienced, as well as their perception about each method of cessation.	Most participants preferred engaging in their own self-defined, alternative smoking interventions, including obtaining nicotine more safely (e.g., vaping, using smokeless tobacco) and using behavioral (e.g., engaging in creative activities and hobbies) and cognitive strategies (e.g., reminding themselves about the positive aspects of not smoking and the negative consequences of smoking). Abrupt, unaided quit attempts were largely unsuccessful. Low n, most participants were not interested in the proposed cessation attempts or suggested their own ways of trying to stop, especially new ways of obtaining nicotine alternatively to cigarettes.
Neisler J et. al., 2018.	**N** = 396; **Age:** mean age = 42.9 years old (SD = 11.8); **Gender:** 64.9% male; 35.1% female; **Setting:** six homeless-serving agencies and/or shelters in Oklahoma City.	Cross sectional.	**Measures:** Enrolled participants completed questionnaires on a tablet computer as items were read aloud to the participants via headphones. **Interventions:** none.	The rate of concurrent nicotine and tobacco use was high - 67.2 %. Participants most frequently endorsed lower cost and a desire to cut down on cigarette smoking as motives for concurrent product use.

(continued)

Table 18.1 Continued

Author and year	Sample	Study type	Methods	Results	Limitations
Lantini R et. al., 2018.	N = 227; **Age**: mean age = 46.2 years old (SD = 12); **Gender**: 55% female; 45% male; **Setting**: -	Clinical trial.	**Measures**: Cigarette scavenging was assessed using three items: a) sharing a cigarette with a stranger; b) smoking a "found" cigarette and c) smoking a previously used cigarette "butt". Participants who endorsed engaging in at least one of these three behaviors were categorized as a scavenger. **Interventions**: Participants were offered cognitive behavioral therapy for smoking cessation plus either yoga or wellness classes.	31.7% of study participants were classified as cigarette scavengers, on top of that, significant differences were observed between the scavengers and the non-scavengers; interventions addressing these behaviors may meet the need of this subgroup of smokers.	The n is composed 100% of smokers trying to quit, and the objective of the study is simply to discover how many of them are scavengers and investigate if this kind of behavior makes them a sub type of smokers (almost 100% of the cigarette scavengers are homeless or incarcerated) that require a different approach on the cessation attempts in order for them to be successful, meaning this study probably applies only to this sub group.
Pinsker EA, et. al, 2017.	N = 430; **Age**: Mean age = 44.4 years old (SD = 9.9); **Gender**: 74% male, 26% female; **Setting**: 8 homeless emergency shelters and transitional housing sites in Minneapolis/St. Paul, Minnesota.	Clinical trial.	**Measures**: Participants were asked to indicate the extent they agreed or disagreed with 10 statements about their smoking urges (e.g., I have a desire for a cigarette right now; I would do almost anything for a cigarette right now). Answer options ranged from 1 (strongly disagree) to 7 (strongly agree). All 10 items were summed to create a scale ranging from 10 to 70, with higher scores indicating greater smoking urges.	Among the full sample, self-efficacy to refrain from smoking increased linearly over time, confidence to quit increased until the midpoint of treatment but subsequently decreased, and smoking urges decreased until the midpoint of treatment but subsequently increased.	

Wrighting Q et. al., 2016.	**N** = 207; **Age**: mean age = 43.04 years old (SD = 11.54); **Gender**: 71.5% male, 28.5% female; **Setting**: Shelter in Dallas, Texas.	Cross sectional.	**Interventions**: Intervention participants received six individual MI counseling sessions each lasting 15-20 minutes, which focused on encouraging smoking cessation and nicotine replacement therapy adherence. Control participants received a one-time advice session on quitting smoking lasting 10-15 minutes. **Measures**: Enrolled participants completed computer-administered questionnaires that allowed them to give self-reported responses via a computer keyboard. **Interventions**: none	Most participants purchased cigarettes by the pack (61.4%), and more than half the sample spent ≤$20 on cigarettes per week. Results indicated that spending less money per week on cigarettes was associated with greater readiness to quit.	Focused only on the purchase pattern.
Maddox S et. al., 2016.	**N** = 104; **Age**: mean age = 50 years old (SD = 13.9); **Gender**: 69.9% male, 30.1% female; **Setting**: The Royal District Nursing Service Homeless Persons' Program (RDNS-HPP) in Melbourne, Australia.	Cross sectional.	**Measures**: Twenty-six nurses completed an anonymous survey describing their attitudes to providing smoking-cessation support, current practices and estimates of client smoking and interest in quitting. Subsequently, nurses administered a survey to determine their smoking prevalence and interest in quitting. **Interventions**: none.	Most clients (82%) smoked, half of these (52%) reported wanting to quit and 64% reported trying to quit or reduce their smoking in the previous 3 months. Nurses approximated clients' smoking prevalence (88% vs 82% reported by clients), but underestimated interest in quitting (33% vs 52% reported by clients).	The study has the objective of comparing the perception that the nurses developed during their time working in the homeless person's program with the perception of the patients themselves.

(continued)

Table 18.1 Continued

Author and year	Sample	Study type	Methods	Results	Limitations
Robinson CD et. al., 2016.	N = 430; **Age**: mean age = 44.3 years old (SD = 10); **Gender**: 74.7% male, 23.3% female; **Setting**: shelters in Minneapolis/St. Paul, Minnesota.	Clinical trial.	**Measures**: enrolled in a smoking cessation study were randomized to Motivational Interviewing (MI) or standard care (SC). **Interventions**: Participants received nicotine replacement therapy and were followed for 26 weeks.	Homeless smokers in the DS group reported higher levels of hopelessness, perceived stress, and craving. There was no effect of DS status on abstinence at week 8 or week 26. There was no significant interaction between depression symptoms (DS vs. Control) and the intervention (MI vs. SC).	Study focused on interventions on the mental health, seeking to use motivation as a tool to help in the cessation process.
Baggett et. al., 2016.	N = 306; **Age**: mean age = 47.6 years old (SD = 10); **Gender**: 74.8% male, 23.6%, 1.6% transgender; **Setting**: 5 clinical sites at Boston Health Care for the Homeless Program.	Cross sectional.	**Measures**: in-person survey, trained interviewers verbally administered the 159-item questionnaire using an electronic tablet. **Interventions**: none.	Eighty-six percent of eligible individuals participated in the survey. In the past month, 37% of respondents used large cigars, 44% used little cigars, 8% used smokeless tobacco, 24% used an e-cigarette, and 68% used any of these products.	*"We did not ask about hookah use or pipe smoking. We also did not assess use of other tobacco products or e-cigarettes among homeless individuals who were not current cigarette smokers. Among participants who had used other tobacco products and e-cigarettes in the past month, we did not assess the frequency of use to identify regular versus non-regular or experimental users. Additionally, we did not ask the reasons for other tobacco product use; as a result, we were unable to determine whether homeless smokers may view these products as less harmful alternatives to conventional cigarettes or as*

Study	Design	Sample	Measures/Interventions	Results	Notes/Limitations
					tools for quitting cigarette smoking. Finally, the small number of individuals who used certain products (e.g. smokeless tobacco) limited our power to detect potentially meaningful correlates of using these products."
Garey L, et. al., 2018.	Cross sectional.	**N** = 465; **Age**: mean age = 43.19 years old (SD = 11.77); **Gender**: 65.1% male, 34.9% female; **Setting**: Shelters to homeless individuals in the Oklahoma City area.	**Measures**: self-report measures of sociodemographic, smoking characteristics, anxiety sensitivity, stress, social support, and the Center for Disease Control (CDC) four-item HRQoL (health-related quality of life) measure. **Interventions**: None	Results suggest that older smokers with greater emotional distress, as evidenced by greater anxiety sensitivity and stress and less social support, may be particularly vulnerable to poorer HRQoL.	The article focuses on the mental health of homeless smokers, it doesn't have the focus on the smoking itself.
Bagget TP et. al., 2016	Cross sectional.	**N** = 306; **Age**: mean age = 44 years old; **Gender**: 75% male, 25% female; **Setting**: Boston Health Care for the Homeless Program.	**Measures**: Interview regarding how much money the surveyed had expended in the last month to acquire their nicotine sources, as well as a fagerstrom questionare for measuring nicotine dependence. **Interventions**: None.	Participants reported spending a mean of $44 (95% confidence interval [CI], $40 to $47) on tobacco in the previous week.	Only appliable in the Boston healthcare for the homeless program, which is much more controlled than the average homelessness scenario.
Pratt R, 2019.	Cross sectional.	**N** = 40; **Age**: mean age = 50.2 years old (SD = 9.2); **Gender**: 72.5% male, 27.5% female; **Setting**: 2 urban homeless shelters in the Upper Midwest.	**Measures**: semi-structured interviews. The interview guide consisted of 17 questions on the topics of the experience of attempting to quit smoking during the study, their experience of the study intervention, and their views on important topics for future research. **Interventions**: None.	Participants described being motivated to quit, and seeing smoking cessation as positively impacting the time and focus they felt they had for finding housing. However, many felt more interested in reducing their smoking, rather than quitting.	Low n.

High smoking prevalence among the homeless was confirmed in all the studied samples, and an increased desire and motivation to quit smoking (8,12) when assessed. Unfortunately, high levels of dependence were observed, with stopping attempts lasting less than 24 hours (8) and a lack of efficient methods in their tries. Sometimes the technique was wholly self-defined and largely unsuccessful (9). Also, some of the main observed goals were simply the attempt to reduce cigarette consumption rather than quitting (11,12), with high levels of failure in that objective as well. Their efforts to obtain cigarettes were considerably high. One study reported a mean of 44 dollars spent on tobacco in the previous week (7). The more they spent on cigarettes, the lower was their expectation of quitting. Another study showed that to maintain their addiction, the scavenging habit was also observed in 32% of the sample (6).

One sensible and important point was the role of their mental health along with their lives and the interaction of this ongoing situation with their tobacco dependence. Feelings of hopelessness, anxiety, and depression-related feelings were observed, directly making it harder for them to quit or even reduce tobacco consumption (3,13,14).

Not only industrialized cigarettes were used as a form to obtain tobacco, but also self-rolled cigarettes (5), as well as any other form of tobacco and nicotine within their reach, such as large cigars, cigars, smokeless tobacco, and e-cigarettes (15–18). Ninety per cent of the tobacco users interviewed in one study reported recent marijuana smoking as well (19).

Discussion and conclusion

Considering the findings of the 19 included studies, we found a higher prevalence of tobacco dependency among the homeless population. Unfortunately, those individuals who wanted to quit faced more substantial barriers in their attempts compared to the general population and there was a high rate of relapse. There has also been a high concomitant use of tobacco and other substances, such as alcohol and cannabis.

This subject is not frequently addressed in the medical literature or clinical practice around the world. Data collection on tobacco smoking is usually part of a more comprehensive questionnaire about substance use and dependence, and harmful habits in a homeless population. More specific studies are needed on this topic.

Also, the homeless population is widely heterogeneous around the world. Their substance use behaviours, including tobacco use, are directly connected to the social environment and the socioeconomic situation of the place in which they live. The approach strategies directed to any studied samples are almost completely individualized and cannot be properly put into practice in a wider scenario. The institutions that develop some type of strategy are usually shelters for the homeless or research centres that survey only the local population within their own area and usually within limited resources, making the studies themselves more limited, even in reference centres.

References

1. **World Health Organization.** Fact sheet: tobacco. 2020. Available from: https://www.who.int/news-room/fact-sheets/detail/tobacco.

2. **Centers for Disease Control and Prevention.** Health effects of cigarette smoking. 2020. Available from: https://www.cdc.gov/tobacco/data_statistics/fact_sheets/health_effects/effects_cig_smoking/.

3. **Melo APS, Lima EP, Barros FCR, Camelo LDV, Guimarães MDC.** Homelessness and incarceration among psychiatric patients in Brazil. Cien Saude Colet. 2018;**23**(11):3719–3733.

4. **Harris T, Winetrobe H, Rhoades H, Wenzel S.** The role of mental health and substance use in homeless adults' tobacco use and cessation attempts. J Dual Diagn. 2019;**15**(2):76–87.

5. **Tucker JS, Shadel WG, Golinelli D, Seelam R, Siconolfi D.** Correlates of cigarette and alternative tobacco product use among young tobacco users experiencing homelessness. Addict Behav. 2019;**95**:145–151.

6. **Lantini R, Sillice MA, Fava JL, et al.** Butt why? Exploring factors associated with cigarette scavenging behaviors among adult smokers enrolling in a clinical trial for smoking cessation. Addict Behav. 2018;**78**:200–204.

7. **Baggett TP, Rigotti NA, Campbell EG.** Cost of smoking among homeless adults. N Engl J Med. 2016;**374**(7):697–698.

8. **Dawkins L, Ford A, Bauld L, Balaban S, Tyler A, Cox S.** A cross sectional survey of smoking characteristics and quitting behaviour from a sample of homeless adults in Great Britain. Addict Behav. 2019;**95**:35–40.

9. **Collins SE, Orfaly VE, Wu T, et al.** Content analysis of homeless smokers' perspectives on established and alternative smoking interventions. Int J Drug Policy. 2018;**51**:10–17.

10. **Pinsker EA, Hennrikus DJ, Erickson DJ, Call KT, Forster JL, Okuyemi KS.** Trends in self-efficacy to quit and smoking urges among homeless smokers participating in a smoking cessation RCT. Addict Behav. 2018;**78**:43–50.

11. **Maddox S, Segan C.** Underestimation of homeless clients' interest in quitting smoking: a case for routine tobacco assessment. Health Promot J Austr. 2017;**28**(2):160–164.

12. **Pratt R, Pernat C, Kerandi L, et al.** "It's a hard thing to manage when you're homeless": the impact of the social environment on smoking cessation for smokers experiencing homelessness. BMC Public Health. 2019;**19**(1):635.

13. **Robinson CD, Rogers CR, Okuyemi KS.** Depression symptoms among homeless smokers: effect of motivational interviewing. Subst Use Misuse. 2016;**51**(10):1393–1397.

14. **Garey L, Reitzel LR, Neisler J, et al.** Health-related quality of life among homeless smokers: risk and protective factors of latent class membership. Behav Med. 2019;**45**(1):40–51.

15. Tucker JS, Shadel WG, Seelam R, Golinelli D, Siconolfi D. Roll-your-own cigarette smoking among youth experiencing homelessness. Drug Alcohol Depend. 2019;**205**:107632.

16. Neisler J, Reitzel LR, Garey L, et al. Concurrent nicotine and tobacco product use among homeless smokers and associations with cigarette dependence and other factors related to quitting. Drug Alcohol Depend. 2018;**185**:133–140.

17. Baggett TP, Campbell EG, Chang Y, Rigotti NA. Other tobacco product and electronic cigarette use among homeless cigarette smokers. Addict Behav. 2016;**60**:124–130.

18. Tucker JS, Shadel WG, Seelam R, Golinelli D, Siconolfi D. Co-use of tobacco and marijuana among young people experiencing homelessness in Los Angeles County. Drug Alcohol Depend. 2020;**207**:107809.

19. Wrighting Q, Businelle MS, Kendzor DE, LeBlanc H, Reitzel LR. Cigarette purchasing patterns, readiness to quit, and quit attempts among homeless smokers. Nicotine Tob Res. 2017;**19**(12):1526–1530.

20. Baggett TP, McGlave C, Kruse GR, Yaqubi A, Chang Y, Rigotti NA. SmokefreeTXT for homeless smokers: pilot randomized controlled trial. JMIR Mhealth Uhealth. 2019;**7**(6):e13162.

Section 5

Services

Chapter 19

Psychosocial treatment for homeless with substance use disorders

Isabel Bernardes Ferreira,
Charles Abrantes Coura,
Angela Bianco Smith, and
Priscila Dib Gonçalves

Introduction

Poverty and social inequality produce experiences of social exclusion, violence, hunger, and unemployment. This lack of resources is present on a large scale in peripheral countries such as Brazil. In addition to these experiences, poverty negatively influences living conditions and increases vulnerability to mental illnesses. In this context, epidemiological data reveal a growing number of people who have experienced some kind of deprivation, and broken social and affective relationships, and moved to the streets and other public spaces (1–3).

A census conducted in Brazil identified 31,922 people over the age of 18 who are homeless, of whom 82% are men, 53% are between 25 and 44 years old, and 67% identified their ethnicity as *Pardo* (mixed-race), or Black. Sixteen per cent reported asking for money as their main mean of survival, 71% had some paid activity (mostly (27%) as a collector of recyclable materials), and 15% said they did not have any formal education. Among the main reasons that led them to homelessness, 35% correspond to the problematic use of alcohol and/or other drugs, 30% to unemployment, and 30% to family conflicts (4,5).

The city of São Paulo has the largest homeless population in Brazil. The latest census survey conducted in 2015 estimated that 15,905 people were staying overnight in the city's reception centres and public places, 32% were aged between 31 and 49 years old, 69% declared themselves as non-white, 10% of respondents who were on the street never went to school, and 82% were men (6). According to the National Policy for the Homeless Population (5):

> The homeless population is considered to be a heterogeneous population group that has in common extreme poverty, broken or weakened family ties, and the absence of regular conventional housing. It uses public places and degraded areas as living spaces. Support, temporarily or permanently, as well as the accommodation units for temporary overnight stays or as temporary housing.

The homeless population is continually undergoing processes of exclusion and marginalization, as well as the violation of fundamental rights such as housing, education, and healthcare. The reasons that led these people to their condition are multifactorial and complex. However, more simplistic explanations tend to blame homeless people for their situation and to link their identity to crime which contributes to the difficulty of inclusion in the work market and promotes isolation of the population (6).

A homeless person lives in a condition characterized by instability: absences of fixed and secure housing, social and family ties, relations, and work. Such determinants generate social vulnerability and health problems. Also, there are real survival issues. Their lives are marked by stigma and negative visibility. This stereotypical view contributes to the perception of the homeless population causing violence and danger rather than mobilizing protection and care for them. Thus, the process of social exclusion is deepened (1,2,6–8).

Several fallacies regarding the homeless population permeate the social imagination, among them, the association between being on the street and the compulsory use of psychoactive substances. Epidemiological data show concerning amounts of drug use by this population, which is a healthcare target; however, such consumption should not be generalized nor naturalized. Thus, it should be the subject of detailed study and careful intervention (2,9).

For example, in the capital of a state in Southeast Brazil (Belo Horizonte), research was conducted on symptoms of depression in the homeless population (10). The results showed that 56% of the people surveyed showed signs of depression; of this proportion, 24% indicated a moderate degree of depression, and 5% had severe symptoms. In another city in the same state (Juiz de Fora), it was found that 10% of homeless people were diagnosed with schizophrenia, which is higher than the general Brazilian population (11,14). In the city of Rio de Janeiro, another survey found that 22% of the people in a hostel had mental disorders, and most reported living with these problems before going onto the streets (12).

In a survey by the Ministry of Health in Brazil (5), 36% of the homeless population reported that alcohol use disorder was one of the main reasons that led them to live on the streets. The survey conducted in 2015 shows that 57% of the homeless population were smokers; 34% consumed alcohol, of whom 18% reported consuming more than three drinks/day; 33% reported using marijuana and 14% inhaled cocaine and crack-cocaine; and 8% of respondents reported using inhalable drugs and 5% injecting drugs (1).

These data highlight the importance of thinking about what sort of psychosocial care it is possible to offer the homeless population with problematic consumption of alcohol and other drugs. The first step should be understanding to what extent a life marked by material deprivation, psychological distress, and difficulty accessing social protection services may result in problematic use of psychoactive substances in this population. The aim here is not to medicalize social issues but to understand and care for them in parallel with health issues, and to do so, it is also necessary to escape from strictly prescriptive approaches and turn to participatory approaches that bring about listening and bonding (13).

Also, to be able to carry out health monitoring with the homeless population, protocols seen in health institutions (especially in hospitals) need to be reformulated, which means establishing an approach so that the person being cared for feels that the healthcare team and the professional genuinely care about them. In this context, the health teams should not only invest in hiring top-level professionals, but also invest in agents who have already had the same experience who are able to offer peer support (12,13). Regular frequency of appointments and keeping the arrangements are the key to strengthening the bond between the client and the health service and, later on, the client with their process of self-care (8).

Health teams should work with a realistic aim, that is, not propose long-term goals or goals that are difficult to achieve in the context of the street and social unprotection. The user should decide whether he/she aims for substance abstinence, and the health professional should assist them; if the person continues to use a substance, the use of harm reduction strategies is a possibility (14).

Harm reduction

Harm reduction is a healthcare strategy that has guided professional practice for many years and has been useful in the context of caring for homeless people (15,16). Harm reduction is the offer of procedures to reduce the harm of psychoactive substance use. There are several harm reduction actions, in addition to the well-known one of exchange of syringes and supplies; for example, individual or group psychosocial interventions and care, provision of consumer safe kits, sexual orientation and education, drug use rooms, planning of substitution of the drug for use with a less harmful one or with less harmful potential in the context of the served user, Housing First programmes, peer support, drug checking, and motivational approaches.

All of these actions are premised on providing knowledge and sharing decisions about the care and treatment process. Health education and the provision of minimum self-care conditions can contribute to the strengthening of autonomy, empowerment, and self-esteem. The definition of what is considered as 'the provision of minimum self-care conditions' varies among societies and governments. For instance, in certain countries, it is guaranteed access to housing, income transfer programmes, work, cultural and leisure activities, and healthcare. The guarantee of such resources contributes to higher treatment adherence, improved quality of life, and decreased consumption of drugs (15,16).

The harm reduction strategy is a public health alternative to the moral/criminal model that aims at punishment as a way to combat drug use and has sustained, for years, the various 'war on drugs' attempts (15,16). It also presents itself as complementary to the model that understands drug use as a brain disease (17). In the first model, the goal is to reduce the supply of drugs and promote a society free of psychoactive substances, while the second model focuses on individuals and seeks to reduce the demand for drugs. In both positions, abstinence becomes the main priority of the treatment.

The harm reduction approach also has the perspective of abstinence. However, it is recognized as an ideal result, and there are other results accepted along the way, building the path to sobriety. Harm reduction aims to reduce the negative consequences of drug use and other risky behaviours, with short goals as the user can endure, one step at a time towards change. The low demands on harm reduction programmes contribute to the development of coping strategies that are more adaptable to the user's reality, promoting increased social support and improving their life context.

Therefore, the emphasis of this approach is on the user and not the drug, so an empathic and supportive attitude is needed. Harm reduction aims to deconstruct labels and stigmas that are generally associated with drug users and thus demystify that the problem drug user is either a patient or an immoral but recognizes him or her as a desiring subject for something risky and these risks will be the central target of interventions (15). For someone to stop wanting to consume things that harm them, among other things, she/he must have the offer of what may do her/him good. Therefore, harm reduction goals also include the promotion of protective and health-promoting factors.

Contingency management

Contingency management (CM) is a psychosocial intervention and bases its principles on fundamental behavioural analysis. CM is based on operant conditioning (creating an association between a specific behaviour and a particular consequence) in which some important factors in developing these connections are the interval between the behaviour and the stimuli, and the magnitude of the reward or punishment (18–21).

CM has been broadly used in treatment for alcohol and substance use disorders, and there is a robust literature supporting its efficacy (18–21). One of the first scientific papers reporting CM and substance use disorders was in the 1990s by Higgins and colleagues (22). More recently, the UK recommends the use of CM for outpatients (23) and the US Department of Veterans implemented CM in 94 clinics with positive outcomes (24).

In the treatment of individuals with substance use disorders, the most common CM methods are voucher based and prize based. In the voucher-based CM approach, participants receive a 'voucher' (exchangeable for goods or services) after providing a negative biological sample (urine or breath) (18–21). In the prize-based approach, also known as the 'fishbowl procedure', participants receive a prize draw ticket (with a chance of winning a prize) after giving an objective proof of recent abstinence (18–21).

A recent meta-analysis reported the increase of short-term cessation after the prize-based CM intervention (18). Also, positive results with the homeless population in smoking cessation, reduction of substance use, and promotion of health behaviours have been reported. A study showed that the benefits of CM were still noted after a 12-month follow-up with a specific population (homeless men who have sex with men). Regarding follow-up effects after CM, the overall positive impact of CM is still noted, although the effects are weaker than during the intervention (19,25,26).

Motivation interviewing

Motivational interviewing (MI) is a *conversation about change* in a non-confrontational manner focused on the client, developed by William R. Miller in collaboration with Stephen Rollnick (27). In MI, the reasons for change are within the client. The professional is the one who is going to direct and guide the client in the process while respecting the client's autonomy. The spirit of MI includes partnership, acceptance, compassion, and evocation. In other words, the professional is going to help the client, not as an expert, but as someone willing to discover what motivates that person to make a change in their lifestyle and commit to this process. Some of the strategies include the use of Open questions, Affirmations, Reflective listening, and Summaries (known as 'OARS') (27).

Initially, MI focused on individuals with problematic drinking; currently, it is used in the treatment of many chronic conditions such as alcohol and substance use disorders, smoking cessation, psychiatric illness, asthma, diabetes, weight loss, and others (27). A study with the young homeless population in Los Angeles, US, showed a reduction in alcohol frequency and lower sexual risk behaviours (28).

Housing First

One of the aggravating conditions of illness and psychological distress among the homeless population is the absence of a fixed dwelling where one can take root and build a sense of belonging and security. The lack of housing and references makes healthcare difficult and the construction and implementation of the singular therapeutic project problematic. Thus, the provision of housing is an essential assumption in the psychosocial care of the homeless population.

Some countries have adopted a programme called 'Housing First', which consists of government actions that provide affordable housing or quality housing for the homeless. Eight principles guide Housing First policies, namely fundamental human rights, respect, host, commitment of the professional team, the separation between the place of treatment and place of residence, user decision power, a sense of self-determination, and recovery and damage reduction.

A Canadian study (16) found that housing programmes produced better responses to psychiatric treatment and reduced the use of alcohol and other drugs.

Assertive community treatment

Assertive community treatment (ACT) is an evidence-based treatment model that was designed to provide community-based psychiatric services, rehabilitation, and support to patients with severe and persistent mental illness. The ACT model of care was created by Arnold Marx, MD, Leonard Stein, and Mary Ann Test, PhD, in the late 1960s. In 1972, the first ACT team was up and running after these doctors closed their hospital ward and provided intensive services, 7 days per week, 24 hours per day, to support patients who were at high risk to be hospitalized, but who could be stabilized with ACT services in the community. The driving force of the ACT model was a realization that many patients were responding well to inpatient hospitalization, only to return shortly after. These founding doctors examined the way they were delivering mental health services and then created a new model to enhance the patient success rate outside the hospital. ACT has been widely implemented in the US, Canada, and the UK. The Department of Veterans Affairs has also performed ACT across the US (29–32).

The ACT model of care is currently operating in Southern California and targets the chronically homeless population while following the Housing First model. The goal of ACT is to provide clients with a higher level of community care. ACT offers an interdisciplinary team approach that encompasses the knowledge and skills of psychiatrists, licensed vocational nurses, registered nurses, mental health professionals in the field of social work or counselling, employment specialists, peer specialists, and substance abuse specialists. Consumers are referred to as clients and receive focused support and assistance to meet basic needs such as food, housing, medication management, and help applying for benefits. Support and assistance are also provided for accessing education, finding employment, and managing activities of daily living. Services are provided in the community rather than in an office or clinic setting, and interventions are integrated through collaboration among team members. The client's responses are monitored during daily case consultation, and the team quickly adjusts interventions to meet changing needs and the client's stage of change. Rather than referring clients to other providers, such as psychiatry, psychotherapy, vocational programmes, and payee-ship services, team members provide an array of treatment and rehabilitation support services.

There are many clients with co-occurring substance use disorders who are referred to ACT; ACT is considered a dual diagnosis treatment approach due to the experience and credentials of the substance abuse specialists. It is not part of the ACT eligibility requirement to have a co-occurring disorder. However, a vast majority of the clients do. Clients have reported feeling less stigmatized receiving ACT services as opposed to outpatient mental health treatment, as a harm reduction model is implemented. It means that clients do not have to be sober or abstaining from substances to receive services. The substance abuse specialist works closely with clients identified as having a substance use disorder and meets with them at least once within 30 days of their enrolment into the programme. ACT services are voluntary and time-unlimited, which allows clients to have freedom of choice in their treatment options. Staff manage their schedules around the needs of the client, provide services in-home, at the client's workplace, and in other settings in the community as identified by the client as the most beneficial to them. The harm reduction model also supports a non-shame-based approach to assessing and safety planning for substance use. Treatment team members validate and recognize the client's mental health diagnosis and substance diagnosis at the same time, working with a small caseload. The client ratio is one to ten, allowing frequent contact with the client to work on harm reduction techniques. It includes limiting substance intake to small amounts each day, keeping a mood log to build insight into substance use effect on mental health symptoms, and implementing the client's relapse prevention plan with 24-hour staff availability.

Intersectionality

The Unified Health System (in Portuguese, Sistema Único de Saúde) is public in Brazil and was established by the Federal Constitution of 1988 through its article 196 of the Social Security chapter. It provides equal and universal access to the entire Brazilian population, directed by the principles of universality, completeness, and equity.

One of the principles of the Unified Health System is integrality, which means healthcare should include the following domains: physical, social, spiritual, mental, and emotional. Thus, it is important to articulate health services with social policies based on an interdisciplinary work developed by a multidisciplinary team to identify the various demands brought by the homeless and make relevant referrals that promote access to healthcare and services. It should be noted that a single healthcare unit cannot be responsible for guaranteeing all rights provided by law to a citizen. It is not responsible for responding to all demands presented by the user; thus, a health unit when identifying other needs should refer them to other sectors such as education, housing, and social assistance. Intersectionality is a way of organizing services and social sectors to bring them closer to the real needs of users and whose demands are not lived and perceived in a compartmentalized way (1,9).

Access

Homeless populations demand specific healthcare because they are exposed to daily risk and vulnerable situations and are deprived of access to goods and services that guarantee minimum living conditions, such as food, water, shelter and protection, medicine, respect, and dignity. The difficulty in promoting self-care and hygiene, for example, reinforces the distance society establishes with homeless people (12,14).

Therefore, enabling constant access promotes a positive impact. Interventions such as active searching, care in the places where they usually stay, and staff availability are ways of adjusting the service to the needs of this population (34–36). They improve the healthcare process: 'the street context is dynamic, and the team must adjust its work to the unexpected' 33.

Street clinics

The first street clinic in Brazil was created in 1999, this pilot project was developed to take care of children and adolescents with problematic drug use living on the streets. In 2004, a street clinic was established at the first Psychosocial Care Center for Alcohol and Drugs in the city of Salvador (2,33).

In 2010, the street clinic was included in the 'Brazilian National Integrated Plan to Fight Crack', to expand access to care services and qualify the care offered to people with alcohol and other drug use. In the current Brazilian health policy, street clinics are part of primary healthcare. They are linked to the basic health units (Unidades Básica de Saúde (UBS)), which are primary care services and a strategic care device that provides the most sophisticated services (33).

In 2011, street advisory teams were established, aiming to increase the access of the homeless population to health services through integral actions of health in partnership with the teams of the UBS, psychosocial care centres (Centros de Atenção Psicossocial (CAPS)), institutions of the Unified Social Assistance System, as well as public and civil society institutions (37).

From this perspective, the street clinic, through primary care, seeks to provide comprehensive care of the homeless population, considering its uniqueness and sociocultural position, providing, as principles, equality, equity, respect for the dignity of the human person, and humanized and universalized care (38).

The teams of street clinics are made up of a range of professionals who develop comprehensive health actions given the needs of this population, and who can be organized into three modalities:

- Modality I: at least four professionals, of whom two must be higher education professionals—nurse, psychologist, social worker, or occupational therapist—and two mid-level professionals.
- Modality II: at least six professionals, of whom three must be higher education professionals—nurse, psychologist, social worker, or occupational therapist—and three mid-level professionals.
- Modality III: compulsorily formed by the same configuration as modality II, plus a physician (37).

Actions and activities with this heterogeneous population are always carried out on an on-site itinerant basis and, when necessary, in partnership with the unit teams: CAPS and UBS component institutions, and services that make up the health and intersectoral network and civil society (37).

The street clinic, along with intersectoral services, promotes health actions using a broad approach, targeting not only health problems but also social problems according to the specificities of each subject. To conclude, the following list includes some actions developed in healthcare, which also enable social inclusion, citizenship recovery, and access to health services, public spaces, and cultural facilities, namely:

- Office Cup at Rua de Futebol (38,39).

- Homeless Women, They are also Divas, an action aimed at rescuing the femininity of homeless women (38,39).

- Boy or girl? Baby Shower, activity developed with the objective of treatment against the chemical dependence of pregnant women and the strengthening of bonds between mother and baby (38,39).

- Preventive screening for sexually transmitted diseases/HIV (38,39).

In general, the actions are strategies created as a way to identify social and health demands, promote the reclamation of citizenship, as well as promote connection with users to enhance the possibility of adherence with therapeutic projects.

In the daily clinical practice of street clinics, there is a psychologist who has a fundamental role. He/she works with the multidisciplinary team articulating with the intersectoral and undersecretary network. His/her purposes are making referrals that enable the mending of broken ties with family members and with society itself.

In this context, the psychologist conducts conversation circles aimed at users of alcohol and other drugs, presenting (a) the effects of these substances on the central nervous system; (b) association with risk behaviour; (c) social, physical, and economic problems related to use; and (d) harm reduction strategies. Also, in individual or group care, the psychologist helps individuals cope with problematic alcohol and other drug use, identifying subjective aspects that directly impact their health, always considering their individuality.

There are also workshops aimed at the transgender population, focused on the reclamation of citizenship through support in the rectification of first names, the recovery of self-esteem, and development of life projects, as well as assistance for hormone therapy through health services as a way of reducing harm. The vast majority of this population makes use of hormones without medical supervision.

The most striking feature of the street clinic is to meet the physiological needs of the reclamation (where and when they can sleep, eat, drink water), or have access to medical treatment. These are the challenges of street care teams: establishing care practices that are not rigid and do not sustain the unpredictability of the streets (33,40).

Conclusion

Psychosocial care for the homeless population that use psychoactive substances is an essential challenge for health teams, especially considering that everyday life is marked by extreme poverty and social vulnerability.

The goal of a psychosocial intervention for the homeless population with alcohol and other drug use should be, first and foremost, to reduce health risks and health problems during substance use and not necessarily to achieve abstinence while the person is unprotected on the street, as it is known that maintaining this condition in a precarious context is difficult to sustain. It is crucial to work for and celebrate small daily achievements, such as improved self-care and self-esteem, reorganization of some everyday tasks, the re-establishment of social and affective bonds, and search for other experiences beyond those established on the street.

Homeless people with substance use disorders are a very heterogeneous population with complex demands which increases the need to develop psychosocial care strategies according to the particular characteristics of each individual, seeking to understand what led to the homeless situation, considering their reference territory, and helping them build a support network that promotes the reduction of their vulnerability.

Psychosocial interventions for homeless people with substance use disorders aiming to reduce vulnerability and provide basic needs, such as harm reduction, Housing First, street clinics, and ACT, are related to better outcomes and could also be combined with psychological approaches such as CM and MI. Finally, when working with this population, the priority is to ensure social minimums and access to intersectoral policies that will promote health and quality of life.

References

1. Barata RB, Carneiro Junior N, Ribeiro MCSA, Silveira C. Desigualdade social em saúde na população em situação de rua na cidade de São Paulo. Saúde Soc. 2015;**24**(Suppl 1):219–232.

2. Borysow IC. O consultório na rua e a atenção básica à população em situação de rua. Doctoral thesis. São Paulo: University of São Paulo; 2018.

3. Castel R. A dinâmica dos processos de marginalização: da vulnerabilidade à "desfiliação". Caderno CRH. 1997;**10**(26/27):19–40.

4. Ministério do Desenvolvimento Social e Combate à Fome, SAGI, SNAS. Rua: Aprendendo a Contar—Pesquisa Nacional sobre a População em Situação de Rua. Brasília: MDS; 2009. Available from: https://www.mds.gov.br/webarquivos/ publicacao/ assistencia_social/Livros/Rua_aprendendo_a_contar.pdf.

5. Presidência da República, Casa Civil, Subchefia para Assuntos Jurídicos. Decreto Nº 7.053, de 23 de dezembro de 2009. Institui a Política Nacional para a População em Situação de Rua e seu Comitê Intersetorial de Acompanhamento e Monitoramento, e dá outras providências. Available from: http://www.planalto.gov.br/ccivil_03/_ato2007-2010/2009/decreto/d7053.htm.

6. FIPE. Censo da População em Situação de Rua da Cidade de São Paulo—Resultados. São Paulo: FIPE, 2015. Available from: https://goo.gl/8GFTnm.

7. **Vannucchi AMC, Barros JO.** População em situação de rua: identificando necessidades para políticas públicas de inclusão social. In: **Silveira C, Carneiro Junior N, Marsiglia RM** (Eds), Projeto Inclusão Social Urbana: Nós do Centro: Metodologia de Pesquisa no Centro da Cidade de São Paulo. São Paulo: Fundação Arnaldo Vieira de Carvalho; 2009:61–90.

8. **Vannucchi AMC.** A população em situação de rua no serviço de urgência psiquiátrica: In: **Baldaçara L, Cordeiro DC** (Eds), Emergências Psiquiátricas. São Paulo: Roca; 2007:215–226.

9. **Hallais JAS, Barros NF.** Street outreach offices: visibility, invisibility, and enhanced visibility. Cad Saude Publica. 2015;**31**(7):1497–1504.

10. **Botti NCL, Castro CG, Silva MF,** et al. Prevalência de depressão entre homens adultos em situação de rua em Belo Horizonte. J Bras Psiquiatr. 2010;**59**(1):10–16.

11. **Heckert U, Amaral AMM, Cunha RCS, Raso DC, Silvia JMF.** Programa de saúde mental para a população de rua: PRORUA. HU Revista. 2001;**27**(1):305–308.

12. **Borysow IC, Furtado JP.** Acesso e intersetorialidade: o acompanhamento de pessoas em situação de rua com transtorno mental grave. Physis. 2013;**23**(1):33–50.

13. **Merhy EE.** Anormais do desejo: os novos não humanos? Os sinais que vêm da vida cotidiana e da rua. In: **Conselho Federal de Psicologia (CFP), Grupo de Trabalho de Álcool e outras Drogas** (Eds), Drogas e Cidadania: Em Debate. Brasília: CFP; 2012:9–18.

14. **Silva FP, Frazaão IS, Linhares FM.** Práticas de saúde das equipes dos Consultórios de Rua. Cad Saude Publica. 2014;**30**(4):805–814.

15. **Marlatt GA.** Redução de Danos: Estratégias para Lidar com Comportamentos de Alto Risco. Porto Alegre: Artmed; 1999.

16. **Rigoni R, Breeksema J, Woods S.** Speed Limits: Harm Reduction for People Who Use Stimulants. Amsterdam: Mainline; 2019.

17. **Goldestein RZ, Volkow ND.** Dysfunction of the prefrontal cortex in addiction: neuroimaging findings and clinical implications. Nat Rev Neurosci. 2011;**12**(11):652–669.

18. **Benishek LA, Dugosh KL, Kirby KC,** et al. Prize-based contingency management for the treatment of substance abusers: a meta-analysis. Addiction. 2014;**109**(9):1426–1436.

19. **Davis DR, Kurti AN, Skelly JM, Redner R, White TJ, Higgins ST.** A review of the literature on contingency management in the treatment of substance use disorders. Prev Med. 2016;**92**:36–46.

20. **Prendegast M, Podus D, Finney J, Greenwell L, Roll J.** Contingency management for treatment of substance use disorders: a meta-analysis. Addiction. 2006;**101**(11):1546–1560.

21. **Rash CJ, Stitzer M, Weinstock J.** Contingency management: new directions and remaining challenges for an evidence-based intervention. J Subst Abuse Treat. 2017;**72**:10–18.

22. **Higgins ST, Delaney DD, Budney AJ,** et al. A behavioral approach to achieving initial cocaine abstinence. Am J Psychiatry. 1991;**148**(9):1218–1224.

23. **Pilling S, Strang J, Gerada C, NICE.** Psychosocial interventions and opioid detoxification for drug misuse: summary of NICE guidance. BMJ. 2007;**335**(7612):203–205.

24. **DePhilippis D, Petry NM, Bonn-Miller MO, Rosenbach SB, McKay JR.** The national implementation of contingency management (CM) in the Department of Veterans Affairs: attendance at CM sessions and substance use outcomes. Drug Alcohol Depend. 2018;**185**:367–373.

25. **Rash CJ, Petry NM, Alessi SM.** A randomized trial of contingency management for smoking cessation in the homeless. Psychol Addict Behav. 2018;**32**(2):141–148.

26. **Reback CJ, Peck JA, Dierst-Davies R, Nuno M, Kamien JB, Amass L.** Contingency management among homeless, out-of-treatment men who have sex with men. J Subst Abuse Treat. 2010;**39**(3):255–263.

27. **Miller WR, Rollnick S.** Motivational Interviewing: Helping People Change (3rd ed). New York: Guilford Publications; 2012.

28. **Tucker JS, D'Amico EJ, Ewing BA, Miles JN, Pedersen ER.** A group-based motivational interviewing brief intervention to reduce substance use and sexual risk behavior among homeless young adults. J Subst Abuse Treat. 2017;**76**:20–27.

29. **Dixon L,** Assertive community treatment: twenty-five years of gold. Psychiatr Serv. 2000;**51**(6):759–765.

30. **Marx AJ, Test MA, Stein LI.** Extrahospital management of severe mental illness: feasibility and effects of social functioning. Arch Gen Psychiatry. 1973;**29**(4):505–551.

31. **Stein LI, Santos AB.** Assertive Community Treatment for People with Severe Mental Illness. New York: WW Norton & Company; 1998.

32. **Borin MES.** Desigualdades e Rupturas Sociais na Metrópole: Os Moradores de Rua em São Paulo. Doctoral thesis. São Paulo: Pontifícia Universidade Católica de São Paulo (PUCSP); 2005.

33. **Londero MFP, Ceccim RB, Bilibio LFS.** Consultation office of/in the street: challenge for a healthcare in verse. Interface. 2014;**18**(49):251–260.

34. **Sarradon-Ecka A, Farnariera C. Hymans TD.** Caring on the margins of the healthcare system. Anthropol Med. 2014;**21**(2):251–263.

35. **Travassos C, Martins M.** Uma revisão sobre os conceitos de acesso e utilização de serviços de saúde. Cad Saude Publica. 2004;**20**(Suppl 2):S190–S198.

36. **Varanda W, Adorno RCF.** Descartáveis urbanos: discutindo a complexidade da população de rua e o desafio para políticas de saúde. Saúde Soc. 2004;**13**(1):56–69.

37. **Ministério da Saúde.** Portaria normativa nº 122, de 25 de janeiro de 2011. Define as diretrizes de organização e funcionamento das Equipes de Consultório na Rua. 2012. Available from: http://bvsms.saude.gov.br/bvs/saudelegis/gm/2012/prt0122_25_01_2012.html.

38. **Ministério da Saúde, Secretaria de Atenção à Saúde, Departamento de Atenção Básica.** Manual sobre o cuidado à saúde junto a população em situação de rua. Brasília: Ministério da Saúde; 2012.

39. **Ministério da Saúde.** Coordenação Nacional de Saúde Mental. Consultórios de Rua do SUS: material de trabalho para a II Oficina Nacional de Consultórios de Rua do SUS. Brasília, DF: EPSJV-Fiocruz; 2010.

40. **Ayres JRCM.** O conceito de vulnerabilidade e as práticas de saúde: níveis de perspectivas e desafios. In: **Czeresnia D, Freitas CM** (Eds), Promoção de Saúde. Rio de Janeiro: Fiocruz; 2003:117–139.

Chapter 20

Homeless persons in rehabilitation

Sarbani Das Roy

Introduction

Psychiatric rehabilitation is to help disabled individuals to establish the emotional, social, and intellectual skills needed to live, learn, and work in the community with the least amount of professional support (1). Recovery, on the other hand, has been defined as 'a deeply personal, unique process of changing one's attitudes, values, feelings, goals, skills, and/or roles. It is a way of living a satisfying, hopeful, and contributing life even with limitations caused by illness. Recovery involves the development of new meaning and purpose in one's life as one grows beyond the catastrophic effects of mental illness' (1). Recovery does not necessarily mean 'clinical recovery' (defined in terms of symptoms and cure). The idea of social recovery is demonstrated in building a life beyond illness without necessarily achieving the elimination of the symptoms of illness. Marginalization due to illness is one of the most disabling factors for people with psychiatric illnesses. Thus, social inclusion is the key to recovery. People with mental health problems should be considered as part of the community, as valued members with access to the opportunities that exist in those communities including being able to contribute to the communities.

The journey of a homeless person with severe mental illness to recovery is a story of rebirth. The home that one is born into has physical, emotional, and societal identities, all woven into one that provides an identity of space, time, and experiences. For homeless persons, this identity blurs or becomes a fond memory as they drift from known to unknown places pressed by poverty, density of population in homes, disability, unemployment, and, for most women, abuse, victimization, vulnerabilities, and violence, to mention a few (2).

Iswar Sankalpa is a non-governmental organization based in Kolkata, West Bengal, India. The organization was formed in 2007 with the aim of reducing the care gap that exists between, on the one hand, the vast number of homeless persons with mental illness in the city and, on the other hand, the meagre resources of psychiatric care available here. Government initiatives for psychiatric care in the city have primarily been through clinical services provided in hospitals. It is striving to build a model of inclusive care for the most vulnerable and least legally protected population, by mobilizing the support of key stakeholders: government, families of the target group, community, law enforcement agency, medical body, civil society, and media. The three main domains in which Iswar Sankalpa works are firstly, reorganization of the power equation and care pathways, within existing systems, that puts the onus of accepting care well within the domain of the recipient; secondly, creation and embedding of a proxy care giving structure around the client built through civil society volunteerism; and thirdly, regaining social capital is prioritized which enhances the 'relationship resources' of the homeless person which they can mobilize for their personal goal and improve their social position.

The person's[1] journey starts from hopelessness, evoked by the pain of symptoms, absence of family or friends, and the total lack of resources to sustain life in an alien geographical landscape, and an unfamiliar cultural milieu. Iswar Sankalpa's interventions with the person has focused to build an affiliative process to break their alienation, and aid clinical and social recovery.

Iswar Sankalpa's values in the work are as follows: firstly, it does not believe in uprooting and institutionalization of people solely in the name of medical service. That to them is neither dignified nor cost-effective, and renders restitution and rehabilitation of people difficult. It believes that a person, even if mentally ill, possesses the right to their self-determination and autonomy, and encourages the practice to negotiate with the person at every step of support and care. Secondly, each person has his or her sense of belonging and possessions. Such belonging may be to a particular corner of the pavement, to a few tattered pieces of cloth, and bits and pieces they possess, and to others who also live on the pavement. While the organization realizes that homelessness is not a self-made choice, it tries to offer alternative forms of living and treatment that are then adapted and adopted according to the individual's preferences and needs. Thirdly, it believes that the intervention, medical or otherwise, should be minimally disruptive to a person's life. Therefore, it provides support and care only as much as desired and accepted by the person. It does not attempt to subsume the person's existential self under the rubric of modern psychiatric discourse. Fourthly, it tries to provide consultation, evaluation, treatment, and care on the pavement and street corners where the person usually sleeps at night. It also

---

[1] A homeless person with severe mental illness has been referred to as person in this text.

tries to mobilize neighbours and local community resources towards providing care to the person.

The affiliative process

In building this affiliative process with the community around them, the person faces an inner block due to the distressful voices, threatening emotions of fear and anxiety, intrusive memories, shame, physical discomfort, hunger pangs, and rough living (3). Many of them speak a different language which may disrupt their urge to communicate with another. On the other hand, there are outer blocks such as persons in the community may harbour mistrust towards this stranger, and harbour fear and anxiety about the seemingly distressed bundle of rags. They may shun the person, and harbour negative views about care for such a person and choose to be indifferent to their situation. All of these or a few of them are real challenges in building a community that cares for the person.

The catalyst and task sharing in the community

The basic building blocks of Iswar Sankalpa's work are the social workers who observe apparently homeless people dwelling on the pavements and make a note of those who appear to have a psychotic condition. In most situations, these persons resent intrusion and try to avoid any direct approach. The social workers gather information about their identity, nutrition and health status, possible symptoms, behavioural oddities, interaction with others, duration of homelessness, and so on from the local people, often shopkeepers, rickshaw pullers, and other street dwellers. During these conversations, local people are sensitized to the plight of these persons and feel more caring towards them. They often express a spontaneous wish to help. The social workers then start to approach the person, striking up a casual conversation, gradually bringing in topics of health and medical care. The next step is for a psychiatrist to visit the person on the street and evaluate, diagnose, and plan treatment. All of this is done with the consent of the person. The social workers negotiate with the person about medication and with the local people about taking care of the person: securing meals, clothing, and giving medicine regularly. Social workers follow up regularly, weekly or fortnightly (4).

The crux of the model is the community caregiver who anchors the process. He supports food and clothes, and bears the responsibility to give medicines daily. His daily conversations with the person increase their social acceptance and increase the person's 'self-esteem'. Spontaneously, the person is absorbed in the caregiver's work or is supported to find employment in the community. The stigma of a severely mentally ill person becoming a lifelong burden is finally broken.

Since its inception, Iswar Sankalpa has been working with voluntary caregivers. They are daily wage earners, small shopkeepers in marketplaces, and tea stall owners—people who live or work in close proximity to the homeless person with mental illness. In 2017–2018, nearly 93 voluntary caregivers invested their time, care, and provision of basic needs for the homeless persons. Out of the 93 caregivers who have assisted the work in 2017–2018, the majority were male; 53% were Muslims and 47% were Hindus. The average income of the 93 caregivers was around 13,522 rupees ($200) per month. Thus, voluntary caregiving and philanthropy is about a 'mindset' and not just wealth and time. The wish to do good makes them feel powerful, they wish to set an example among peers, to do as per religious guidelines, to help so that they too will be blessed by God, and to do good as it is their duty are some of the shared inspirations and motivations of the struggling philanthropists in our society. Some of the challenges of the model are that the caregiver may forget or neglect his duties, some may lose or sell the medicines kept in custody, and the priorities may change in certain circumstances. To address these, we usually try to tag an additional co-caregiver per patient.

Mr P's story

In February 2011, a social worker from Iswar Sankalpa met Mr P, a 30-year-old male, at the Salvation Army Unit in Beniapukur, Kolkata, from where he used to collect his lunch every day. Self-laugh, irrelevant talk, and blunt affect were observed. His treatment started in August 2011.

With regular intervention, Mr P opened up to the social worker and in a few weeks' time, the social worker had traced his family. Mr P had a mother, brother, sister-in-law, and niece in his family, but he stayed away from them on the street close to their house. The death of his sibling had precipitated his problem.

Initially, Mr P did not accept medicines. For about a month, constant efforts to build a rapport with him earned his trust. Once on regular treatment, he improved rapidly. After about 6 months, he started working at a nearby sweet shop (Fig. 20.1). Right from the onset, the shop owner was very caring and helpful towards Mr P. He cared for him like a family member. Mr P earned 1500 rupees (roughly $20) a month. The shop owner had arranged a place for him to stay, but Mr P preferred to stay on the street near his home. The income brought with it new challenges, especially because on the street there was no place to keep the money safe. Mr P had started drinking alcohol and chewing tobacco. He was counselled to control and give up his addictive urges.

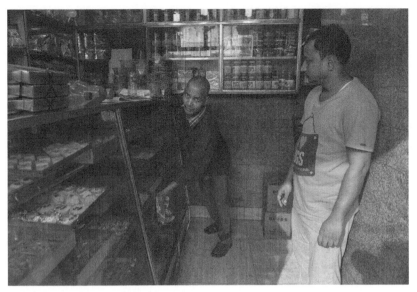

Fig. 20.1 Mr P and his community caregiver.

Presently, Mr P is working well, earning, and saving money. He travels independently within the city to bring goods for the shop, and manages the cash counter. Last Christmas, from his savings he purchased clothes for himself. In 2018, Sankalpa arranged a PAN[2] card, and opened a savings bank account for Mr P. He now keeps his money in the bank and has savings of 8000 rupees ($120). From a man, loitering aimlessly on the street, queuing up for free lunches, to a life of dignity, Mr P's recovery in reference to his disability scores (shown in Table 20.1) is a result of both treatment and affiliative processes in the community who appreciated his transformation at every milestone.

Odd jobs in the community

There are 212 persons registered in the community outreach programme of Iswar Sankalpa. Out of them, 59 persons are involved in odd jobs found in the locality where they live with the support of their caregiver and friends in the community. Among them, 50 persons are male and nine are female. The age group of 20–30 years comprises ten persons; 31–40 years, 22 persons; 41–50 years, 19 persons; and 50+ years, nine persons. Of the 59 homeless persons

---

[2] A PAN is a unique identifier issued to all judicial entities identifiable under the Indian Income Tax Act, 1961.

Table 20.1 Mr P's global disability score

Baseline, January 2012	10
July 2012	6
October 2012	4
April 2013	9
October 2013	6
April 2014	6
October 2014	4
April 2015	3
April 2016	3
June 2017	3
June 2018	3

employed in odd jobs, there are 38 persons diagnosed with schizophrenia, seven diagnosed with psychosis, and six diagnosed with schizoaffective disorder. Additionally, there is one person with cannabis-induced psychosis, two persons with paranoid schizophrenia, one person with undifferentiated schizophrenia, one person with intellectual disability, and two persons who have intellectual disability along with psychoses. One client is still under observation.

There are three main categories of employment in which the homeless persons are supportively occupied: 14 persons are working as daily labour, 14 persons are working as hotel assistants, and 16 persons are working as shop assistants. The other types of work in which they are involved are varied. One person works as a clinic attendant, seven persons as rag pickers, one person as a rickshaw puller, one person as a security guard, one as a tea stall assistant, while another works as a tea stall assistant as well as a van pusher, There is an individual who pushes vans for a living as well as selling fruits on the roadside. Finally, there are also two persons selling vegetables in the market.

Looking at the two groups of unemployed homeless persons with mental illness and the ones employed in the community, a t-test was done to determine if there is a significant difference between the means of their global disability score within the two groups which could throw light on the effect of habilitation avenues accessed. We found there is a significant difference (t stat = 3.85) between the group that was employed (M = 4.04) and the group with no employment (M = 1.61) (Table 20.2).

Table 20.2 T-test: two sample assuming unequal variances

	Variable 1	Variable 2
Mean	4.035714286	1.610687023
Variance	16.72597403	12.85496183
Observations	56	131
Hypothesized mean difference	0	
Degrees of freedom	93	
t stat	3.849697824	
P(T<=t) one-tail	0.000108453	
t critical one-tail	1.661403674	
P(T<=t) two-tail	0.000216907	
t critical two-tail	1.985801768	

Work has strengthened the affiliative processes in the community besides enabling economic empowerment for persons with severe mental illness, who were homeless, and leads to better recovery chances—both social and clinical.

Addressing aspirations

The outreach programme offered jobs to persons, but in some cases it failed to address the aspirations of a better life that they harboured despite the debilitating effects of their condition.

Long years on the street resulted in physical ill health due to prolonged malnutrition. The majority had experienced penury throughout their lives. Access to education had been a challenge and often they had poor communication skills and a low self-esteem. Those who were employed were perceived by their employers as unreliable due to their mood fluctuation. The shelters for the homeless provided uncertified vocational skills that at best benefitted therapeutic outcomes but did not enhance employability. All these factors and more contributed to the 'unemployability' of the person.

One of Iswar Sankalpa's aim has been to create an ecosystem that showcases the talent and workmanship of persons with psychosocial disability.

The first step was choice making. Of the 80 residents at the shelter for homeless women, 20 expressed their wish to learn to make cakes. They were divided into groups of five women and training started under the tutelage of experienced chefs from the Culinary Institute and Hotel, Kolkata. The course included soft skills and training on etiquette and functional literacy on a par with industry standards. Visits were undertaken to cafes and eateries for a first-hand experience. For most of the trainees, sitting inside a cafe and being served food as they peered out of the glass onto the very streets and pavements that held their torturous memories, was a defining moment. Indeed, they had come far. A mock cafe with in-house customers and friends of the organization was then set up. This helped the trainees build up their confidence and practise their newly learnt skills. Finally, 'Crust & Core', a cafe was started. This bears the signature of homeless persons with psychosocial disability. Here, talent is celebrated, and myths that homeless persons with mental illness were a burden to the society are shattered.

There were challenges too, but these were opportunities to fine-tune work. The staff working had fluctuating energy levels. This proved a challenge in an organized activity that had time-bound deliverables. The model attempted to match the energy level with the task. A person feeling low, with a low energy level, was given the task of layering a cake, or making shells for tarts and quiches; those with high energy levels were involved in dough making, carrying goods, and cleaning the utensils and kitchen. Fluctuating motivation and high sensitivity to perceived failure were addressed through affirmations and negotiations, at regular intervals. The confectionary trade demands long hours of standing (Fig. 20.2). The trainees, with their history of malnutrition, and rough living on the streets, found it difficult to meet the physical stamina demanded

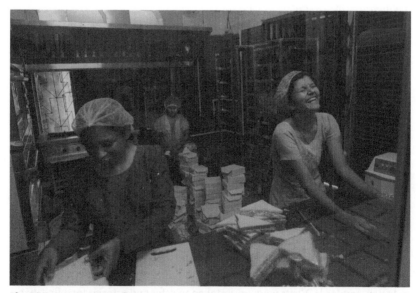

Fig. 20.2 Training in confectionary.

by the trade. The training sessions were therefore made shorter, with longer breaks. This helped to accommodate more trainees in groups.

A phoenix rises

In 2016, a woman evidently suffering from malnutrition was referred by the Garden Reach Police Station to Iswar Sankalpa's Women's Shelter. She was wearing a school uniform and had poor hygiene. She kept sobbing and did not interact with anyone at all. She was apparently of 30 years of age and active social avoidance was profound in her behaviour. She remained mostly preoccupied, and displayed restricted shallow affect with absence of eye contact. After a few days, she said her name was Ms C. Over time, with treatment and other therapeutic interventions, she began to participate in activities of the shelter and her rapport with others gradually improved.

It was only after a few months that she shared that her real name was not Ms C but Ms SM and that she was from Karnataka. She recollected that her alcoholic husband and father-in-law were physically abusive and that she had to return to her maternal home. But soon she had felt restless at home due to her symptoms and left the house. Smilingly, she said that earlier she did not trust anyone in the shelter, and so did not want to reveal her real name.

She had studied until the first year at college, but had forgotten most of it. At the shelter, she was enrolled into functional literacy classes and soon she took the National Institute of Open Schooling exams. She wanted to get involved with the kitchen work and so became a part of the Mousumi Staff Canteen[3] and served everyone with a smile. During a choice-making session, Ms SM shared her interest in the cafe project and was enrolled in it. She has since been a contributing member to the cafe. Besides preparing and serving delicious confectioneries, the cafe has helped her with a job opportunity. She often shares that she wants to learn to work better, become financially independent, and then return home to her mother and daughter. Working in the cafe requires her to maintain proper hygiene, interact with team members and customers regularly, understand various instructions and follow recipes, take initiatives, and be efficient, all of which facilitate recovery in the mentioned domains of the Indian Disability Evaluation and Assessment Scale (IDEAS) as illustrated in Table 20.3.

Ms SM has presently saved enough to plan her visit to her family. She is taking pleasure in buying gifts and negotiating with her family, who are eager to know how much money she has saved. Ms SM shared that she will visit her family and

---

[3] Mousumi Staff Canteen is a tiffin service run by a self-help group of homeless women recovering from severe mental illness within the office premises of Iswar Sankalpa.

Table 20.3 Ms SM's IDEAS score over 2 years

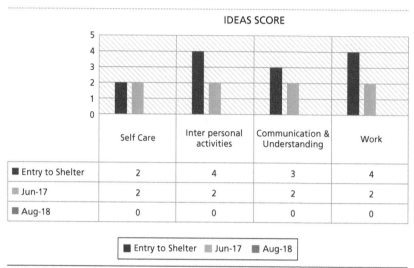

	Self Care	Inter personal activities	Communication & Understanding	Work
■ Entry to Shelter	2	4	3	4
▨ Jun-17	2	2	2	2
■ Aug-18	0	0	0	0

■ Entry to Shelter   ▨ Jun-17   ■ Aug-18

then come back to Kolkata again, as she needs to practise her chosen trade in future.

Rehabilitation for the homeless persons with severe mental illness: back to the soil

The mission of Iswar Sankalpa has been to offer choices to homeless individuals with severe mental illness for rehabilitation and reintegration with society and to support them through this process. Over the years, the experience has shown that beyond the catastrophic effects of mental illness the individual finds it a challenge to rise and become a 'productive' citizen once again. In order to prevent 'institutionalization' of long-stay persons who may never be able to return home, our team discovered that many of them had previous experience of agriculture and animal rearing as a form of livelihood.

Amid the green fields of Uttar Kashipur, Shanpukur Panchayat in the South 24 Parganas district, Iswar Sankalpa dreamt of building a new social and ecological justice-based village programme—Nayagram. Here, a few women would live life at their own pace, follow their own routine, work with the soil, sell the produce in the local market, keep accounts, pay for their own expenses, live in rented accommodation, pay its rent, work in the rural economy, and mingle with people, with little oversight by Iswar Sankalpa from Kolkata. It was the closest they could feel to returning to their families. Iswar Sankalpa identified Mr Ganguly, a local anchor. He was a respected community member, a good

Samaritan, and the headmaster of the local school at Kashipur under whose caring eye the small commune flourished.

Living in and as a commune of women offered the women a graded exposure to independent living, a promotion of self-regulation and discipline, with minimum supervision, and facilitated an 'affiliative process' in community participation which fostered a sense of belonging in persons who had lost every other bond in their lives.

Twenty-five women chose to move to Nayagram. Since then, a few have gone back to their families, and a few others found it difficult to cope with the work and life offered in Kashipur, and returned to the women's shelter in Kolkata. Twelve women continue to stay there, constantly trying to rebuild their lives in an open community (Fig. 20.3).

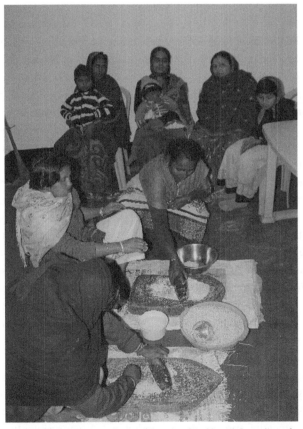

Fig. 20.3 Nayagram commune work—making sundried lentil dumplings for sale with community women.

The journey from homelessness to survival on the streets, to a life in a shelter, and finally to community living is one of many struggles, abuses, and reclamations. This journey is marked by care, nurturance, and friendships. The kinship and affection that is developing between the residents and the village community at Nayagram is evident. The community has connected to them to the extent that when the residents had gone to the city for a fortnight, the villagers kept asking where they were and when would they return back. A sense of familial affection has emerged with the community people gifting them their home-grown vegetables, unused jewellery, and even bringing back mementos from their holidays. The care giving is mutual. So, the residents even lent money to their anchor Mr G when he needed 500 rupees in an emergency situation. In case of any crisis, the neighbours consult in a group for problem-solving. They take it upon themselves to devise methods to mediate and resolve disputes. The community people are organizing a folk and food festival and it was decided to involve the residents of Nayagram in a cultural performance during the occasion.

The challenges have been aplenty depending on the phase of settling in to the new life. During the first 3 months of their stay at Nayagram, the entry phase, there is some discomfort with the new environment where the comforts of the former shelter are missed and residents experience a conflict between comfort and independence. There is an undeniable power dynamic within the commune, and subgroups are quickly formed. To maintain continuity with treatment, and maintenance of personal hygiene, supervision was required. Participation in regular work required constant coaxing.

After the first 3 months until about the end of the first year, a middle phase is observed, marked by relative independence of the women. It brings with it an increased vulnerability and feelings of desire and inappropriate behaviours begin to surface. As the sense of agency arises, interpersonal conflicts increase within the commune alongside high expressed emotions. This is indeed a very tricky phase. After the end of the first year, in the so-called late phase, women show evidence of increased authority and a sense of control over surroundings. This leads to an increased sense of independence and a challenging of authority structures. Subgroups and interpersonal conflicts increase but at the same time, coping mechanisms strengthen.

The rewards have been significant for the individuals, the organization, and for the society as a whole. Persons who were earlier considered a 'burden' on the society are now cultivating and producing vegetables that reach our tables (Fig. 20.4). Taking care of the cattle has been therapeutic and has inculcated an element of 'empathy' and 'care' in each individual. A new script is being written by this commune—the dignity of being able to sustain oneself on the earnings

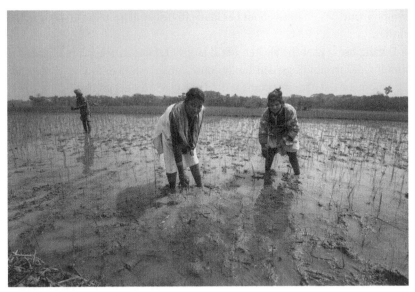

Fig. 20.4 Cultivation by Nayagram women.

from one's own labour. The community around them has offered 'kinship' and embraced the 'otherness' of women who may speak a different language and walk a different path and yet are a part of the life of the community.

A story of hope

Ms Z was identified during a medical camp organized by Iswar Sankalpa at Dhakuria, South Kolkata. West Bengal. She was first seen loitering in the Tollygunge Metro Station area with a few bags stuffed with paper pieces, torn clothes, and calendars. She was continuously muttering to herself as she walked around aimlessly. When she was approached to get into the ambulance for a doctor's check-up, she readily accepted the offer. Though unkempt and untidy, Ms Z was in a better hygienic condition than many others. She constantly complained of filth and foul smells from another person in the ambulance. At the medical camp, she cooperated with the staff of Sankalpa, took a bath, got her nails clipped, put on some new clothes, and sat down to eat. She properly divided the food and ate slowly and neatly. When offered a place at the shelter, Ms Z, though constantly preoccupied and muttering to herself, immediately agreed.

Ms Z was evidently malnourished. She kept muttering to herself continuously, was disoriented, did not keep eye contact, had disorganized thoughts, had a tendency to hoard things, and talked irrelevantly, or, in short, was highly symptomatic. Ms Z talked about her home in Belbandi from the first day in the shelter.

During her stay at the shelter, Ms Z largely remained preoccupied and un-mindful of surroundings, constantly complaining of filth or foul smells. As her treatment started, the symptoms started to subside quite rapidly. She improved remarkably within a short period of time. She now always complimented anyone wearing an embroidered dress. Hence, she was involved in stitching activities in vocational training classes.

She soon recalled her family who were then quickly traced by the restoration team at Iswar Sankalpa. Her younger brother and father informed the team that Ms Z was tortured and abandoned by her husband and in-laws after giving birth to three daughters and soon she started showing symptoms of a mental disorder. Ms Z came back to stay with her younger brother and father but then wandered out on quite a number of occasions from the house and was brought back every time. But the last time she went out, she could not be traced and had been missing for about 3 years. The family had a very humble background and they were amazed to see the remarkable progress in her health and socialization skills. The brother said Ms Z did not do any work at home and since they lived in a very remote village, it was next to impossible for a woman to get a job. They re-quested Iswar Sankalpa to continue with Ms Z's treatment for few more months at the shelter itself, where they knew she was safe and improving.

Accordingly, a progressive plan was made for Ms Z. She stated that she had studied in school but did not remember much about how to read or write. She was enrolled in the functional literacy classes and in a few months showed tremendous progress. She is due to take her National Institute of Open Schooling exams.

She is involved in daily household chores and has joined a 6-month long sewing/stitching training programme at a local institute. The goal is to make her capable and self-sufficient in order to make a living back at her home when she returns.

In 2018, Ms Z went to Nayagram. In the span of 10 months, she improved further, especially in interpersonal activities. She had lived in a village all her life and after being homeless for quite some time, she was recovering quite well in the shelter. But perhaps the desire to return to her village and work in the fields like before led her to choose Nayagram. And this could be a contributing factor in her recovery.

The graphs in Fig. 20.5 of Ms Z's IDEAS scores show as the first bars the condition in which she was initially found and entered the shelter, the second as the condition during which she chose to leave the shelter to go to Kashipur, and the third as the condition she is presently in after 10 months in the rural community.

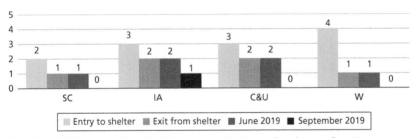

Fig. 20.5 IDEAS scores of Ms Z. C&U, communication and understanding; IA, interpersonal activities; SC, self-care; W, work.

Conclusion

Through all three interventions, we conclude that along with basic living support and treatment, the two integral processes of affiliation and affirmation have been of paramount importance in finding a new meaning in and purpose of a person's life after the disastrous effects of homelessness and severe mental illness. Rehabilitation is not just about transfer of a skill set or ensuring economic gains but of developing confidence in the ability of oneself to trust and have faith in the significant others of the new world.

References

1. **Anthony WA.** Recovery from mental illness: the guiding vision of the mental health service system in the 1990s. Psychosoc Rehabil J. 1993;**16**(4):11–23.
2. **Ravi M, Ravikanth L, Das Roy S.** India Exclusion Report: Urban Homeless People with Mental Illness. Delhi: Books for Change; 2018.
3. **Braehler C, Gumley A, Harper J, Wallace S, Norrie J, Gilbert P.** Exploring change processes in compassion focused therapy in psychosis: results of a feasibility randomized controlled trial. Br J Clin Psychol. 2013;**52**(2):199–214.
4. **Chatterjee D, Das Roy S.** Iswar Sankalpa: experience with the homeless persons with mental illness. In: **White RG, Jain S, Orr DMR, Read U** (Eds), The Palgrave Handbook of Sociocultural Perspectives on Global Mental Health. London: Palgrave Macmillan; 2017:751–777.
5. **Anthony WA.** Principles of Psychiatric Rehabilitation. Baltimore, MD: University Park Press; 1979.

Chapter 21

Mental health services for homeless people

Philip Timms

Introduction

Over the last 40 years, health services for homeless people, including specialist mental health services for homeless people, have been established all over the US, Australia, and Europe. But why should this be so? Why should one need to even contemplate a specialist service for homeless people? There are no mental disorders unique to the homeless population. There are the obvious barriers that arise in a fee-for service, or insurance-based system, but such services develop even in countries with universal health coverage, free at the point of delivery (1). The major drivers of homelessness are political and social more than medical or psychiatric (see Chapter 2). Nevertheless, these specialist services continue to exist—I myself worked in one for nearly 30 years.

Specialist mental health services for homeless people first emerged in the mid-1980s in the US, a response to the growing numbers of severely mentally unwell homeless people on the streets. This was widely seen as a result of rapid deinstitutionalization of mental health services, with meagre replacement provision of community services following the closures of state mental hospitals. A similar process happened in the UK, when a majority of mental hospitals were closed. However, in reality, this was related more closely to the wholesale closures of hostels for the homeless across large British cities (2). Similar services sprang up in Europe from the early 1990s, stimulated, at least in part, by the burgeoning American literature on the subject. Most of these services have been focused on psychosis.

Of course, a homeless person may be found in a range of unsatisfactory situations—from sleeping out on the street, to sleeping on the sofa of a friend or relative. However, the health profile of those who 'sofa surf' tends to be less extreme and marginalized than that of those living in formally homeless situations, such as hostels, night shelters, or on the street. I am going to focus on those services targeted at people in the latter category, whose health needs tend to be more extreme.

Few, if any, homeless services have been centrally planned and organized. They have usually arisen from the efforts of local enthusiasts engaging with the practicalities of the situations they have witnessed in a pragmatic way, rather than being directed by a clear theoretical model or political imperative. However, several themes have emerged from these services, overlapping considerably with the psychiatric literature on assertive outreach. I will look at some established models of approaching homeless people with severe mental illness, but also at some more recent developments in psychological services, which seek to address issues of addiction and personality disorders by using a model of multiple trauma. I will also address the thorny issue of collaborative versus enforced treatment and what the future might hold for such services.

But might there be a distinctive theoretical model to employ? An overarching notion of inclusion health practice has been established to characterize models of service that might best meet the needs of any socially excluded population—including homeless people.

Inclusion health

This term has been coined to describe services and policies that aim to prevent and redress health and social inequities among the vulnerable and excluded populations (3). Homeless people are one such excluded group, experiencing significant barriers to adequate health care—but, why should this extra effort be necessary?

Even if a health service is free at the point of access, homeless people can find it hard both to register with a primary care service (being sometimes illegally refused registration) as they may not be able to give a residential address, and, even when registered, to get an adequate service from such services (4). In Europe, researchers have noted little involvement of mental health staff, with low levels of active outreach and case finding. Services can also exclude homeless people because of their specific inclusion criteria. There is often significant prejudice in health services towards homeless people as well as those who have mental illness, thus creating a double exclusion. Services do not coordinate well with each other and, in an insurance-based system, there may be difficulties in obtaining health insurance (5).

Five themes inform such work:

Equity

A distinguished general practitioner (GP), Julian Tudor Hart, noticed that disadvantaged populations seem to have less access to health and social services rather than more. His inverse care law (6) suggests that this is more or less universal—those most in need get the fewest services. So, the over-riding principle of inclusion health is that of social equity—that everyone, no matter what their situation, should have access to the health services that they need. Healthcare is viewed not as a commodity, but as a right. This is not a value that underpins every healthcare system, but it does seem to be something that most health professionals feel in their bones—whether or not they believe that it is practical or economic to do so. However, at least in Europe, there is some legal backbone to this idea. Article 35 of the Charter of Fundamental Rights of the European Union (7) states:

> Everyone has the right of access to preventive health care and the right to benefit from medical treatment under the conditions established by national laws and practices.

There are, of course, multiple obstacles to achieving such equity of access and health provision. These can be political decisions, structural problems within services, practitioner attitudes, and barriers felt by the deprived individuals themselves.

Moreover, while the less well-off have less access to mainstream services, this seems to be matched by their increased use of emergency services, such as ambulances and accident and emergency departments (8). This results in unhappiness all round. These acute services are not set up to deal with the sort of chronic and multiple problems experienced by deprived populations—and stigmatizing attitudes towards homeless patients can develop in such services (9).

Multiple morbidities

Homeless people are not just at the lower end of the social ladder—they have fallen off the bottom rung. And for all disadvantaged populations, 'When sorrows come, they come not single spies, but in battalions' (10). Social deprivation is generally associated with worse health and lower life expectancy—and so it is for those who have lost contact with supportive social networks and helping agencies (11). Multiple morbidity is the norm rather than the exception, often at a level which would be normal for those many decades older (12). Physical and mental health problems coexist with multiple emotional, social, and financial problems. This does not fit well with traditional models of health provision, which (with the honourable exception of general practice) divide practitioners according to the organ or system in which they specialize. This has tended to stimulate the development of homeless services that are both multidisciplinary and include non-health personnel.

Outreach

Echoing Tudor Hart's observations of low-income populations, many surveys of homeless populations have found very high levels of physical and mental pathology, but have recorded a correspondingly low level of service use. Cynics may put this down to a capricious refusal of services by the fecklessness of the homeless people concerned. But, mysteriously, such people appear to be quite happy to use services that are delivered in a less formal way, in or close to their usual surroundings (13). Much of the theory and practice underpinning this approach was based on the assertive outreach literature. This acknowledged the fact that, at some points in a person's illness trajectory, they may become less able to make informed decisions—or to initiate the actions that are needed to ensure their safety or well-being. Hence the need, sometimes, to approach a person less as a consumer or client and, perhaps, more as a patient whose capacity is compromised. I will explore this further in a later section which explores street assessments.

Engagement

Health providers can often be frustrated by the fact that many people who are homeless seem to find it hard to engage with them—or, indeed, with any other helping personnel—even though doing so would be to their benefit. At the same time, there is little or no attention given in medical and nursing training to the issue of how to engage a prospective patient in a therapeutic relationship. That is to say, one that is helpful, supportive, and enables recovery. This relationship issue seems to be independent of the practical problems described previously and has recently been explored within the developing notion of multiple trauma.

Multisectoral collaborative working

The multiple deficits that exist in a homeless person's life are not susceptible to a single model of intervention from a single profession or service. Therefore, services for homeless people tend to be much more actively cross-sectoral than other mental health services. This type of collaboration is easy in theory but can be problematical in practice. Different sectors may have conflicting priorities and values even though they all wish for an improvement in a person's welfare (14).

Practical features of such services

So, how might these work out in practice? Let's start with the characteristics of assertive outreach services, set up to approach those with severe and enduring mental illness who do not, for whatever reason, engage well with standard services (15). They should:

◆ Be multidisciplinary—including doctors, nurses, and social workers as a minimum, but also with psychologists, housing workers, vocational trainers, and peer support workers, as necessary.

◆ Accommodate caseloads of less than ten clients per case worker.

◆ Provide intensive frequency of client contact, up to four times per week.

◆ Emphasize the process of engagement and creating a therapeutic relationship.

◆ Impose no time-limit on services.

◆ Provide or access specific evidence-based treatments.

◆ Work with clients in their own environment and with their social network.

◆ Provide support for team members.

These are similar, but not identical, to the characteristics of homeless mental health services—with the exception of caseload size. In the UK, I have never come across a homeless mental health service where workers had a caseload of ten or less. But, otherwise, they seem to be pretty comparable. I will consider these, and other characteristics, many of which were set out in the 1980s (16).

Outreach

Traditional assertive outreach services strive to engage better with those who are not doing well with an existing service. Homeless services, on the other hand, are usually trying to engage with those who have *no* contact with existing health or social services. And so a major task is that of the initial approach to the homeless person. And this will differ according to the type, or level, of outreach that is offered. Homeless populations generally have high levels of psychosis, and so this will be a major focus for specialist mental health services. An Edinburgh survey in the 1970s suggested that, while homeless people with alcohol and personality problems tended to present themselves to services, those with psychosis did not (17). I have constructed a rough classificatory system for outreach services, each level being dependent on the local ecosystem of statutory and voluntary sector providers.

Primary

A specialist mental health service approaches and engages directly with the potential service user—on the street, in hostels and night shelters, or in day centres. And, of course, such services are usually the only ones prepared to carry out an assessment in such settings. Given the episodic nature of medical attention, such activity will usually be concerned with assessment. Project Help, in New York, US, reported such assessments as being conducted in emergency situations (18) -and highlighted some difficulties. These included little knowledge of the potential patient's history, little or no privacy in the course of the assessment, unwanted interference from passers-by, and, sometimes, agitation and distress on the part of the person concerned. Such assessments were often heavily weighted in favour of observation over conversation with the patient.

Secondary

A mental health service works collaboratively with another organization (usually voluntary sector) delivering direct services to homeless people, such as a street outreach team. The mental health service can take advantage of:

1. The relationship of trust already established between the partner organization and their homeless clientele. So, the initial approach may not be so threatening for the client. A voluntary sector outreach organization, who will usually know the person best, can provide some background knowledge of the person and a longitudinal perspective on their predicament. By being already known to the person involved, their participation can smooth the first contact and any actual assessment.

2. The range of physical and practical support services offered by the voluntary sector.

Subsequently, the partner organizations can support each other in continuing work. This approach makes particular sense when a street assessment is not so much an emergency, but part of a process (often over several weeks or months) of attempted engagement with a vulnerable person (19).

Tertiary

A specialist mental health facility is set up within a hospital clinic, or hospital structure, to focus on the mental needs of homeless people. This can certainly work for some, but does tend to select a better-engaged subgroup of homeless people (20).

Accessibility

This can be geographical, temporal, or cultural. A homeless person will often not have the resources to be able to travel to a clinic or hospital, so a service provided within the local milieu will clearly be more accessible. Extended opening hours, or flexible appointment times, will be easier to use—and, sometimes, may be the only way of establishing and maintain contact. For example, one may only be able to find a person at their sleeping site out of normal working hours. A less formal way of working can help to bridge the social distance that inevitably exists between the homeless person and the service provider.

Flexibility

Every service likes to say that it is flexible, but such flexibility is often constrained by structural limitations—clinic times, availability of senior staff, set working hours, and so on. This may not matter so much with a domiciled population with some flexibility of its own and the resources to get to (sometimes geographically remote) health services. However, those without the ability to get around are less likely to use services. A Bristol outreach clinic commented that, although they had had some success in providing a service for local homeless people, they were seeing a highly selected group who had managed, for example, to register with a GP (20). And registering with a primary care provider is still a significant barrier to homeless people in accessing healthcare, both in the UK and elsewhere (21,22).

Integration with other provider systems

This has often been a thorny problem—agencies are run from different budgets and can have different priorities and targets. However, there is some evidence that more integrated services can work better, even than 'parallel' services which, on paper, deliver the same components of service (23).

Generalist

In an age where specialization of teams and service providers has tended to become the norm (24), homeless services are more often generalist in nature. This means that the individual service user does not have to go from one service to another to get the help that they need. It is also much easier to form a trusting relationship with one service rather than several. An indirect benefit is that one is not constantly having to turn down referrals from (say) voluntary sector agencies because they do not fit a particular diagnostic profile. And in homeless populations, where multimorbidity is the norm, it maynot be clear, at a particular point in time, which issue should be assigned highest priority.

Relationship-focused provision

In a sense, this is forced upon any effective homeless service as the service user will often have had poor experience with services in the past. He or she may be, at best, ambivalent, at worst hostile, to the idea of engaging with any such service again. On the other hand, if the service provider can demonstrate that they are a safe and competent presence, then a fruitful relationship can be established, which seems to improve outcomes (25). Such a way of working takes time—hence the benefit of small caseloads.

Multiskilled/resourced services: moving beyond psychosis

This notion makes perfect sense in many service milieux—but particularly so in homelessness, where individuals usually present with multiple needs in different domains at a single point in time. This can be achieved by incorporating other disciplines within a single team, by close collaboration with other agencies, or by physically basing a range of services in a single geographical location, or by some mixture of these approaches. The Compass Centre, in Bristol, UK, is hosted by St Mungo's, a voluntary sector provider—but contains a number of National Health Service (NHS) and non-NHS services, including primary care, addictions, sexual health, counselling, and mental health services (26). But why no formal provision of housing or social services? Our experience in South London suggested that organizational barriers can often interfere with such active interagency working (14). And while most outreach services for homeless people have been focused on psychosis, attention usually needs to be paid, at the same time, to several other areas of need.

Use of peer advocates

This was pioneered in the US and the Netherlands but has recently become a common feature of services in the UK (27).

Most of the attributes described previously would actually be used by many mainstream services to describe how they work. So, what does make homeless services different? There is surprisingly little reference to this in the literature but, to me, certain characteristics stand out, more by emphasis than by absolute difference.

Continuity

One characteristic that goes against the grain of current service provision, at least in the UK, is that of continuity over time—or, as it has been described, as a continuous-relationship model of service (28). This refers to a service which is continuous from the initial point of contact, on the street or in some other homeless milieu, to the point at which the individual is firmly established in permanent accommodation and so can be safely referred to a mainstream service. This eliminates the need for changes in team as a person moves (at least in the traditional way) from the street, to temporary accommodation, and then to permanent accommodation.

Relationship building

The establishment and maintenance of a trusting and meaningful relationship between outreach worker and client. This includes five common tasks:

- Establishing contact and credibility.
- Identifying people with mental illness.
- Engaging clients.
- Carrying out assessments and treatment planning.
- Providing a longer-term, continuing service.

Throughout all these phases, several things are going on at the same time. Both practical and psychological tasks can be ways of establishing oneself—and one's team—as a safe, helpful presence in a person's life.

So, at first, the emphasis will often be on sorting out some basic practical issues for the person, while demonstrating one's reliability and safety. This is done by turning up on time, listening, not promising more than the worker or team can offer, trying to attend to the patient's priorities, as far as possible, and not meeting rejection with rejection. Other issues to grapple with include:

- The apparently paradoxical task of responding supportively to dependency needs while, at the same time, helping the person to become more independent.
- Setting clear and firm limits while maintaining flexibility.
- Acknowledging and dealing with resistance (the refusal or avoidance of assistance and treatment)—without rancour or rejection (29).

Critical time intervention

Susser and his colleagues in New York (30), provided extra time and input to clients who were in the process of moving from one form of accommodation to another—usually from a large night shelter to a single-room occupancy hotel. This substantially reduced both the dropout rate from services and the nights spent homeless by two-thirds. Gains over the control group (receiving normal services) were maintained over the 18 months following the withdrawal of the critical time intervention service.

One might argue that this is just good practice anyway, but doing it in a planned and structured way did seem to make a significant difference to the levels of engagement and outcomes. It involved home visits, individual support, support for caregivers, and negotiation and mediation with caregivers when problems arose. Long-term plans were constructed and formal handovers to local agencies were negotiated. This period of increased support lasted from 7 to 9 months and caseloads for critical time intervention workers were typically held at 15 or less.

Why should such an intervention be necessary? During a period of transition, clients typically have to negotiate a complex and fragmented system of care (31). Both the positive and negative symptoms of psychosis are likely to impair their ability to understand such systems and to be able to form and maintain the relationships necessary to negotiate them. Another important factor may have been that the critical time intervention process fostered the establishment of a new system of necessary dependencies for the client. This meant that the withdrawal of the original service provider, on which the client had become dependent, would have less impact.

Some new models of service

Psychologically informed environments

A model of psychologically integrated services has recently emerged from the homeless sector and the Royal College of Psychiatrists (32). The basic problem it seeks to address is the very high levels of psychological problems (not just mental illness) in the various settings in which homeless people are served or accommodated. And the logic goes—why not introduce sophisticated psychological expertise to these environments? By so doing, individual and group therapy can be offered to service users, but also staff can be encouraged to practise more reflectively, with regular staff meetings with a psychologist. In many ways this is an outgrowth of the work of the therapeutic community movement. An online guide is available to facilitate the development of such projects (33). Although this approach makes perfect sense, outcome data is, as yet, sparse.

Trauma-informed care

This addresses the issues of the (often multiple) traumas that occur in the early lives of both homeless people and those with mental health problems. We know that people who are homeless are likely to have had some form of previous trauma. Homelessness can, itself, be traumatic, and being homeless increases the risk of further victimization and trauma. As a consequence, many homeless people can find it hard to engage with services because of lack of trust and rekindling of previous traumatic experiences. Problems with managing emotions and adhering to social norms can create problems in living and in moving to settled housing, where some contact with other people is unavoidable. Trauma-informed care is not a separate 'therapy' but seeks to embed an awareness of these issues in a range of services, from mental health to housing (34).

Enhanced access to psychotherapy

This has been piloted in central London, UK (35), by the Lifeworks project, which provided psychodynamic psychotherapy services under the umbrella of St Mungo's, a voluntary sector housing provider. For the sake of confidentiality, these services were provided in GP surgeries, offices, and in some daycentres. Again, a major principle has been to maximize access—by eliminating acceptance criteria, apart from the desire of the client to come to therapeutic sessions. Outcomes seem to have been generally good—including reduced use of emergency services. It even appears to be economically effective.

For people still sleeping out, or not engaged with other housing services, a 'pre-treatment' approach has been taken (36) by providing a twice-weekly drop-in service at a specialist GP surgery for homeless people. This focuses on providing the necessary elements of any sort of therapy—safety, a trusting relationship, speaking the same language, and establishing clear boundaries. These tentative, 'getting to know one other' contacts can then progress to more formal psychotherapy sessions. They also run an open, drop-in discussion/anger support group and offer telephone and email support between sessions.

Enhanced capacity assessments

Most mental health services for homeless people aim to increase access to services and to reduce social exclusion—with the active participation of the client. Collaboration and increasing autonomy are seen as desirable.

However, situations do arise where decisions made by the individual seem to imperil their health, their safety, and (rarely) the safety of others. The presence of a significant mental illness may mean that, although therapeutic input, physical healthcare, and practical assistance have already been offered on the street, this has not resulted in the establishment of a meaningful therapeutic relationship or change.

Workers with such teams are then faced with a dilemma. How far should they compromise their client's autonomy in order to safeguard them, or to promote their recovery and journey from homelessness (37)? In extreme cases, this can involve the choice to over-ride an individual's autonomy and safe their life—or, by not doing so (and given the extreme conditions faced by homeless people), to let them die (38). This clash of professional impulses can create real problems, leading to no decisions being made and no action being taken.

In the UK, the legislation governing mandatory hospital admission and treatment (39) demands that signs and symptoms of mental disorder are identified by the assessors. However, the experience of many street outreach teams has been that such symptoms can be hard to elicit clearly when meeting with someone on the street. So, individuals who seem to a have an obvious impairment to those who know them best, do not get the assessment and treatment they need.

One way forward may be to not focus on the presence or absence of clear psychiatric symptoms alone. Instead, one can explore the capacity of the individual to make a specific and significant informed choice—such as whether to stay on the street or not. A capacity assessment can demonstrate that a person is unable to make a choice of a particular sort for themselves at a particular point in time. It does not substitute for an assessment of psychiatric symptoms, but complements it. The underlying assumption is that if an individual's capacity seems to be significantly compromised vis-à-vis an important decision concerning their health and well-being, they should, perhaps, be given a period of assessment in hospital, even if they are unwilling or unable to give consent for this. A consortium of agencies in London has created a guide for such assessments to be used by non-medical as well as medical workers in this area (40).

Effectiveness of services

It's all well and good discussing ways of helping a particular clientele. But the acid test is, does a service actually help? It must be more than a sentimental response to the guilty cry of 'something must be done about this'. There is evidence for a range of interventions for homeless people with mental health problems, even though most studies use proxy measures rather than direct assessments of mental state or functionality.

What does work?

Assertive outreach

Assertive outreach for domiciled people has not been found to be particularly helpful in UK community populations (41). This may have been due to lack of fidelity to the assertive outreach model and comparison services already having some of the characteristics of assertive outreach teams. However, the situation does seem to be different with homeless people. A well-randomized study in Missouri, US (42), found that homeless people who received assertive community treatment seem to gain accommodation more quickly than those who received brokered case management, outpatient treatment, or services from a drop-in centre. More assistance in finding and maintaining housing were especially predictive of shorter homeless spells.

A comparison with standard services in Baltimore (43) found that assertive community treatment for homeless people was both more cost-effective than a standard service and 'significantly more effective in producing more days of stable housing ... at significantly lower in-patient and emergency room costs and significantly higher out-patient costs'. So, here the balance of cost was shifted to community services from hospital services.

What is the effect of a specialist community team on hospital admission?

A comparative survey in Birmingham, UK, compared hospital admissions of homeless people over two time periods—one before, and one after the introduction of a specialist (44) mental health team for homeless people. The actual number of admissions remained much the same. Although the team felt that they prevented many admissions, there was a much higher rate of compulsory admissions, possibly suggesting that the team was identifying people with severe mental illness on the street who had been overlooked prior to the introduction of their service. The rate of follow-up post discharge was also significantly higher—but usually by the homeless team itself, suggesting that pickup by local mainstream services continued to be problematical. The team focused on psychosis and commented that 'The patients who seemed to gain least from the specialist team homeless were those with non-psychotic disorders, predominantly personality and substance use disorders'. So, here is a clue that one size does not fit all, and that a range of provision is needed to match the range of presenting needs.

Does admission to hospital help?

In spite of a therapeutic pessimism noted by many of those who work in this area, there is evidence of the effectiveness of psychiatric interventions in homeless populations, albeit usually with small-scale studies. A small London study in 1999 (45) noted the pessimism felt by staff towards street-sleeping people with mental health problems. Staff believed that 'admission would be difficult, the psychiatric outcome poor and that people would return to the streets soon after discharge'. However, over 90% of those with psychosis were able to remain in touch with mental health teams—admittedly, the small number of patients involved ($n = 12$) meant that all this study could be was a proof of principle. Against this was the poor outcome of those who were admitted, but did not have a psychosis—again a small and skewed sample, with four cases of psychiatric Munchausen's. But, overall, a small glimmer of hope in an area deemed hopeless.

Another small study (n = 24) at Bellevue hospital in New York (46) demonstrated significant symptom reduction between admission and discharge from hospital. There were no follow-up data but a comment that 'homeless people frequently make choices and refuse medication and psychotherapy', in a world where 'most people cannot be trusted'. This highlighted a feature of homelessness that only started to be formally addressed with the introduction of trauma-based approaches (see earlier in chapter).

More recently, in 2017 the START team, in London (47), looked at 37 consecutive compulsory hospital admissions of people living on the street—and asked what was happening a year later. Seventy-five per cent of those detained and treated were still in touch with psychiatric services, 70% were still in accommodation, and most were now registered with a GP. These can be seen as proxy measures to be sure, but they remain significant ones. However, two problems were noted. The fact that a small number of patients had had to be admitted twice, because on the first occasion the ward staff did not view the individual as being sufficiently mentally ill. The second was that most of this cohort were still being looked after by the specialist homeless team. As had been found in Birmingham, the objective of handing over clients to local services proved difficult.

Prevention

It can be argued that, as the principal drivers of homelessness are outside the control of mental health services, then there is nothing to be done about primary or secondary level prevention by such services. Certainly, mental health was only a very small part of a recent review of homelessness prevention (48). However, there are hints that there is work to be done in tertiary prevention. A London homeless service (START team) looked at 3 months of its referrals and found that 60% of them had had previous contact with the local mental health trust (49). Moreover, this contact had often been substantial. On average, they had had contacts with four separate trust services, 35 contacts (face-to-face/phone triage), and had spent 65 days as an inpatient in the local hospital service. This suggests that there are significant problems with the way that mainstream services deal with homeless people—but also that this could be a useful focus for service improvement.

What doesn't work?

An early overview of a range of services in the US (50) found that many services 'typically spent the majority of their time and effort on screening and identifying mentally ill homeless persons in need of mental health and other human services; clients were generally provided with verbal referrals, but little follow-up assistance'. And that such services were ineffective. Simple sign-posting is beloved of service planners because it seems both to be cheap, and to make the best use of existing resources. However, services that focus exclusively on assessment, and then only provide (usually verbal) referrals to other services, just don't seem to work very well for homeless people (50). This is not surprising. The offer of advice/signposting assumes that the homeless person will have the necessary resources to take advantage of such information—and often they do not.

Conclusion

In spite of the numbers of homeless people with severe mental illness, the active provision of psychiatric services to homeless people did not develop until the mid-1980s. Such services have survived, in many places, but have generally been unable to make any substantial change in the surrounding conditions that have created the problem in the first place. Social determinants such as inequality (51), poverty, and discrimination are the main drivers of homelessness (52) and these are beyond the immediate sphere of influence of health providers. So, what is the point of such services? It is worth noting that even countries with less inequality and poverty still have a problem with people with mental disorders who become homeless. So there still seems to be an international problem with how mental health services are organized.

Although most homeless services started as psychosis services, it has become clear that there are many other people who are homeless who can benefit from a wider range of provision. And some novel psychological initiatives, described earlier, have emerged to meet this need.

One can look at such services as fulfilling a moral imperative—to ensure that no one who requires treatment and support is denied it. But one can also look at homeless services in a more technical sense—as pioneers of different models of mental health practice, including models of assertive outreach, psychologically informed environments, and more accessible models of psychological intervention. And, via their much deeper levels of collaboration with non-medical and psychological organizations, as pioneering a different way to provide mental health services. Operating as part of a greater whole, better able to meet an individual's several needs in a comprehensive and coordinated way.

All effective treatment programmes have involved psychiatric provision as a coordinated part of more general provision of housing and social services. In many ways, they have anticipated the needs-led assessment, case management, and service coordination that have developed as part of community psychiatry programmes in many countries. It can be argued that most of the characteristics of these services are really nothing more than the requirements for an effective, non-institutional community psychiatry, whether the recipients of such a service are domiciled or not. And these technical innovations are combined with an acute awareness of the reality and impact of social exclusion, and a determination to maximize social inclusion.

As to what needs to change—further integration of primary care and substance abuse services, or at least the incorporation of such expertise into services for homeless people.

Given that the drivers of homelessness and social exclusion are unlikely to disappear in the foreseeable future, I would expect such services to continue from necessity, but also to provide models for positively inclusive, comprehensive mental health services for all.

References

1. **Brandt P.** Homelessness and mental illness in Denmark: focus on 'street-dwellers'. Int J Ment Health. 2001;**30**(3):84–92.
2. **Craig T, Timms P.** Out of the wards and onto the streets? Deinstitutionalization and homelessness in Britain. J Ment Health. 1992;**1**(3):265–275.
3. **Luchenski S, Maguire N, Aldridge RW,** et al. What works in inclusion health: overview of effective interventions for marginalised and excluded populations. Lancet. 2018;**391**(10117):266–280.
4. **Eavis C.** The barriers to healthcare encountered by single homeless people. Primary Health Care. 2018;**28**(1):26–30.
5. **Réamonn Canavan R, Barry MM, Matanov A,** et al. Service provision and barriers to care for homeless people with mental health problems across 14 European capital cities. BMC Health Serv Res. 2012;**12**:222.
6. **Tudor Hart J.** The inverse care law. Lancet, 1971;**297**(7696):405–412.
7. **European Union.** Charter of Fundamental Rights of the European Union. 2000. Available from: https://www.europarl.europa.eu/charter/pdf/text_en.pdf.
8. **Ní Cheallaigh C, Cullivan S, Jess Sears J,** et al. Usage of unscheduled hospital care by homeless individuals in Dublin, Ireland: a cross-sectional study. BMJ Open. 2017;**7**:e016420.
9. **Jeffrey R.** Normal rubbish: deviant patients in casualty departments. Sociol Health Illn. 1979;**1**(1):91–107.
10. **Shakespeare W.** Hamlet, Act IV, Scene V. 1602.
11. **Fazel S, Geddes JR, Kushel M.** The health of homeless people in high-income countries: descriptive epidemiology, health consequences, and clinical and policy recommendations. Lancet. 2014;**384**(9953):1529–1540.
12. **Queen AB, Lowrie R, Richardson J, Williamson AE.** Multimorbidity, disadvantage and patient engagement within a specialist homeless health service in the UK. BJGP Open. 2017;**1**(3):0641.

13. **Morse G, Calsyn RJ.** Mentally disturbed homeless people in St. Louis: needy, willing but underserved. Int J Ment Health. 1986;**14**(4):74–94.

14. **Timms P.** Partnership and conflict: working relationships between voluntary and statutory agencies providing services for homeless people. In: **Cowan D** (Ed), Housing: Participation and Exclusion. Collected Papers from the Socio-Legal Studies Annual Conference. London: Routledge; 1998:68–83.

15. **Sainsbury Centre for Mental Health.** Assertive Outreach. London: Sainsbury Centre for Mental Health; 1971.

16. **Breakey WR.** Treating the homeless. Alcohol Health Res World. 1987;**11**(3):42–47.

17. **Priest RO.** The homeless person and the psychiatric services: an Edinburgh survey. Br J Psychiatry. 1976;**128**:128–136.

18. **Tsemberis S, Cohen NL, Jones RM.** Conducting emergency psychiatric evaluations on the street. In: **Katz SE, Nardacci D, Sabatini A** (Eds), Intensive Treatment of the Homeless Mentally Ill. Washington, DC: American Psychiatric Press; 1993:71–89.

19. **Barreto E, Bento A, Leonori L,** et al. Dignity and Well-Being: Practical Approaches to Working with Homeless People with Mental Health Problems. Brussels: SMES Europa; 2019.

20. **Tomison AR, Cook M.** Rootlessness and mental disorder. Br J Clin Soc Psychiatry. 1987;**5**(1):5–8.

21. **Burrows M, Edgar R, Fitch T.** More than a Statistic. London: Healthy London Partnership; 2016.

22. **Health Quality Ontario.** Interventions to improve access to primary care for people who are homeless: a systematic review. Ont Health Technol Assess Ser. 2016;**16**(9):1–50.

23. **McHugo GJ, Richard R, Bebout RR,** et al. A randomized controlled trial of integrated versus parallel housing services for homeless adults with severe mental illness. Schizophr Bull. 2004;**30**(4):969–982.

24. **Laughnarne R, Thompson M, Srivastava A,** et al. Getting a balance between generalisation and specialisation in mental health services: a defence of general services. Bulletin BJPsych. 2018;**42**(6):229–232.

25. **Chinman MJ P, Rosenheck R, Lam JA.** The case management relationship and outcomes of homeless persons with serious mental illness. Psychiatric Serv. 2000;**51**(9):1142–1147.

26. **The Compass Health Centre.** Homepage. Available from: https://www.compasshealthbristol.co.uk/

27. **Barker SL, McGuire N.** Experts by experience: peer support and its use with the homeless. Comm Ment Health J. 2017;**53**(5):598–612.

28. **Morse GA, Calsyn RJ, Miller J, Rosenberg P, West L, Giuiland J.** Outreach to homeless mentally ill people: conceptual and clinical considerations. Community Ment Health J. 1996;**32**(3):261–274.

29. **Kuhlman T.** Psychology on the Streets. New York: Wiley; 1994.

30. **Susser E, Valencia E, Conover S,** et al. Preventing recurrent homelessness among mentally ill men: a "critical time" intervention after discharge from a shelter. Am J Public Health. 1997;**87**(2):256–262.

31. **Dorwart R, Hoover CW.** A national study of transitional hospital services in mental health. Am J Public Health. 1994;**84**(8):1229–1234.

32. **Johnson R, Haigh R.** Social psychiatry and social policy for the 21st century: new concepts for new needs—the 'enabling Environments' initiative. Ment Health Soc Incl. 2011;**15**(1):17–23.

33. **Keats H, Maguire N, Johnson R, Cockersall P.** Psychologically informed services for homeless people. Good practice guide. **Department of Communities and Local Government**; 2012. Available from: https://eprints.soton.ac.uk/340022/.

34. **Hopper EK, Bassuk E, Olivet J.** Shelter from the storm: trauma-informed care in homelessness services settings. Open Health Serv Policy J. 2010;**3**(2):80–100.

35. **Cockersell P.** Applying psychology as a response to the impact of social exclusion. in social exclusion, compound trauma and recovery. In: **Cockersell P** (Ed), Applying Psychology, Psychotherapy and PIE to Homelessness and Complex Needs. London: Jessica Kingsley Publishers; 2018:80–106.

36. **Conolly J.** Pre-treatment therapy approach for single homeless people. in social exclusion, compound trauma and recovery. In: **Cockersell P** (Ed), Applying Psychology, Psychotherapy and PIE to Homelessness and Complex Needs. London: Jessica Kingsley Publishers; 2018:109–133.

37. **Michael Rowe M, Frey J, Bailey MSW,** et al. Clinical responsibility and client autonomy: dilemmas in mental health work at the margins. Am J Orthopsychiatry. 2001;**71**(4):400–407.

38. **Cournos F.** The case of Miss Joyce Brown. Hosp Commun Psychiatry. 1989;**40**(7):736–740.

39. **Legislation.co.uk.** Mental Health Act 1983. 1983. Available from: https://www.legislation.gov.uk/ukpga/1983/20/contents.

40. **Clowes E, Timms P, Bax A,** et al. Mental Health Service Assessments for Rough Sleepers: Tools and Guidance. London: Pathway; 2017.

41. **Killaspy H, Kingett S, Bebbington P,** et al. Randomised evaluation of assertive community treatment: 3-year outcomes. Br J Psychiatry. 2009;**195**(1):81–82.

42. **McBride TD, Calsyn RJ, Morse GA,** et al. Duration of homeless spells among severely mentally ill individuals: a survival analysis. J Community Psychol. 1998;**26**(5):473–490.

43. **Lehman AF, Dixon L, Hoch JS,** et al. Cost-effectiveness of assertive community treatment for homeless persons with severe mental illness. Br J Psychiatry. 1999;**174**:346–352.

44. **Commander M, Odell S, Sashidharan S.** Psychiatric admission for homeless people: the impact of a specialist community mental health team. Psychiatr Bull. 1997;**21**(5):260–263.

45. **Graham, ZC, Salton-Cox FS, White PD.** The outcome of rough sleepers with mental health problems admitted to a psychiatric ward. Psychiatr Bull. 1999;**23**(3):164–166.

46. **Caro Y, Nardacci D, Silbert H,** et al. Hospital assessment. In: **Katz S, Nardacci D, Sabatini A** (Eds), Intensive Treatment for the Homeless Mentally Ill. Washington DC: American Psychiatric Press; 1993.

47. **Timms P, Perry J.** Sectioning on the street—utility or futility? Br J Psych Bull. 2016;**40**(6):302–305.

48. **Pleace N.** Preventing Homelessness: A Review of the International Evidence. Dublin: Simon Communities of Ireland; 2019.

49. **Timms P, Craig T.** Deinstitutionalisation, prison and homelessness. Br J Psychiatry. 2016;**209**(4):349–350.

50. **Hopper K, Mauch D, Morse G.** The 1986–1987 NIMH-Funded CSP Demonstration Projects to Serve Homeless Mentally Ill Persons: A Preliminary Assessment. Rockville, MD: National Institute of Mental Health; 1990.

51. **Pleace N.** Homelessness and inequality. In: **Anderson I, Sim D** (Eds), Housing and Inequality. London: Chartered Institute of Housing; 2011:187–204.

52. **Schinn M.** Homelessness, poverty and social exclusion in the United States and Europe. Eur J Homelessness. 2010;**4**:19–44.

Chapter 22

Service experiences and perceptions of people experiencing homelessness

Nick Kerman and John Sylvestre

Introduction

People who are homeless are a highly vulnerable and quite diverse population, often having unmet needs across many domains. Although the fundamental need they share is housing, many people also struggle with food insecurity, unemployment, insufficient social support, and a range of complex health problems, including chronic medical conditions, substance use, and severe mental illness (1–5). Given the many challenges they face, the lives of people experiencing homelessness are filled with services. In many communities, people access emergency shelters to sleep, soup kitchens and meal programmes multiple times per day to eat, drop-in centres for warmth and social connection, and emergency departments to address urgent health problems. In short, many people experiencing homelessness go to bed and wake up in service settings and spend their days traversing from one service to another. Moreover, many of the services they access daily do not permanently resolve the foundational need for housing. Instead, they offer temporary solutions to manage urgent problems.

Despite the many health, social, and community services that exist for people experiencing homelessness, a proportion of the homeless population does not use services. In some instances, this is a personal choice (e.g. not accessing healthcare because it is not seen as needed, sleeping on the streets to avoid the shelter system), but for others, the issue is service accessibility (6–8). Many studies have sought to better understand the factors associated with service use and non-use. Although this research has yielded insights into specific factors that may increase or decrease the likelihood of service use, a clear picture of the factors that predict service use remains elusive. This may be due to the heterogeneity of the homeless population (e.g. predictors of service use for homeless youth may differ from those for homeless veterans), differences between services (e.g. factors associated with use of emergency departments may minimally overlap with those related to case management or counselling), and geographical and contextual variation (e.g. policy and service availability differences). Taken together, research predicting service use by people experiencing homelessness may not be generalizable beyond the types of services used, the homeless subpopulation studied, and the region where the research was conducted. Given the challenges with predicting service use, the perceptions and experiences of this population are critical to understanding service use and improving service delivery to this population.

Positive service experiences are instrumental to quality healthcare (9,10) and the same can be said of social and community service delivery. The importance of experience is perhaps even greater for people experiencing homelessness as they commonly report negative experiences, which can lead to service discontinuation and exacerbation of health problems (11,12). As such, considerable research has been conducted to understand the perspectives and experiences of people who are homeless with the objective of improving the provision of treatment and care. This chapter reviews the evidence on the experiences and perspectives of the homeless population when using services. Much of the evidence comes from qualitative studies that foreground the voices of people experiencing homelessness, though other methodological approaches have also been used. Findings are categorized according to seven factors (Table 22.1), which can be multifaceted and interrelated. Implications for service delivery are subsequently discussed.

Accessibility

Access to services for people experiencing homelessness has been extensively researched, with many studies highlighting the range of accessibility challenges encountered by this population. Service accessibility for people experiencing homelessness includes issues of location and mobility; flexibility; capacity and eligibility, including service bans and refusals; coordination; and affordability. Beginning with location and mobility, studies have found that the scattering of services around a city can make it difficult for people experiencing homelessness to access them (13–18). Limited income for public transportation required to access services is a prominent contributor to accessibility problems (15,16,18). In contrast, mobile outreach teams and multiservice agencies that act as one-stop shops can enhance accessibility and are perceived positively (11,14,19).

Table 22.1 Factors contributing to service experiences for people experiencing homelessness

Factor	Components	Reflective considerations for improving service delivery
Accessibility	Location and mobility; flexibility; capacity and eligibility; service coordination; affordability	How far are service users typically travelling to use the programme?
		Does the programme prevent or make it more difficult for service users to meet their other needs (e.g. attending other appointments, accessing shelter and food)?
		If service users are banned or ineligible for the programme, how are they supported to address their needs elsewhere in the community?
		How does the programme work with service users and other organizations in the community to coordinate and facilitate needed care?
Personal beliefs	Perceived level of need; help-seeking adaptations; self-stigma	What personal beliefs may prevent people from accessing or remaining engaged with the programme?
		What information do service users need to address any beliefs (e.g. self-stigma, feeling the need to withhold information) that could lead to negative experiences using the programme?
Organizational policies and procedures	Rigidity of rules, record-keeping. and mandatory reporting	Are organizational rules preventing service users from meeting their housing and health needs?
		Are service users informed about how their personal health information is stored?
		What accommodations are available to service users who do not feel comfortable with certain information being recorded in an organizational record (e.g. patient chart)?
Interactions with service providers	Characteristics and approach of service provider; perception of service user; consistency and continuity	How do service users rate the quality of their working relationships with service providers?
		If service users have a primary provider (e.g. case manager, housing worker) with whom they do not have a good working relationship, are they able to change workers?
		Is the approach to service provision recovery oriented and strengths based?
Sense of safety and welfare	Violence and thefts; other harms (i.e. racism, homophobia, transphobia, substance use); women-only services	How safe do service users feel when using the programme? Consider rates and reports of assault, theft, racism, homophobia, and transphobia.
		How does the programme treat substance use so that service users who use substances are not stigmatized or discriminated against while those in recovery are also not triggered?

(continued)

Table 22.1 Continued

Factor	Components	Reflective considerations for improving service delivery
Service environment and quality	Atmosphere; privacy; size of space; quality of provided services	How do service users describe the atmosphere and environment of the programme?
		If the programme is an emergency shelter: how much privacy is there and do service users have access to a secure place to store possessions?
		How satisfied are service users with the treatment and care provided to them?
Outcomes and follow-up	Basic needs (i.e. housing, health, and food); social support and connection	Are challenges associated with homelessness addressed sufficiently so that basic needs of service users are met?

Service flexibility is another critical component of accessibility that contributes to people's experiences using services. Paperwork required to access a service, including a lack of assistance in completing forms, has often been found to contribute to a more negative experience (15,17,18,20,21). Paperwork that is difficult to understand or that requires information that service users do not have can produce feelings of frustration and exasperation that lead to service discontinuation or non-use (17,18,20). Moreover, the importance of providing assistance with paperwork is even greater among people with cognitive impairments who are over-represented in the homeless population (22).

Inflexible hours of operation can be another accessibility barrier. Few services are available 24/7 and 9-to-5 hours of operation are perceived as accommodating the schedules of the people providing the services rather than those using them (12). Flexible scheduling of appointments that is respectful to homeless people's other engagements and responsibilities, as well as leniency with the consequences of missed appointments, may improve service retention (19,23). Additional considerations related to service flexibility include the development of pet-friendly and low-barrier policies and availability of interpretation services (13,17,24,25).

Even after people experiencing homelessness reach a service and navigate a complex maze of paperwork, they may still encounter problems related to service capacity and eligibility. Many services have a limited capacity to meet the level of demand. People experiencing homelessness commonly experience long waiting times and delays, including for outcomes (e.g. awaiting the results of an assessment needed to access disability income supports) (6,8,11,14,16–18,26,27). The consequences of having to wait for services are not only non-use but also difficulties with addressing other basic needs (e.g. food and shelter) and exiting homelessness (14,27). As for ineligibility, service bans and refusals (e.g. due to diagnosis, substance use, medication non-adherence, homelessness, and legal involvement) are frequent barriers reported by people experiencing homelessness (11–13,15). Feelings of hopelessness and abandonment have been linked to service bans and refusals (11); however, beyond this, their consequences remain largely unknown.

The other two components of accessibility are service coordination and affordability. Service coordination refers to the continuity of service systems and information available about services. Given the complex needs of the homeless population, it is common for people to need support from multiple service systems. However, the fragmentation that exists between systems can lead to frequent referrals from one agency to another (16,28). Because of the complexity and fragmentation of service systems, people experiencing homelessness report valuing information about what is available to them and assistance with navigation (11,19). In addition, to facilitate engagement, it is vital to provide information on what a service entails, such as psychotherapy (29). As for affordability, health services that are free or covered by insurance are highly valued, whereas people's inability to access unaffordable services can worsen self-esteem (11,13,15,18,21).

Personal beliefs

The personal beliefs of people experiencing homelessness can have an important role in how they engage with services, or whether or not services are used at all. When problems are not perceived to be sufficient to warrant treatment or support, people are unlikely to seek care (16,21,29). These decisions are not always the result of people considering only their own needs but also those of others. For example, some people experiencing homelessness report that they delay treatment-seeking because they do not want to waste the time of doctors who could be treating other people who are sicker (21). Such a view may lead to a deterioration in health and a more severe presentation when people ultimately do seek care—a common occurrence with the homeless population (30). A second personal belief that can affect service experiences is feeling the need to hide parts of one's life to receive treatment. Two studies have found that people experiencing homelessness may adapt their help-seeking by not reporting their homelessness or substance use to health providers as a means of increasing the likelihood of access or improving the quality of their care (14,16). Lastly, self-stigma about help-seeking may prevent people experiencing homelessness from accessing services or contribute to a more complicated experience (29).

Organizational policies and procedures

Services often have policies and procedures to which people experiencing home-lessness must adhere. Similar to accessibility, when these rules and regulations are rigid and inflexible, the services are perceived negatively (8,11,12,17,31). Emergency shelters are described as being particularly rule-bound. For ex-ample, people may need to line up to get a bed and go to sleep at designated times (8,11,25,32). Requirements to receive treatment and care, such as needing a mental health diagnosis to obtain housing or having to attend a religious ser-vice to receive a meal, may yield resentment and prolong homelessness (12,17). Record-keeping and mandatory reporting policies and procedures can also prevent people from opening up with service providers as these practices may be seen as undermining confidentiality (11,31). Further, people experiencing homelessness may have concerns about how their disclosed personal health information, particularly when written in their patient chart, will affect their treatment and care in the future (e.g. fear that reporting substance use during a hospital visit may lead to discrimination and withholding of needed pain management medication in the future). In contrast, organizations that have less bureaucracy and place lower demands on service users are perceived more positively (11,31).

Interactions with service providers

Human interaction is at the core of medical, behavioural health, social, and community service use. Because of this, paramount contributors to service experiences are the characteristics and approach of the people who provide the services, how (and if) service users feel they are being perceived, and the consistency and continuity of service provision. Because people experien-cing homelessness access a range of services, they are able to compare and contrast between providers who they view positively and those they do not. The evidence is clear that people experiencing homelessness highly value service providers who are non-judgemental, compassionate, respectful, understanding, and encouraging (11,12,14,17,19,28,32–34). Working with such service providers can facilitate trust, enhance service engagement, and yield more positive perceptions of service effectiveness (28,33). However, experiences with service providers who are disrespectful, insensitive, un-caring, and impersonal are commonly reported by the homeless population and can lead to service avoidance (6,11,12,15–17,21,31,34,35). These service providers are often perceived as being untrustworthy and only there for their pay cheques (11,12).

The approach of service providers is also key to service experiences. Opportunities to talk and be heard, as well as a sense of control and collaboration in treatment and care, are seen as particularly important (8,29,34). The significance of these factors may be heightened given that people experiencing homelessness often feel subjected to paternalistic care or are excluded from decision-making (11,12,17). Use of recovery-oriented and strengths-based approaches, providers who are not strictly 'by the book', and the involvement of people with lived experience in service delivery are also perceived positively (12,17,19).

People learn a lot about whether or not they are valued when using services from how those services are delivered to them. In short, people experiencing homelessness want to be seen as people (14,34). However, experiences of discrimination, labelling, and poor-quality care are common and yield perceptions that service providers do not see them as human. Instead, service users can feel they are reduced to their presenting problems (e.g. homelessness, mental illness, and substance use), a statistic or number, or not seen at all (14,21,28,35). Youth experiencing homelessness have the added problem of being viewed as children, who are not autonomous, mature, or smart (17).

Due to homeless people often having previous experiences of discrimination and poor treatment, consistency and continuity of service provision are beneficial for developing good working relationships (13,14,31). For individuals who may not be ready or are initially resistant to accessing support, consistent offers of help, without obligation, provide people experiencing homelessness with the agency to make their own decisions regarding treatment and care (29). Staff turnover can undermine service provision continuity and team cohesion (31,36).

Sense of safety and welfare

Homelessness is a traumatic experience in which people's bodily integrity and welfare are continually under threat. Given this reality, services can be places of risk or refuge. Concerning the former, many studies have found people using homeless sector services report concerns and experiences of violence, thefts, and other forms of victimization (11,17,20,25). Other threats to safety and welfare include negative influences on recovery (i.e. visible substance use by other service users), racism, homophobia, and transphobia (11,12,37). Factors that positively affect a sense of safety have been minimally studied, with only access to women-only services and female providers being identified as a significant contributor (11,14,19).

Service environment and quality

In addition to influencing perceptions of safety, service spaces can also contribute to service experiences in other ways. Emergency shelters are often described as chaotic and stressful environments, where overcrowding and limited space are common (11,25,31,32). In contrast, services that offer privacy, have environments that are calm and quiet, and allow service users to move around as if it were their own home are perceived more positively (11,20,35). Experiences are also contingent on the perceived quality of the services that are provided. Poor-quality meals and uncleanliness in homeless services are notable grievances (11,17,20). As for medical and mental health services, a treatment that is rushed or does not sufficiently explore symptoms may yield perceptions of poor-quality care (16,21,28).

Outcomes and follow-up

Service experiences and perceptions are not limited to the time that people spend using a service. The outcomes and follow-up from service use, particularly whether people meet their basic needs and have opportunities for social support and connection, are important contributors to service experiences. Regarding basic needs, services that effectively address issues of housing and shelter, health, and food security are viewed positively (8,11,12). However, health professionals must be attentive to the challenges brought on by homelessness that can complicate the provision of effective treatment (e.g. inability to fill prescriptions due to cost) (18,27). Social support and connection is another important outcome of service use for people experiencing homelessness, though not for all. Although services can be places to socialize with other people and even develop friendships (11,14,20), some people prefer to keep to themselves as a way of preventing any victimization. As such, social support and connection that is found in service settings may be contribute to a positive perception but is also not devoid of risk.

Conclusions and implications for service delivery

The health, social, and community services used by people experiencing homelessness are instrumental in addressing their complex needs. However, research on this population's service experiences and perceptions demonstrates that service use can be a series of challenges and frustrations rather than a straightforward means to better health and housing. People can face numerous barriers before a service is even used. When a service is accessed, it may come at a price.

People may be required to comply with rules and procedures that make it difficult to address other concurrent problems, such as their health or housing. The setting in which services are delivered may be unsafe and put people at risk of being victimized. The service providers with whom they interact are also a gamble; they could be non-judgemental and compassionate or disrespectful and unhelpful. People who are fortunate to work with a supportive service provider one day may have to work with someone new the next due to shift work or staff turnover. By the end, people may have exited homelessness, they may still be right where they started, or they may be worse off and avoid the service system altogether.

To improve service provision to people experiencing homelessness, it is critical to first consider and value their experiences and perceptions. From this vantage point, critical questions can then be asked about the extent to which services are designed and delivered with service users in mind. Table 22.1 provides a starter list of reflective questions to improve service delivery to people experiencing homelessness that programmes can consider. At the core of these questions is the necessity of asking: at what cost do services help? By considering how services may make life more difficult for people experiencing homelessness, opportunities for small changes that may have big impacts can be identified. Strengthening capacity within homeless sector services to conduct formal programme evaluations that include meaningful participation by people with lived experience of homelessness would also be helpful in strengthening the delivery of person-centred treatment and care.

The review findings also suggest that staffing issues and training deficits among service providers may have problematic trickle-down effects on service experiences. For example, burnout and trauma symptoms, which are common among service providers working in the homeless service system, are negatively associated with compassion satisfaction (38). As people experiencing homelessness are highly attentive to the characteristics and approach of service providers, those struggling with burnout and trauma may be perceived by service users as being less compassionate. Thus, promotion of the health and well-being of service users requires promotion of the health and well-being of service providers (39). A range of staffing best practices for homeless sector services may be useful to prevent issues related to burnout and trauma. These include use of multidisciplinary teams with diverse expertise; individual and team supervision; formal staff supports, such as peer support and critical incident debriefing; informal staff supports, such as social outings; and provision of training, including trauma-informed care (40).

References

1. **Baggett TP, Singer DE, Rao SR, O'Connell JJ, Bharel M, Rigotti, NA.** Food insufficiency and health services utilization in a national sample of homeless adults. J Gen Intern Med. 2011;**26**(6):627–634.

2. **Barman-Adhikari A, Bowen E, Bender K, Brown S, Rice E.** A social capital approach to identifying correlates of perceived social support among homeless youth. Child Youth Care Forum. 2016;**45**(5):691–708.

3. **Eyrich KM, Pollio DE, North CS.** An exploration of alienation and replacement theories of social support in homelessness. Soc Work Res. 2003;**27**(4):222–231.

4. **Fazel S, Geddes JR, Kushel M.** The health of homeless people in high-income countries: descriptive epidemiology, health consequences, and clinical and policy recommendations. Lancet. 2012;**384**(9953):1529–1540.

5. **Poremski D, Distasio J, Hwang SW, Latimer E.** Employment and income of people who experience mental illness and homelessness in a large Canadian sample. Can J Psychiatry. 2015;**60**(9):379–385.

6. **Applewhite SL.** Homeless veterans: perspectives on social services use. Soc Work. 1997;**42**(1):19–30.

7. **Donley AM, Wright JD.** Safer outside: a qualitative exploration of homeless people's resistance to homeless shelters. J Forensic Psychol P. 2012;**12**(4):288–306.

8. **Ogden J, Avades T.** Being homeless and the use and nonuse of services: a qualitative study. J Community Psychol. 2011;**39**(4):499–505.

9. **Kerman N, Kidd SA.** The healthcare triple aim in the recovery era. Adm Policy Ment Health. 2020;**47**(4):492–496.

10. **Whittington JW, Nolan K, Lewis N, Torres T.** Pursuing the triple aim: the first 7 years. Milbank Q. 2015;**93**(2):263–300.

11. **Kerman N, Gran-Ruaz SM, Lawrence M, Sylvestre J.** Perceptions of service use among currently and formerly homeless adults with mental health problems. Community Ment Health J. 2019;**55**(5):777–783.

12. **Voronka J, Wise Harris D, Grant J, Komaroff J, Boyle D, Kennedy A.** Un/helpful help and its discontents: peer researchers paying attention to street life narratives to inform social work policy and practice. Soc Work Ment Health. 2014;**12**(3):249–279.

13. **Bhui K, Shanahan L, Harding G.** Homelessness and mental illness: a literature review and a qualitative study of perceptions of the adequacy of care. Int J Soc Psychiatry. 2006;**52**(2):152–165.

14. **Bungay V.** Health care among street-involved women: the perpetuation of health inequity. Qual Health Res. 2013;**23**(8):1016–1026.

15. **Nickasch B, Marnocha SK.** Healthcare experiences of the homeless. J Am Acad Nurse Prac. 2009;**21**(1):39–46.

16. **Reid P, Klee H.** Young homeless people and service provision. Health Soc Care Community. 1999;**7**(1):17–24.

17. **Thompson SJ, McManus H, Lantry J, Windsor L, Flynn P.** Insights from the street: perceptions of services and providers by homeless young adults. Eval Program Plann. 2006;**29**(1):34–43.

18. **Wise C, Phillips K.** Hearing the silent voices: narratives of health care and homelessness. Issues Ment Health N. 2013;**34**(5):359–367.

19. **David DH, Rowe M, Staeheli M, Ponce AN.** Safety, trust, and treatment: mental health service delivery for women who are homeless. Women Ther. 2015;**38**(1–2):114–127.

20. **Daiski I.** Perspectives of homeless people on their health and health needs priorities. J Adv Nurs. 2007;**58**(3):273–281.

21. **Martins DC.** Experiences of homeless people in the health care delivery system: a descriptive phenomenological study. Public Health Nurs. 2008;**25**(5):420–430.

22. **Stone B, Dowling S, Cameron A.** Cognitive impairment and homelessness: a scoping review. Health Soc Care Community. 2019;**27**(4):125–142.

23. **Stanhope V, Henwood BF, Padgett DK.** Understanding service disengagement from the perspective of case managers. Psychiatr Serv. 2009;**60**(4):459–464.

24. **Kerman N, Gran-Ruaz S, Lem N.** Pet ownership and homelessness: a scoping review. J Soc Distress Homeless. 2019;**28**(2):106–114.

25. **McCormack RP, Hoffman LF, Norman M, Goldfrank LR, Norman EM.** Voices of homeless alcoholics who frequent Bellevue hospital: a qualitative study. Ann Emerg Med. 2015;**65**(2):178–186.

26. **Brown M, Mihelicova M, Lyons J,** et al. Waiting for shelter: perspectives on a homeless shelter's procedures. J Community Psychol. 2017;**45**(7):846–858.

27. **Kidd SA.** Street youth: coping and interventions. Child Adolesc Soc Work J. 2003;**20**(4):235–261.

28. **Darbyshire P, Muir-Cochrane E, Fereday J, Jureidini J, Drummond A.** Engagement with health and social care services: perceptions of homeless young people with mental health problems. Health Soc Care Community. 2006;**14**(6):553–562.

29. **Chaturvedi S.** Accessing psychological therapies: homeless young people's views on barriers and facilitators. Counsell Psychother Res J. 2016;**16**(1):54–63.

30. **Hwang SW, Weaver J, Aubry T, Hoch JS.** Hospital costs and length of stay among homeless patients admitted to medical, surgical, and psychiatric services. Med Care. 2011;**49**(4):350–354.

31. **De Rosa CJ, Montgomery SB, Kipke MD, Iverson E, Ma JL, Unger JB.** Service utilization among homeless and runaway youth in Los Angeles, California: rates and reasons. J Adolesc Health. 1999;**24**(6):449–458.

32. **Thompson SJ, Pollio DE, Eyrich K, Bradbury E, North CS.** Successfully exiting homelessness: experiences of formerly homeless mentally ill individuals. Eval Program Plann. 2004;**27**(4):423–431.

33. **Sosin M, George C, Grossman S.** Service content as a determinant of homeless adults' perceptions of program efficacy. J Community Psychol. 2012;**40**(2):249–263.

34. **Wen CK, Hudak PL, Hwang SW.** Homeless people's perceptions of welcomeness and unwelcomeness in healthcare encounters. J Gen Intern Med. 2007;**22**(7):1011–1017.

35. **Hoffman L, Coffey B.** Dignity and indignation: how people experiencing homelessness view services and providers. J Soc Sci. 2008;**45**(2):207–222.

36. **Kidd SA, Miner S, Walker D, Davidson L.** Stories of working with homeless youth: on being "mind-boggling". Child Youth Serv Rev. 2007;**29**(1):16–34.

37. **Ecker J, Aubry T, Sylvestre J.** A review of the literature on LGBTQ adults who experience homelessness. J Homosex. 2019;**66**(3):297–323.

38. **Waegemakers Schiff J, Lane AM.** PTSD symptoms, vicarious traumatization, and burnout in front line workers in the homeless sector. Community Ment Health J. 2019;**55**(3):454–462.

39. **Bodenheimer T, Sinsky C.** From triple to quadruple aim: care of the patient requires care of the provider. Ann Fam Med. 2014;**12**(6):573–576.

40. **Olivet J, McGraw S, Grandin S, Bassuk E.** Staffing challenges and strategies for organizations serving individuals who have experienced chronic homelessness. J Behav Health Serv Res. 2010;**37**(2):226–238.

Special groups

Chapter 23

LGBT homelessness and mental health

Marcos Roberto Vieira Garcia

Introduction

The issue of 'mental health and homelessness', which is central to the present book, refers to 'vicious circle' logic: becoming mentally ill makes people vulnerable, and, therefore, predisposes them to homelessness (or keeps them in this condition), while homelessness generally damages mental health (or maintains it in a poor condition). This 'circle' has also been described in studies that specifically refer to homeless LGBT[1] people's mental health, especially that of young people.

In order to specifically address the topic of the present chapter, the context of discrimination and its effects on the lives and mental health of the LGBT population in general needs to be analysed, since this helps in understanding the course of homeless LGBT young people's lives. Following this, the specificity of this segment of society and some specificities regarding the transgender segment, and the intersectionality with racial issues, are explored.

Discrimination against LGBT youth and homelessness

LGBT youth are disproportionally represented among the homeless youth population in the US (1–6). It has been estimated that between 20% and 40% of

---

[1] The term LGBT, which encompasses lesbians, gays, bisexuals, and transgender people, is used in the present chapter. However, some studies that are cited also include the letter Q ('queer'), which encompasses people of both genders who present a variety of sexual orientations, preferences, and habits; in other words, a neutral word that can be used for all supporters of this movement; I ('intersex'), that is, people who do not have exclusively male or female sexual characteristics; and A ('asexual'), that is, people who are not sexually attracted towards either men or women or who do not present a defined sexual orientation. Sometimes the symbol '+' is added, meaning that other similar possibilities are left open.

homeless youth identify themselves as LGBT, while they comprise 5–8% of the entire young population in the US (2,7). A recent report estimated that the risk of becoming homeless among LGBT youth is 120% higher than the risk among cisgender and heterosexual youth (8). Likewise, non-white youth, and specifically black youth, are at higher risk of becoming homeless and are over-represented both among the overall homeless youth population and among homeless LGBT youth (2,4). Homeless LGBT youth are also over-represented in governmental programmes (9) and in child welfare systems. A report in 2014 revealed that almost 20% of young people in the Los Angeles child welfare system identified as LGBT (10).

The main explanations for the high percentage of LGBT young people in homeless situations involve heterosexism[2] (related to heteronormativity[3]) and cisgenderism[4] that are present in the family, school, and work spheres. Lack of family support leads many LGBT young people to leave their original families or to be expelled by them, which often brings difficulties regarding housing (13,14). When LGBT young people come out to their families and friends, they often face rejection and physical and emotional abuse that forces them to move to the streets. A report has indicated that 40% of LGBT youth are homeless mainly as a result of family rejection (2).

LGBT youth also face adversities at school, relating to their gender identity and/or sexual orientation (15). According to the Gay, Lesbian & Straight Education Network (16), in a 2011 survey approximately 64% of lesbian, gay, and bisexual (LGB) students and 44% of transgender students reported a sense of insecurity in the school environment, which ought to be a place of welcoming and safety regarding differences (16). For many of them, schools are a place of bullying and harassment (17,18), and this has a severe negative impact on their mental development. LGBT youth also often face obstacles relating to jobs and experience generalized discrimination and incomprehension from service providers and other users of these services (19–23). Young people from

---

[2] The expression 'heterosexism' refers to the systematic marginalization of lesbian, gay and bisexual people, and to the structural favouring of heterosexual people and relationships (11).

[3] 'Heteronormativity' describes how social norms, discourse and practices build heterosexuality as being superior to all other expressions of sexuality (12). Within a heteronormative society, gender expression of men as male and women as female is naturalized and has preference (2).

[4] According to Ansara and Hegarty (12), cisgenderism is 'the ideology that invalidates or pathologizes self-designated genders that contrast with external designations'. Intolerance within society of gender self-awareness, also known as self-designated gender, can also contribute towards family rejection.

this segment of society are also more likely to experience violence than their heterosexual peers. They are three times more likely to report being raped than heterosexual young people (16% versus 5%) (24).

Discrimination against homeless LGBT youth on the streets and in institutions

Homeless LGBT youth are at high risk of sexual victimization and exploitation. The fact that they resort to survival sex often contributes towards these situations of violence, and this brings significant psychological consequences (25). Homeless people generally face higher risks of contracting sexually transmitted infections through their involvement in riskier sexual intercourse, such as unprotected sex and sex worker activities in exchange for shelter and food (26), which is frequently worsened in cases of LGBT young people.

Another survey observed a higher tendency among LGBT youth to remain unaccompanied on the streets because of the prejudice that is reproduced in daily life there, which makes them even more vulnerable to situations of violence (27).

Discrimination is also reproduced in assisted housing. There is a higher tendency among LGBT young people for them to move around various institutions (28,29). Congregate care systems are often unsafe for this segment of society because they make these individuals more susceptible to victimization (30).

It has also been indicated in the literature that discrimination against homeless LGBT young people due to their sexual orientation and/or gender identity is also reproduced in shelters (4). In these facilities, service providers and caregivers frequently control young people's gender behaviour (26,31), thus reproducing prejudicial attitudes.

Life in foster homes may also be unsafe for LGBT youth. In a focus group study conducted among 25 foster parents, they revealed that they feared that an adopted LGBT child could make other children in their homes non-heterosexual and/or could abuse them (32). This frequently led to these young people being transferred to other facilities, thus illustrating what was mentioned previously regarding higher mobility of LGBT youth among institutions for homeless people (33).

Mental health of LGBT youth

LGBT people are generally more likely to present with substance abuse and to suffer from mental illness (17,18). They often face higher rates of emotional and psychological problems (26). The combination of seeking sexual identity and experiencing harassment and discrimination has the potential to put LGBT youth at higher risk of several mental health issues, such as depression and suicidal ideation, compared with their heterosexual peers (34). Regarding mental health, it has been estimated that the LGBT population is 2.5–3 times more susceptible to suffering from major depression or general anxiety, and is four times more likely to attempt suicide (age group 10–24 years) than their heterosexual peers (21,35). Thirty per cent of LGBT teenagers have experienced clinical levels of mental disorders such as anxiety, depression, and post-traumatic stress disorder (PTSD), and almost 32% of LGBT teenagers may attempt suicide (36,37).

A longitudinal cohort study conducted in New Zealand found associations between LGB sexual orientation and suicidal ideation, suicide attempts, depression, generalized anxiety disorder, and conduct disorder (38). Sexual minorities presented a higher prevalence of PTSD than the reference group ('heterosexual people without sexual contact with people of the same sex') in the Growing Up Today Study, and higher exposure to child abuse explained higher rates of PTSD (39). In another study comparing sexual minorities and their heterosexual peers, sexual minority status was predictive of suicidal ideation and suicide attempts, self-mutilation behaviour, and histories of psychotherapy and psychiatric medication (40). LGB young people were also more likely to present with longer depressive episodes (41.3%), PTSD (47.6%), and suicidal ideation (73.0%) than their heterosexual peers (28.5%, 33.4%, and 53.2%, respectively) (14).

One of the factors that explain the high rate of mental illness among LGBT youth is parental rejection, which can increase the prevalence of depression and suicide attempts. LGBT youth are six times more likely to suffer from depression (41) and are four times more likely to attempt suicide than heterosexual people (27). These disparities may have a severe and deadly impact on the LGBT population, and are made even more complicated and confounded through the fact that homosexuality was considered to be an illness until the 1970s (42), thus severely limiting mental healthcare services for LGBT people.

The LGBT population is 200% more likely to smoke tobacco and is 25% more likely to present alcohol abuse than the overall population. In addition, gay men are 2.5 times more likely to smoke marijuana, 2.2 times more likely to use amphetamines, and 9.5 times more likely to use heroin than heterosexual men (18,42). Regarding the high propensity towards abuse of both licit and illicit drugs, three non-exclusionary hypotheses can be formulated, as analysed in a previous study (43):

1. High propensity to use drugs because of the places frequented. The lack of acceptance by families that is often experienced makes these young people proportionally more likely to seek alternative socialization spaces, especially within nightlife, where there is higher availability of both licit and illicit drugs.

2. Drug abuse as a way of dealing with situations of anxiety that are caused by lack of personal and social acceptance of their divergent sexual orientation and/or gender identity. However, seeking 'immediate relief' for mental distress often leads to harmful use of these substances.

3. Breaking away from social norms relating to heteronormativity and cisgenderism may lead some LGBT people to start living with other marginalized groups, such as drug users. The tendency among groups of 'outsiders' for them to come together was described by some classics of sociology (44,45).

Mental health of homeless LGBT youth

After becoming homeless, LGBT young people present an increased risk of becoming physically and mentally ill, compared with heterosexual teenagers (46). Homeless LGBT young people experience adverse mental issues, such as depression, PTSD, and suicidal ideation, compared with homeless heterosexual young people (22). This group is more likely to report having higher levels of depressive symptoms than heterosexual young people (47). Homeless LGB young people also present a higher likelihood of seeking hospital treatment for emotional disorders, suicidal ideation, and suicide attempts, and of having depression, compared with homeless heterosexual people (7).

A study on service providers for homeless youth sought to identify the experiences of homeless LGBT youth (1). The service providers were asked to compare the state of mental health of LGB, heterosexuals, transgender, and cisgender young people (the response options included 'much worse', 'a little worse', 'more or less the same', and 'a little better'). The interviewees reported that the state of physical health of LGBQ young people was the same as that presented by heterosexual people, while transgender people presented worse physical health than cisgender people. Likewise, the service providers reported that the state of mental health of the LGBTQ group was worse than what was observed among their heterosexual and cisgender peers. The interviewees were more likely to report that the state of mental health among transgender people was worse.

The mental health of homeless LGBT youth cannot be dissociated from their physical health. This segment of society is more involved in risky behaviour, such as drug abuse and survival sex, which are linked to high rates of HIV infection (26). The emotional consequences of homelessness are also associated with drug abuse, which serves as a coping mechanism for the stress caused by homelessness (48). In a study on social workers, 53% of homeless LGBT people reported having histories of alcohol or substance abuse (2).

The mental problems of homeless LGBT youth are not necessarily related to individual claims of LGBT identity but, rather, are the result of social structures (e.g. heterosexism of families and schools, and taking homeless people for granted, among other causes) that marginalize these individuals. These factors exacerbate the vulnerability of this segment of society, threaten these individuals' physical and mental health, and have an impact on their long-term economic and job prospects (49).

It is essential to highlight that studies have shown that family acceptance is associated with positive self-esteem and overall good health. Therefore, this is a protective factor against mental health problems such as depression, abuse of recreational drugs, and suicidal behaviour (50).

Lastly, the situation of homeless LGBT youth should be considered not only from the perspective of victimization, given that at some level, there is a 'choice' in taking the freedom of the streets rather than going to foster homes or other facilities (51). Likewise, many homeless LGBT young people are able to overcome prejudice and discrimination, to fully embrace their stigmatized identities and thus become an example for other homeless LGBT young people to work to improve their own situations of life (7).

The specificity of transgender people

Transgender people form a disproportionally high percentage among the homeless population, even compared with the cisgender LGB youth. It is much more common for transgender young people to experience homelessness in their lives. In shelters, they also frequently face harassment and discrimination (17,52,53).

Some transgender young people, like many people living on the streets, resort to illegal economic activities to survive, such as prostitution or drug selling (54). This puts them at risk of violence and exposes them to sexually transmissible diseases (in the case of those who have sexual intercourse with men), especially AIDS (55). Transgender people are significantly more likely to be HIV positive than their cisgender peers (1). Local initiatives to deal with HIV are crucial for homeless transgender populations, who face high exposure rates and have limited healthcare options.

Mental health issues, particularly suicidal ideation, are common findings in studies on transgender people. One study (56) found that most transgender youth subjectively fought against their gender expression before coming out to their friends and family. Mental health issues and substance abuse, which are prevalent among homeless transgender youth (56–58), may derive from how they subjectively deal with their divergent gender expression, while other causes of mental angst originate from harassment or lack of comprehension from other people.

Homeless transgender youth are subject to strong social stigma, harassment, and risk of death due to their transition (59,60). Change, in its physical and/or legal aspects, is generally undertaken without many resources (money, social support, or health insurance). Transgender youth often enter the social care system, but find specific difficulties in institutions within the child and youth welfare system. Mental health treatments and other behavioural modifications can be used against these young people to try to modify their gender expression (61,62).

The lack of professional training and policies relating to transgender identities brings further disadvantages to these young people. Even the training offered to healthcare and assistance workers, focusing on diversity in general, usually does not include issues relating to transgender people (63). This leaves workers in these institutions with the responsibility of deciding which shelters they should use to accommodate transgender people, despite not fully understanding the specific needs of this group. Bad experiences with social workers serve to further discourage transgender youth from seeking help from governmental institutions that act within the social protection network.

Intersectionality with race and class

According to Brah and Phoenix (64), the concept of 'intersectionality' means:

> (T)he complex, irreducible, varied and variable effects which ensue when multiple axes of differentiation—economic, political, cultural, mental, subjective and experiential—intersect in historically specific contexts. The concept emphasises that different dimensions of social life cannot be separated out into discrete and pure strands. (p. 76)

In this regard, understanding the way in which the racial and class dimensions intersect with gender and sexuality is crucial for enabling an analysis of the specificities of homeless LGBT youth.

Black and/or poor people may experience heterosexism and transphobia differently, thus demonstrating how discrimination against gender and sexuality intersects with discrimination against race and class. In addition, black youth, especially children and young people from economically disadvantaged families, are disproportionally represented within child welfare systems (10,65).

Youth assistance systems (in other words, relating to housing, healthcare, education, and employment) often do not have the capacity to recognize and respond to the needs of young adults whose lives are affected by multiple layered stigmas resulting from racism, classism, heterosexism, and cisgenderism (66). A large proportion of recent studies have evaluated the needs of LGBTQ people as a broad group, which has often masked the variability of the experiences of the subgroups within it. More recent studies have evaluated homeless LGBT youth subpopulations, including Hispanic gay and bisexual young men (67) and black LGBT young people (68,69). Nonetheless, very few studies have used an intersectional lens to examine how marginalized multiple identities contribute towards experiences of shelters and the lives of homeless LGBT youth.

Another study (50) aimed to understand the impact of family acceptance or rejection between Hispanic and white non-Hispanic LGBT young adults whose sexual orientation was known to at least one of their parents. This study showed that family acceptance was more dependent on family dynamics than on the sexual orientation or gender identity of the young people. Parents from the Hispanic community, with low socioeconomic status and religious affiliation, and who were immigrants, were less receptive.

Black LGBT young people experience systemic racism and its subsequent effects, such as police and community harassment, and racial microaggressions (68). In many cases, this intersects with divergent sexual orientation and gender identity. Black LGBT young people experience double discrimination within child welfare systems, which shape how the behaviour of some young people, including their gender behaviour, is monitored and disciplined (61).

Some reflections on mental healthcare for homeless LGBT youth

Caregiving practices within an intersectional perspective assume, above all, reflection on the specificity of each segment within a broader group. If the specificity of homeless LGBT youth in relation to homeless youth as a whole is emphasized in the present chapter, this consideration also encompasses the necessity of addressing the needs of each of the subgroups that comprise homeless LGBT youth: lesbians, gays, bisexuals, and transgender people, who also all have intersections with class and racial issues.

Another important element to be highlighted is the impossibility of addressing caregiving within an individualized perspective, without considering oppression mechanisms such as heterosexism, cisgenderism, and systemic racism. These mechanisms, as discussed in this chapter, are directly responsible for many difficulties that homeless LGBT youth experience over the course of their lives, which often leads them to homelessness and/or becoming mentally ill. This is, therefore, a matter of understanding mental health as a process that is deeply linked to current forms of social oppression and the ways of coping with them.

Within this perspective, and from the reference point of Paulo Freire (70), it is essential to establish a horizontal relationship with the group with which dialogue is conducted or the institution in which interventions take place. Interventions should start from a posture of humility, relating to acknowledgement that one does not know better than the people themselves do, regarding their own lives and the difficulties they have experienced. Thus, interventions in which outsiders impose their values and certainties end up implicitly depreciating the existing local knowledge. This leads not only to a high risk of low effectiveness of the intervention, since the reading of the group's problems is impaired, but also to detachment regarding the group's members because posture adopted depreciates other people.

In dealing with homeless LGBT people, this posture is particularly risky, especially if these individuals' behaviour diverges from what is socially considered to be 'normal'. For example, a study that the present author conducted in São Paulo, Brazil (43), demonstrated this conflict between institutions' desire for normalization in relation to their users and the way of life of homeless LGBT youth. That study dealt with conflicts that were described in various city shelters regarding the existence of homoerotic sexual practices in the bathrooms of these facilities. The predominant institutional justification was that shelters were a place 'to sleep' and not to have sexual intercourse. On the other hand, the LGBT users of these spaces referred to the constant use of public toilets, and not only the bathrooms in shelters, as a reference point for sexual practices. This conflict, which was reproduced in several shelters, showed the impossibility of establishing a dialogue regarding this issue that could result in compromise solutions that would take into consideration users' wishes, such as establishment of spaces where homoerotic sexual practices would be accepted in shelters, thus avoiding 'hidden' activities. There are countless challenges in developing effective forms of shelter for this segment of society, such as the case of the use of social names, dormitories, and bathrooms according to gender identity, among other examples.

Lastly, it can be understood that caregiving practices should be established from the reference point of promotion of healthcare, which encompasses mental health and has been described as a healthcare model that extrapolates medical assistance, bringing back the concept of health as a social product

(71,72). Among the critical components of this process are dissemination of information and education, which enable individuals and communities to assume greater control over the personal, socioeconomic, and environmental factors that affect health (73). Underlying this approach are concepts of empowerment and promotion of emancipation and autonomy of social groups. These are concepts that frequently overlap in different attitudes towards community practice management. To reflect on these concepts within the field of sexual and reproductive rights, it is necessary to take a critical procedure within these concepts, both regarding proposals for universalizing interventions and regarding the individualizing notions of subject that are often present (74). If healthcare promotion presupposes prevention, based on the concept of risk or the likelihood of becoming ill, it also transcends this, as the focus moves from illness to the sociocultural factors that intersect with it.

References

1. **Choi SK, Wilson BDM, Shelton J, Gates G.** Serving Our Youth 2015: The Needs and Experiences of LGBTQ Youth Experiencing Homelessness. Los Angeles, CA: Williams Institute with the True Colors Fund; 2015.

2. **Durso LE, Gates G.** Serving Our Youth: Findings from a National Survey of Service Providers Working with LGBT Youth Who Are Homeless or at Risk of Becoming Homeless. Los Angeles, CA: Williams Institute with True Colors Fund and The Palette Fund; 2012.

3. **Lankenau SE, Clatts MC, Welle D, Goldsamt LA, Gwadz MV.** Street careers: homelessness, drug use, and sex work among young men who have sex with men (YMSM). Int J Drug Policy. 2005;**16**(1):10–18.

4. **Maccio EM, Ferguson-Colvin KM.** Services to LGBTQ runaway and homeless youth: gaps and recommendations. Child Youth Serv Rev. 2016;**63**:47–57.

5. **Quintana S, Rosenthal J, Krehely J.** On the streets: the federal response to gay and transgender homeless youth. Center for American Progress; 2010. Available from: https://www.americanprogress.org/issues/lgbt/reports/2010/06/21/7983/on-the-streets/.

6. **Van Leeuwen JM, Boyle S, Salomonsen-Sautel S,** et al. Lesbian, gay, and bisexual homeless youth: an eight-city public health perspective. Child Welf. 2006;**85**(2):151–170.

7. **Ray N.** Lesbian, Gay, Bisexual and Transgender Youth: An Epidemic of Homelessness. New York: National Gay and Lesbian Task Force Policy Institute, National Coalition for the Homeless; 2006.

8. **Morton MH, Dworsky A, Matjasko JL, Curry SR, Schleuter D, Farrell AF.** Prevalence and correlates of youth homelessness in the United States. J Adolesc Health. 2017;**62**(1):14–21.

9. **Van Leeuwen JM, Boyle S, Salomonsen-Sautel S, Baker DN.** Lesbian, gay, and bisexual homeless youth: an eight-city public health perspective. Child Welf. 2006;**85**(2):151–170.

10. **Wilson BDM, Cooper K, Kastanis A, Nezhad S.** Sexual and Gender Minority Youth in Foster Care: Assessing Disproportionality and Disparities in Los Angeles. Los Angeles, CA: The Williams Institute; 2014.

11. **Ansara YG, Hegarty P.** Cisgenderism in psychology: pathologizing and misgendering children from 1999 to 2008. Psychol Sex. 2012;**3**(2):137–160.

12. **Warner M.** Fear of a Queer Planet: Queer Politics and Social Theory. Minneapolis, MN: University of Minnesota Press; 1993.

13. **Cochran BN, Stewart AJ, Ginzler JA, Cauce AM.** Challenges faced by homeless sexual minorities: comparison of gay, lesbian, bisexual, and transgender homeless adolescents with their heterosexual counterparts. Am J Public Health. 2002;**92**(5):773–777.

14. **Whitbeck LB, Chen X, Hoyt DR, Tyler KA, Johnson KD.** Mental disorder, subsistence strategies, and victimization among gay, lesbian, and bisexual homeless and runaway adolescents. J Sex Res. 2004;**41**(4):329–342.

15. **Lindsey RB, Diaz RM, Nuri-Robins K, Terrell RD, Lindsey DB.** A Culturally Proficient Response to LGBT Communities: A Guide for Educators. Thousand Oaks, CA: Corwin Press; 2013.

16. **Gay, Lesbian & Straight Education Network.** National school climate survey. 2011. Available from: http://www.glsen.org/press/2011-national-school-climate-survey.

17. **Cray A, Miller K, Durso L.** Seeking shelter: the experiences and unmet needs of LGBT homeless youth. Center for American Progress; 2013. Available from: https://cdn.ameri canprogress.org/wpcontent/uploads/2013/09/LGBTHomelessYouth.pdf.

18. **Kaiser Family Foundation.** Health and access to care and coverage for lesbian, gay, bisexual, and transgender individuals in the U.S. 2018. Available from: http://files.kff. org/attachment/Issue-Brief-Health-and-Access-to-Care-and-Coverage-for-LGBT-Indi viduals-in-the-US.

19. **Abramovich A.** Understanding how policy and culture create oppressive conditions for LGBTQ2S youth in the shelter system. J Homosex. 2016;**64**(11):1484–1501.

20. **Shelton J.** Transgender youth homelessness: understanding programmatic barriers through the lens of cisgenderism. Child Youth Serv Rev. 2015;**59**:10–18.

21. **Cochran SD, Sullivan JG, Mays VM.** Prevalence of mental disorders, psychological distress, and mental health services use among lesbian, gay, bisexual adults in the United States. J Consult Clin Psychol. 2003;**71**(1):53–61.

22. **Gangamma R, Slesnick N, Toviessi P, Serovich J.** Comparison of HIV risks among gay, lesbian, bisexual and heterosexual homeless youth. J Youth Adolesc. 2008;**37**(4):456–464.

23. **Gattis MN.** An ecological systems comparison between homeless sexual minority youths and homeless heterosexual youths. J Soc Serv Res. 2013;**39**(1):38–49.

24. **US Centers for Disease Control and Prevention.** Sexual identity, sex of sexual contacts, and health risk behaviors among students in grades 9–12: youth risk behavior surveillance, selected sites, United States, 2001–2009. 2011. Available from: https:// www.cdc.gov/mmwr/pdf/ss/ss6007.pdf.

25. **Rew L, Whittaker TA, Taylor-Seehafer MA, Smith LR.** Sexual health risks and protective resources in gay, lesbian, bisexual, and heterosexual homeless youth. J Spec Pediatr Nurs. 2005;**10**(1):11–19.

26. **Keuroghlian AS, Shtasel D, Bassuk EL.** Out on the street: a public health and policy agenda for lesbian, gay, bisexual, and transgender youth who are homeless. Am J Orthopsychiatry. 2014;**84**(1):66–72.

27. **Corliss HL, Goodenow S, Nichols L, Austin SB.** High burden of homelessness among sexual minority adolescents: findings from a representative Massachusetts high school sample. Am J Public Health. 2011;**101**(9):1683–1689.

28. **Elze D.** LGBTQ youth and their families. In: **Mallon GP, Hess PM** (Eds), Child Welfare for the 21st Century: A Handbook of Practices, Policies, and Programs. New York: Columbia University Press; 2014:158–178.

29. **Mallon GP, Aledort N, Ferrera M.** There's no place like home: achieving safety, permanency, and well-being for lesbian and gay adolescents in out-of-home care settings. Child Welf. 2002;**81**(2):407–439.

30. **Jacobs J, Freundlich M.** Achieving permanency for LGBTQ youth. Child Welf. 2006;**85**(2):299–316.

31. **Saewyc EM, Skay CL, Pettingell SL,** et al. Hazards of stigma: the sexual and physical abuse of gay, lesbian, and bisexual adolescents in the United States and Canada. Child Welf. 2006;**8**(2):195–213.

32. **Clements JA, Rosenwald M.** Foster parents' perspectives on LGB youth in the child welfare system. J Gay Lesbian Soc Serv. 2007;**19**(1):57–69.

33. **Wilson BDM, Kastanis AA.** Sexual and gender minority disproportionality and disparities in child welfare: a population-based study. Child Youth Serv Rev. 2015;**58**:11–17.

34. **Woodford MR, Han Y, Craig S, Lim C, Matney MM.** Discrimination and mental health among sexual minority college students: the type and form of discrimination does matter. J Gay Lesbian Ment Health. 2014;**18**(2):142–163.

35. **Lick D, Durso LE, Johnson KL.** Minority stress and physical health among sexual minorities. Perspect Psychol Sci. 2013;**8**(5):521–548.

36. **Mustanski B, Andrews R, Puckett JA.** The effects of cumulative victimization on mental health among lesbian, gay, bisexual, and transgender adolescents and young adults. Am J Public Health. 2016;**106**(3):527–533.

37. **Mustanski B, Liu RT.** A longitudinal study of predictors of suicide attempts among lesbian, gay, bisexual, and transgender youth. Arch Sex Behav. 2013;**42**(3):437–448.

38. **Fergusson DM, Horwood LJ, Beautrais AL.** Is sexual orientation related to mental health problems and suicidality in young people? Arch Gen Psychiatry. 1999;**56**(10):876–880.

39. **Roberts AL, Rosario M, Corliss HL, Koenen KC, Austin SB.** Elevated risk of posttraumatic stress in sexual minority youths: mediation by childhood abuse and gender nonconformity. Am J Public Health. 2012;**102**(8):1587–1593.

40. **Balsam KF, Beauchaine TP, Mickey RM, Rothblum ED.** Mental health of lesbian, gay, bisexual, and heterosexual siblings: effects of gender, sexual orientation, and family. J Abnorm Psychol. 2005;**114**(3):471–476.

41. **Hunt J.** Why the gay and transgender population experiences higher rates of substance abuse. Center for American Progress; 2012. Available from: https://cdn.americanprogress.org/wp-content/uploads/issues/2012/03/pdf/lgbt_substance_abuse.pdf.

42. **Wyatt-Nichol H, Naylor LA.** Liberty and equality: in defense of same sex marriage. Public Integr. 2015;**17**(11):117–130.

43. **Garcia MRV.** Homeless people, nomadism and contexts of vulnerability to HIV/AIDS. Temas Psicol (Ribeirão Preto). 2013;**21**(3):1021–1034.

44. **Becker HS.** Outsiders: Studies in the Sociology of Deviance. London: Free Press of Glencoe; 1963.

45. **Goffman E.** Stigma: Notes on the Management of Spoiled Identity. Englewood Cliffs, NJ: Prentice-Hall; 1963.

46. **Safren S, Heimberg R.** Depression, hopelessness, suicidality, and related factors in sexual minority and heterosexual adolescents. J Consult Clin Psychol. 1999;**67**(6):859–866.

47. **Noell JW, Ochs LM.** Relationship of sexual orientation to substance use, suicidal ideation, suicide attempts, and other factors in a population of homeless adolescents. J Adolesc Health. 2001;**29**(1):31–36.

48. **Toolis EE, Hammack PL.** The lived experience of homeless youth: a narrative approach. Qual Psychol. 2015;**2**(1):50–68.

49. **Tam TW, Zlotnick C, Robertson MJ.** Longitudinal perspective: adverse childhood events, substance use, and labor force participation among homeless adults. Am J Drug Alcohol Abuse. 2003;**29**(4):829–846.

50. **Ryan C, Russell ST, Huebner D, Diaz R, Sanchez J.** Family acceptance in adolescence and the health of LGBT young adults. J Child Adolesc Psychiatr Nurs. 2010;**23**(4):205–213.

51. **Forge N, Ream GL.** Homeless lesbian, gay, bisexual and transgender (LGBT) youth in New York City: insights from the field. Child Welf. 2014;**93**(2):7–22.

52. **Mottet L, Ohle J.** Transitioning our shelters: making homeless shelters safe for transgender people. J Poverty. 2006;**10**(2):77–101.

53. **Yu V.** Shelter and transitional housing for transgender youth. J Gay Lesbian Ment Health. 2010;**14**(4):340–345.

54. **Gwadz MV, Gostnell K, Smolenski C,** et al. The initiation of homeless youth into the street economy. J Adolesc. 2009;**32**(2):357–377.

55. **Tyler KA.** Homeless youths' HIV risk behaviors with strangers: investigating the importance of social networks. Arch Sex Behav. 2013;**42**(8):1583–1591.

56. **Olson J, Schrager SM, Belzer M, Simons LK, Clark LF.** Baseline physiologic and psychosocial characteristics of transgender youth seeking care for gender dysphoria. J Adolesc Health. 2015;**57**(4):374–380.

57. **Clements-Nolle K, Marx R, Katz M.** Attempted suicide among transgender persons: the influence of gender-based discrimination and victimization. J Homosex. 2006;**51**(3):53–69.

58. **Grossman AH, D'Augelli AR.** Transgender youth and life-threatening behaviors. Suicide Life Threat Behav. 2007;**37**(5):527–537.

59. **Badgett MVL, Durso LE, Schneebaum A.** New Patterns of Poverty in the Lesbian, Gay, and Bisexual Community. Los Angeles, CA: University of California, Williams Institute; 2013.

60. **Stotzer RL.** Violence against transgender people: a review of United States data. Aggression Violent Behav. 2009;**14**(3):170–179.

61. **Mallon GP, DeCrescenzo T.** Transgender children and youth: a child welfare practice perspective. Child Welf. 2006;**85**(2):215–241.

62. **Marksamer J.** A Place of Respect: A Guide for Group Care Facilities Serving Transgender and Gender Non-Conforming Youth. San Francisco, CA: National Center for Lesbian Rights; 2011.

63. **Taylor JK.** Transgender identities and public policy in the United States: the relevance for public administration. Admin Soc. 2007;**39**(7):833–856.

64. **Brah A, Phoenix A.** Ain't I a woman? Revisiting intersectionality. J Int Womens Stud. 2004;**5**(3):75–86.

65. **Roberts D.** Shattered Bonds: The Color of Child Welfare. New York: Basic Books; 2003.

66. **Olivet J, Dones M.** Intersectionality and race: how racism and discrimination contribute to homelessness among LGBTQ youth. In: **Price C, Wheeler C, Shelton J, Maury M** (Eds), At the Intersections: A Collaborative Report on LGBTQ Youth Homelessness. New York: True Colors Fund and the National LGBTQ Task Force; 2016:56–59.

67. **Castellanos HD.** The role of institutional placement, family conflict, and homosexuality in homelessness pathways among Latino LGBT youth in New York City. J Homosex. 2016;**63**(5):601–632.

68. **Gattis MN, Larson A.** Perceived microaggressions and mental health in a sample of Black youths experiencing homelessness. Soc Work Res. 2017;**41**(1):7–17.

69. **Gattis MN, Larson A.** Perceived racial, sexual identity, and homeless status-related discrimination among Black adolescents and young adults experiencing homelessness: relations with depressive symptoms and suicidality. Am J Orthopsychiatry. 2016;**86**(1):79–90.

70. **Freire P.** Pedagogy of the Oppressed. Harmondsworth: Penguin; 1972.

71. **Sícoli JL, Nascimento PR.** Promoção de saúde: concepções, princípios e operacionalização. Interface (Botucatu). 2003;**7**(12):101–122.

72. **Souza EM, Grundy E.** Promoção da saúde, epidemiologia social e capital social: interrelações e perspectivas para a saúde pública. Cad Saude Publica. 2004;**20**(5):1354–1360.

73. **World Health Organization.** Health Promotion Evaluation: Recommendations to Policymakers. Copenhagen: European Working Group on Health Promotion Evaluation; 1998. Available from: https://apps.who.int/iris/bitstream/handle/10665/108116/E60706.pdf?sequence=1&isAllowed=y.

74. **Paiva V.** Sexualidades adolescentes: escolaridade, gênero e o sujeito sexual. In **Parker R, Barbosa R** (Eds), Sexualidades Brasileiras. Rio de Janeiro: Relume-Dumará, ABIA, IMS/UERJ; 1996:213–235.

Chapter 24

Why and how should we care about homeless youth suffering from severe mental illnesses?

Amal Abdel-Baki, Raphaël Morisseau-Guillot, Hubert Côté, Julie Marguerite Deschênes, Virginie Doré-Gauthier, and Isabelle Sarah Lévesque

The phenomenon of youth homelessness

Youth homelessness is defined as the situation of youth 'who are living independently of parents and/or caregivers, but do not have the means or ability to acquire a stable, safe or consistent residence' (1). The definition of 'youth' varies from including adolescents from the ages of 13 up to 25 years old to the early thirties (1,2). Youth homelessness represents a continuum of housing instability (3), ranging from being unsheltered, that is, absolutely homeless and sleeping on the streets or parks, to emergency sheltered or also precariously housed, for example, so-called sofa surfing, and youth at risk of homelessness. It entails a breakage in important relationships during a pivotal period of development that hinders a gradual, harmonious transition into adulthood and its challenges (4), a process sometimes referred to as early adultification (5).

Extent of the phenomenon

Over 12 months, nearly 3.5 million youths experienced homelessness in the US (6), while it was estimated that over 83,000 youths had used homeless services, and 1.3 million have slept rough or in an unsafe place in the UK (7). In Canada, approximately 6000–7000 youths experience homelessness daily (3), and 40% of homeless youth (HY) are younger than 16 years when they first experience homelessness (8). This subgroup is much more likely to go through multiple episodes of homelessness with even more precocious involvement with child protection (8).

Some minority groups, such as newcomers, indigenous people, and lesbian, gay, bisexual, transgender, and queer/questioning (LGBTQ) people, are over-represented within the HY population. For instance, between 20% and 40% of HY identified as LGBTQ in Canada, the US, and the UK (8–10); for them, sexual identity or orientation has often been a cause of homelessness, typically because of negative reactions of parents (11,12). In Australia, 42% of the Indigenous homeless population was 18 years old or younger, roughly twice the rate of non-Indigenous homeless people (13). In Canada, while Indigenous people represent 4.3% of the general population, Indigenous youth make up 30% of the homeless population (8). In Australia, the risk of homelessness was six to ten times higher in young refugees than Australian-born youth (14).

In Canada, almost one-third of HY had been uninterruptedly homeless for a year; of those, 60% had been homeless for at least 3 years (8). For others, the trajectory into homelessness is not linear. It consists of multiple episodes of varying degrees of precariousness, including being transiently homeless, and therefore these HY are particularly challenging to help and account for (7,8). In comparison with the overall homeless population, HY are more likely to experience 'hidden homelessness', making them more vulnerable since they are less likely to receive help from typical service provision models (15) especially when homelessness is experienced at an earlier age. By the time youth do access homelessness services, they have often experienced multiple episodes of instability over many years (8).

Before becoming homeless: factors associated with youth homelessness

Although, for a minority, homelessness is the consequence of a personal choice for youth who, to express their independence, purposefully decide to run away from their home, a growing body of literature is pointing at much more diverse and complex causes of youth homelessness that involve individual factors, but also systemic shortcomings (4).

A problematic familial environment is a key factor preceding homelessness for many youth (4,16–18). Either because of physical, sexual, and/or emotional abuse, violence, or transitions (divorce, moving, introduction of step-parents) (8,19–22), homes can seem no longer welcoming or safe for youth. Even when removed from a problematic environment to be placed in child protection settings, placement can often be perceived by youth as uncaring and unwelcoming, therefore causing further traumatic experiences (23). This explains why the street can be perceived as relatively safer and more appealing for youth experiencing such a predicament (23,24). On an individual level, mental health problems (including substance use disorders (SUDs)), learning difficulties, academic derailment, and misdemeanour have also been associated with youth homelessness (25). These personal factors are, however, difficult to distinguish from familial factors (26), including parental SUD (27) and mental illness (28), or socioeconomic status (29), that have also been associated with youth homelessness.

Risks and consequences associated with youth homelessness

Youth homelessness is associated with significant deleterious consequences. Already vulnerable because of pre-existing risk factors, youth face further adversity when entering the streets. Moreover, this takes place during a pivotal period of personal and social development with milestones like the transition into adult healthcare (1).

Homelessness also has severe consequences for physical health of youth: rates of hepatitis B, hepatitis C, HIV infections, as well as pregnancies in HY are higher compared to housed youth and are often linked to substance use, associated with promiscuity behaviours, including prostitution (30). The mortality rate in HY was found to be 11 times higher than the expected rate, with suicide and drug overdose being the leading causes of death (30). In this key period of physical development, nutritional deficiencies are also endemic (31). HY are also more likely to suffer from various forms of violence (30), including sexual exploitation (32,33), but this violence is less likely to be addressed than in domiciliated youth (34). The disproportionately high rate of school dropouts in this population limits work opportunity and renders providing for oneself particularly challenging (4,34). HY may therefore resort to offences like theft or drug selling to survive and are at risk of involvement with the justice system (8,35,36).

Lastly, HY are much more likely to be victims of crimes than their stably housed counterparts (8,37). An American study conducted in 2013 also found that after committing crimes and being released from the judicial system, 26% of youth were homeless over a 12-month follow-up period, further compounding the risk of recidivism and poor outcome in terms of mortality and morbidity (38).

Coping with adversity: youth homelessness and severe mental illness

Beyond these various consequences, perhaps the most striking impact of homelessness on youth is mental illness. Eighty-five per cent of HY report high levels of psychological distress and poor psychological health, as well as single or multiple suicide attempts in 42% (8,39). There is a complex interplay between homelessness, and trauma and mental illness, both being a potential trigger or exacerbating factor for the other (8). Moreover, trauma during childhood increases risks of homelessness (40,41), substance misuse (42), and psychosis (43,44). Therefore, trauma and mental illness are both contributing causal factors and consequences of homelessness in youth (45–47). While it is recognized that mental health problems often precede homelessness (46,48), the precarity of the street is known to exacerbate pre-existing disorders (49–51), including severe mental illness, which in turn further complicates transitioning into stable living circumstances (49).

Mental disorders are more prevalent in HY than in domiciliated youth (52,53), including alcohol and drug abuse (42% and 39%, respectively), post-traumatic stress disorder (36%), major depression (31%), and personality disorder (19%) (53,54), while concurrent disorders are frequent (60%) (55–57). When homelessness is first experienced at a younger age, it is associated with more severe symptoms and substance misuse, poorer quality of life, and higher suicidality (8).

Severe mental illness rates such as for psychosis vary greatly between studies (58). The relative paucity of data can be explained by the fact that homelessness and severe mental illness render research participation difficult often because of disorganization. In HY, psychosis is likely significantly more prevalent, especially when associated with drug use such as methamphetamines (55). Longitudinal studies of youth with first-episode psychosis (FEP), report a history of homelessness in up to 26% of FEP youth (59) either before or during a 2-year follow-up period in an Early Intervention in Psychosis Programme (EIPP) (60). HY with FEP are more likely to have a SUD, lower educational achievement, more legal problems, and poorer symptomatic and functional outcomes despite treatment, compared to stably housed FEP patients (61). Homelessness is also associated with the persistence of SUD in FEP, in turn linked with poor outcomes (62). This is of great importance: not only are HY with FEP more vulnerable at admission to EIPPs, compared to stably housed youths because of their medical and psychosocial history, but they are more vulnerable and have poorer outcomes despite treatment (including more hospitalizations and emergency visits than housed youth) possibly because of their ongoing precarious status, hence the need for specific interventions targeting HY.

Personal and societal costs of homeless youth

Despite this dire situation, outpatient mental healthcare utilization remains limited for HY (58,63,64). While some youth may purposefully choose not to access care, data indicate that a majority of HY coping with mental illness would like to have better access to services (65).

Specifically targeting youth homelessness is pivotal because evidence indicates that for many chronically homeless adults, the path to precarious housing started when they were young (66,67). Because HY are particularly at risk of academic derailment and social disaffiliation, homelessness can have profound effects on their overall life trajectory and the importance of rapid interventions cannot be overstressed. While coping with pre-existing severe disorders and facing the plight of homelessness that can exacerbate symptoms or create new problems like substance use, HY are at greater risk of becoming entrenched in street life (23). In those with severe mental illness, it is even more important to prevent delays in accessing care, since longer duration of untreated psychosis is associated with poorer prognosis (68).

Australian data from 2016 estimate that youth homelessness costs roughly $750 million per year to the country's economy (69). These costs are then duplicated when HY become chronically homeless adults, because of costly, reactive care instead of preventive healthcare services as well as involvement in the legal system and welfare with loss of productivity.

Barriers to mental health services access for homeless youth with mental illness

HY with mental illness face many barriers to mental health services use, which results in suboptimal utilization of existing resources.

Suboptimal utilization of existing resources

Suboptimal integration of services

Many Western health and social systems organize their services by specific problems or diagnoses which complicates access to the appropriate care for HY since they might not 'fit' any specific 'category' because most have concurrent disorders and/or because mental illnesses symptomatology are often non-specific in their early course (70).

Accessing services needed by HY is therefore complex since community organizations and public health institutions usually have their locations, schedules, and mandates. For the youth, it can become difficult to plan and prioritize appointment schedules and transportation, while confronted with limited financial resources and limited time to fulfil their basic needs, often at the disadvantage of their mental health follow-ups. The fragmentation and specialization of services results in the multiplication of service providers and the lack of communication and partnership between the different providers results in silo work. The lack of collaboration and sharing philosophy of intervention might result in a lack of consistency between services which can reduce the impact of each approach as they interfere with each other: an example would be the harm reduction approach compared to approaches advocating abstinence in SUD. Moreover, there often is a lack of integration of mental health and addiction rehabilitation services (71,72).

Lack of continuity and poor transition between services

Continuity refers to how care should be considered, with philosophical consistency and with the same actors over time (73). This is an essential matter for HY with mental illness, as they are often facing complex issues and their difficulties in engaging with caregivers are often an important challenge because of personal histories of abandonment or negligence. The duration in time as well as the constancy of the treatment team members would allow the development of a therapeutic trusting relationship and the subsequent involvement of the youth in their treatment.

Various situations of breakage of continuity of care are problematic in the typical trajectory of HY suffering from severe mental disorders. The break in continuity between youth and adult services is indeed a potential cause of youth homelessness. Indeed, more than 40% of HY have had involvement with foster care or group homes (74–77). Because of underdeveloped living skills, low education level, lower levels of physical and emotional well-being, and lack of support and resources, many youth who leave child protection care (whether it is a choice or because they reach 18 years old and must leave their placement) fail to make the transition to independent living (78). Furthermore, the organization of public and community services available for HY is, for the most part, short-term emergency services where the youth is rushed to an independent lifestyle (76,79–85), which would be unable to guarantee a return to housing stability for many youths after an initial episode of homelessness. Evidence from Australia, the UK, the US, and Canada indicates that youth typically 'age out' of youth health and social services arbitrarily when entering 'legally defined adulthood', meaning that they no longer have access to minimal safety nets provided by youth protection or social and healthcare services (86–88). The absence of an adequate transition into adult services leaves the most vulnerable youth without a home to return to, and no services to help them solve their social and mental health issues, which perpetuates their homeless status. However, disengagement of the treatment teams is often seen (89) with homeless patients after a hospitalization, based on the patient's refusal of conventional psychiatric follow-up, which is often not tuned with that population's specific needs. Indeed, when homeless patients with schizophrenia and comorbidities are hospitalized, they are often discharged from hospitalization with inadequate planning (90). For example, it might be impossible for a patient to fill a discharge medication prescription without the necessary healthcare card and to attend subsequent appointments if basic needs, such as housing and transportation costs, were not adequately tackled during hospitalization.

The delays of transfer between the various mental health services, hence between initial evaluation and treatment, are also occasions for continuity breaks, undermining youth engagement.

Continuity challenges for young people at discharge from psychiatric hospitalization can be solved by assertive and rigorous follow-ups by treatment teams to initiate and maintain contact (91), these being more likely to engage HY with severe mental illness in treatment (92).

To address mental health services' lack of continuity, experts thereby recommend smoother transition programmes to adulthood (e.g. 15–25 or 14–30 years) and joint programmes between child psychiatry and adult psychiatry (93–96).

Youths not seeking help

No perception of need

Determinants of the use of mental health services include the capacity for perceiving one's own needs and the ability to be aware of the presence of a problem (97). Young people report that awareness, involving the level of knowledge about mental health and the ability to find and use information about services (98), is an incentive to use the services and provides motivation to consult a therapist (91), a key factor to accessing mental health services (99).

The lack of perceived needs for mental health services, especially in HY with severe mental illness such as psychosis where insight into illness is affected by the illness, is a barrier to accessibility (100,101). Besides the resistance of youth to 'accept' mental illness, refusing it 'as if it was suggested to be a part of their identity' during the developmental turning point of transition to adulthood (102,103), HY with severe mental illness face further stigmatization (linked to homelessness), deterring them from seeking services. Moreover, subgroups like LGBTQ people, substance users, and visible minorities, when homeless, are further marginalized making them less likely to adhere to what they perceive as further 'stigma'-related services (1,104).

Self-healing

Even when youth recognize their mental health problems, they may still not use the appropriate services: indeed, they are less likely to seek treatment than older age groups and more likely to attempt to manage mental health challenges on their own (105), which might be an attempt at affirming their need for independence (106). The main reasons given for not accessing mental health services would be the desire to solve one's problems by oneself (107) while in other cases, they may believe that their mental distress is temporary and tend to normalize it (102).

More urgent needs: finding shelter, food, and so on

HY report competing demands with mental health issues as a barrier to the utilization of mental health services (100). Indeed, mental health issues may not be prioritized in the hierarchy of their needs, the primary need being related to obtaining a clean and safe place to sleep or live (108). For instance, it might be difficult for youth coping with active psychiatric symptoms and little organizational aids (no agenda, no phone) to attend follow-ups scheduled at inconvenient times and requiring transportation fees when they face conditions of insecurity, such as insufficient financial resources to secure basic needs or the obligation to secure a bed or a meal at a shelter at a certain hour.

Lack of guidance from a trustworthy adult or 'role model'

HY, particularly in the presence of a severe mental illness, widely experience the breakdown of family ties and lack a sufficient support network. Social isolation increases the risk of being homeless during unplanned or stressful events. As advice on one's mental health and navigation in the health system can be more easily received from a trustworthy adult (109), HY may lack support in their search for mental health treatment.

Mistrust towards institutions secondary to previous experiences

The high prevalence of childhood traumas in HY (110,111), and HY with severe mental disorders, affects their ability to build and maintain a long-term relationship (112). It thereby influences their interaction with adult service providers (113) and slows the engagement process. Previous difficult or traumatic experiences with the institutional setting may induce reluctance to engage with the public system services because of mistrust, fear of judgement, and therefore the desire to be released from services (113). Indeed, having a history of involuntary placements or hospitalizations (common in HY with severe psychiatric illnesses) can deter young people from seeking help. Subsequently, many young people refuse mental health support and receive services only during crises in emergency room or hospitalization, therefore repeating negative and potentially traumatic experiences (114), and preventing the provision of adequate services.

Not youth-friendly services or not adapted to special needs because of settings or staff's attitude

Feeling judged or discriminated against and perceiving the treatment teams as not understanding, or having an authoritative communication style, as well as one-way communication, are barriers to the utilization of existing services (115–117).

Health facilities are often focused on speed and efficiency, with a high patient-to-clinician ratio resulting in the need for rapid interventions, which are not adapted for this vulnerable population. The gap between youth expectations, often related to obtaining immediate support (e.g. housing support), and traditional services offered, undermine the use of mental health treatment, stressing the need for flexible integrated services adapted to a wide range of medical and psychosocial needs.

Finally, HY view homeless adults as having more severe and chronic mental illnesses and personal hygiene issues (118) and have often experienced harassment or prior violence from homeless adults in adult shelters (119), making them uncomfortable to share waiting rooms or housing facilities with them.

Suboptimal access

Not adapted to youth experiencing homelessness and mental illness issues

Despite identified needs among HY, they are less likely to be referred to specialists (91). Moreover, some specific specialized mental health services (e.g. programmes for severe personality disorders) might simply not exist or are not accessible for HY because of strict eligibility criteria (104).

Services should be obtained rapidly, without intermediary steps, once the youth formulates a demand for mental health help. Long waiting lists (115,120,121), leading to a lack of timely care, are barriers to accessibility, especially for HY as they often try to engage with service providers in crisis situations (121). Moreover, being on a waiting list leads them to think that they are not important (91) and reinforces their perception of their stigmatization.

The lack of awareness of available services (91,97,120,122), which are often limited and not youth oriented (99), remains another challenge to service accessibility for HY. Although trust in treatment provider competency is crucial (99), service providers may lack specific training about over-represented homeless populations (LGBTQ, aboriginals, immigrants), trauma, post-trauma, and family interventions, as well as awareness of homelessness community resources (123,124), which can prevent optimal access to care adapted to their needs.

Complicated administrative process

HY describe a sense of being overwhelmed and lost in the healthcare system. Service providers themselves also describe the system as complex, segregated, and difficult to navigate. Appropriate referral pathways lack clarity, especially for this population, and the follow-up of referrals is often problematic (125). The presence of numerous agencies and their bureaucratic requirements involving interagency referrals, the need for identification cards or proof of residence (immigrants being over-represented in the population of HY with severe mental disorders), the ability to be contacted by telephone or mail, and time-consuming paperwork represent structural barriers to mental healthcare for HY (118), particularly if already disorganized as a result of severe mental disorders. In countries without universal healthcare, a lack of a private health insurance plan will often result in service inaccessibility. In that sense, mentors helping the youth navigate this system and encourage treatment are facilitators to mental health treatment (118).

How to help them?

Overview of interventions aimed at homeless youth and related populations

Although the limited available research reported worse clinical and social outcomes in HY, few studies addressing interventions for HY with severe mental health disorders were conducted.

Different approaches such as assertive community treatment, critical time intervention, 'Housing First' programmes, and integrated treatment for addiction and psychiatric disorders (126,127), resulted in good outcomes in homeless adults with severe mental illness such as a reduction in alcohol misuse, psychiatric symptoms, and length and frequency of hospitalizations; improvement in independent living capacity, housing stability, as well as quality of life; while preventing homelessness or facilitating the exit of homelessness (128–142).

While case management led to positive outcomes on substance misuse, mood and anxiety symptoms, and delinquent behaviour in HY without a diagnosed psychiatric disorder (143), EIPPs can improve involvement in work or school, engagement in treatment, and reduce positive and negative symptoms severity and hospitalizations (144), therefore preventing the negative impact of a long duration of untreated psychosis (145–147) in youth with emerging psychosis.

Therefore, essential principles emerge from these interventions developed for homeless populations and are described in the following sections: the importance of an early and intensive follow-up, with outreach interventions, targeting housing issues early on, and integrating treatment for SUD and mental illness.

Case management and outreach interventions

Since most HY typically have multiple psychosocial and medical needs that require services from more than one agency, the case manager can serve as a unifying coordinator enabling communication between services (143), including mental and physical health, residential, financial, and vocational services, and facilitating access through outreach interventions in the community.

Assertive community treatment is a model of case management that distinguishes itself by the integration of a multidisciplinary team, a lower client/case manager ratio (allowing a more intensive follow-up), 24-hour coverage by the treatment team, and community-based services directly provided through outreach interventions, rather than brokered to other organizations (128).

Early and intensive follow-up

In addition to intensive approaches allowing regular contact and outreach interventions, as well as acute crisis management, the timing of intervention is critical, highlighting the importance of offering services early on and at specific times to improve clinical outcomes.

Critical time intervention aims to prevent recurrence of homelessness and other adverse outcomes after discharge from the hospital by maintaining continuity of care during this critical transitional period, strengthening the individual's long-term ties to their social network and to service providers while providing emotional and practical support (134).

EIPPs have been developed over the last 30 years in efforts to prevent the negative impact of a long duration of untreated psychosis (145–147). These interventions based on friendly, community outreach approaches and vocational rehabilitation, aim to engage youth in treatment early in the course of their illness (148).

Housing support

The core feature of the Housing First approach is the immediate provision of permanent housing and support to people experiencing homelessness and severe mental illness. Housing First consists of immediate access to housing with no housing readiness conditions, consumer choice and self-determination, recovery orientation (including harm reduction), individualized and person-driven supports, and social and community integration (138).

Integrated treatment for SUD and mental illness

Integrated treatment approaches for addiction and psychiatric disorders which integrate mental health treatment, substance use counselling, and housing services through a single organization have shown positive outcomes (126).

Addressing barriers to mental health services for homeless youth

Youth-friendly services adapted to HY special needs

Youth-exclusive clinics, shelters, and other service agencies allowing HY to avoid contact with older homeless adults which makes them uncomfortable, may be a facilitator to access. Youth-friendly environments are recognized as prerequisites to HY engagement with mental health treatment teams. Such environments are influenced by the attitude and type of approach of services' staff, the diversity of treatment options, and the physical settings themselves. Client-centred responses from service providers, as well as staff attitudes based on trust, respect, empathy, and being non-judgemental, friendly, and understanding, allow for therapeutic relationships with HY with mental health problems, especially with psychotic patients who might be harder to engage in treatment (125,149). The consideration of the youth's perception of their needs and their preferences in treatment options will contribute to the engagement process. The diversity of treatment options (e.g. outreach, home-based, phone, and street clinic) (99), free services with extended opening hours (91), and physical environments for service provision based in local communities whose atmosphere is relaxed and open (91) are seen as facilitators by HY, who prefer healthcare services to be delivered at familiar and accessible places such as drop-ins with an open-door policy (150), already frequented by HY to which they are already acculturated to, and/or where assistance with transportation needs is offered when referral or outside care is needed (118). Flexibility is imperative, as required by frequent appointment cancellations and unforeseen circumstances due to their instability. Assertive follow-ups therefore must acknowledge that instability through efforts at initiating and maintaining contact with the youth.

Service organization

Multiple barriers prevail in current systems of mental healthcare, demanding a major transformation for young people with severe mental disorders to be able to access services, especially HY and those at risk of homelessness. A systemic response would require a modification of service organization, starting with the elimination of the rupture of care from the child/adolescent to adult health system and its associated risk of disengagement of services. Child/adolescent and adult services professionals should be merged into a single team targeting the 11–30-year-old population (151) offering transdiagnosis services since the clinical picture is often heterogeneous and non-specific early in their evolution. They should be delivered in community-based, youth-friendly physical environments, along with alternative activities and holistic support groups targeting this culturally diverse population. These services should be accessible, hence obtained rapidly after an initial contact, and flexible, allowing for extended contact hours through diverse contact modalities with services providers, unscheduled appointments for crisis intervention, and based on outreach approaches, addressing practical obstacles relative to their financial difficulties and psychosocial instability. Emphasis should initially be on accessibility and the resolution of that instability (e.g. through housing services), with further positive results on engagement in treatment.

Current systems of care fail to engage many youths with mental disorders, particularly so for HY. Australia's national youth mental health initiative *Headspace* (93,152) was created in 2006 to tackle the need for transformational change in mental health services, followed by its Irish counterpart in 2007, *Headstrong* (94) (renamed *Jigsaw* in 2016) and the pan-Canadian programme, ACCESS Open Minds (151) with its specific HY site ACCESS Open Minds–RIPAJ Montreal Homeless Youth Network (153,154) reinforcing partnerships between existing institutional and community organizations. All these initiatives shared universal principles, revolving around early identification and early intervention in emerging mental disorders with rapid access to assessment and appropriate care; creation of youth-friendly environments; accessibility of coordinated, integrated, and evidence-based interventions adapted to the youth needs without a child–adult services break of continuity; engagement of young people in programme design and planning; implementation of educational and training programmes for service providers; and promotion of community-wide awareness of youth mental health.

Although the typical care provision models do not allow for addressing the complex psychiatric and psychosocial problems of HY (155), the availability of unique settings where HY can receive both health and social services is an interesting solution to overcome the lack of coordination between service providers, which was identified as an important barrier to accessibility and engagement in services (118). Integration of services implies the 'incorporation of educational, social, physical and mental health services into "one-stop distribution points" where educators, social workers, and physical health stake-holders collaborate to deliver personalized services' (156).

Solutions for HY with severe mental illnesses

To tackle HY with severe mental illness difficulties in engaging in treatment, efforts should be directed towards the inclusion of HY and their significant others in the assessment, goal setting, and treatment planning, but also in the development and delivery of services. HY involvement, through the resultant empowering and the elaboration of youth-friendly services taking their specific needs into account, would result in the appropriation and improved utilization of services, as would the implication of relatives in treatment, also resulting in enhanced social support.

The inclusion of peer workers in treatment teams and in community organizations can alleviate HY distrust of mental health services through the creation of an alliance based on shared experiences. Initiation of contact could be smoother and better received, therefore facilitating the engagement process with treatment teams. The establishment of a relationship with a mental health professional before treatment initiation, facilitated by a regular presence in youth-oriented community organizations, would allow for an optimized utilization of services by youth during crisis periods.

It is also stressed that further training is needed for staff members working in institutional and community settings. Training should focus on mental health assessment skills to improve early case identification and on existing homelessness resources and mental health resources to establish contact and transition with the appropriate service providers according to the youth's needs. Information transmission about reference processes and services to HY should also be optimized. Moreover, as stigmatization is an important barrier to service access for HY with severe mental illness, training related to over-represented homeless subgroup realities can improve access to care, being more oriented to HY needs. More globally, professionals should be trained to establish an empathic, non-judgemental initial contact and adopt a securing, supporting attitude to facilitate youth engagement in services.

The Canadian example: EQIIP SOL

Considering the factors that prevent HY from accessing mental healthcare and engaging with service providers, as well as the literature supporting effective interventions addressed to HY and related populations, an intensive outreach team (Équipe d'intervention intensive de proximité (EQIIP SOL)) was created in 2012 at the Centre Hospitalier Universitaire de Montréal.

Based on interventions that showed significant improvements in clinical and functional outcomes in HY and related populations (128–142), EQIIP SOL improves accessibility to appropriate psychiatric and addiction services, to facilitate the exit of homelessness and to promote social integration through supported employment interventions (adapted for youth including accessing education). It offers adapted intensive case management for HY with FEP and addiction, integrating early intervention for psychosis and addiction (mainly harm reduction and motivational) interventions, as well as specialized housing support into a single team, offering a high intensity of services (early when discharged from hospital or during crisis periods) and outreach interventions. Its target population is HY or youth at risk of homelessness aged between 18 and 30 years with FEP and comorbid problematic substance use.

Three psychiatrists (part-time) and three full-time social workers contribute to the team. Outreach interventions are achieved through a partnership developed with the community and institutional organizations working with HY in Montreal, Canada (emergency shelters, drop-in day centres, supported housing organizations for HY or for people with mental illnesses, organizations offering addiction services or 'Housing First' programmes). The low case manager-to-patient ratio (1:10) allows flexibility for these outreach interventions, as well as high intensity and frequency of follow-up. In case of an urgent event or crisis, the great availability of case managers allows youth and community workers to have direct and rapid access to EQIIP SOL to avoid psychosis relapse or a slip into homelessness. Furthermore, EQIIP SOL professionals are present regularly in the main community organizations for HY and, as needed, also offering training sessions. Regular meetings for sharing administrative and clinical information (if authorized by the youth) allows the establishment of a community of practice, through which a strong therapeutic alliance built on trust can be developed with the youth.

The evolution of youth followed by EQIIP SOL from its creation in February 2012 was recently published (157). At baseline, HY with FEP and addiction showed poor prognosis factors: cluster B personality traits or disorder, childhood trauma, legal problems, lower educational level, and SUD. The main positive outcome of the EQIIP SOL intervention is the decrease in homelessness. Indeed, the addition of this intervention was associated with an increased likelihood of attaining housing stability and attaining housing stability faster than the EIPP only. Both interventions showed drastic reduction of homelessness, with only 10% of the participants in both groups still being homeless at 12 months.

Regarding emergency and hospitalization use, EQIIP SOL participants spent fewer days hospitalized during follow-up than EIPP participants. The number of participants living in autonomous accommodation increased significantly compared to institutionalized accommodation. The attainment of early housing stability was facilitated by the partnerships developed by EQIIP SOL with the community organizations offering supervised housing and Housing First support, offering opportunities (including emergency supervised apartments) to end homelessness early in follow-up. The need for supervised housing remains prevalent in HY with FEP and addiction over an autonomous living, likely explained by factors such as the great social disaffiliation, the weak family support, the low level of functional autonomy, the high prevalence of SUDs, and the legal history in this population, making living autonomously difficult. Functional and clinical outcomes with EQIIP SOL did not differ from the EIPP; however, a significant reduction in alcohol use disorder and any SUD (at least one substance) was shown over the follow-up period.

Conclusion

HY with severe mental illness have specific needs that can be addressed by specific teams dedicated and trained to integrate the interventions needed by this population. Without such teams, the complexity of their past and current situations often results in a long duration of untreated illness and its deleterious consequences. Promising interventions have been developed (77,157). However, further research is needed to see whether these interventions are replicable in other sociopolitical cultures and other health and social services organizations.

References

1. **Canadian Observatory on Homelessness**. Canadian Definition of Youth Homelessness. Toronto: Homeless Hub; 2016.
2. **Quilgars D**. Youth homelessness. In: **O'Sullivan E, Busch-Geertsema V, Quilgars D, Pleace N** (Eds), Homelessness Research in Europe. Brussels: FEANTSA; 2010:187–210.
3. **Canada Without Poverty**. Youth Rights! Right Now! Ending Youth Homelessness: A Human Rights Guide. Toronto: Canadian Observatory on Homelessness; 2016.
4. **Gaetz S**. Coming of Age: Reimagining the Response to Youth Homelessness in Canada. Toronto: Canadian Observatory on Homelessness; 2014.
5. **Schmitz RM, Tyler KA**. Growing up before their time: the early adultification experiences of homeless young people. Child Youth Serv Rev. 2016;**64**:15–22.
6. **Morton M, Dworsky A, Matjasko J**, et al. Prevalence and correlates of youth homelessness in the United States. J Adolesc Health. 2018;**62**(1):14–21.
7. **Clark A, Burgess G, Morris S, Udagawa C**. Estimating the scale of youth homelessness in the UK. Cambridge: University of Cambridge; 2015.
8. **Gaetz S, O'Grady B, Kidd S, Schwan K**. Without a Home: The National Youth Homelessness Survey. Toronto: Canadian Observatory on Homelessness Press; 2016.

9. **Price C, Wheeler C, Shleton J, Maury M.** At the Intersections: A Collaborative Report on LGBTQ Youth Homelessness. New York: True Colors Fund and the National LGBTQ Task Force; 2016.

10. **The Albert Kennedy Trust.** LGBT Youth Homelessness: A UK National Scoping of Cause, Prevalence, Response & Outcome. London: The Albert Kennedy Trust; 2015.

11. **Cull M, Platzer H, Balloch S.** Out On My Own: Understanding the Experiences and Needs of Homeless Lesbian, Gay, Bisexual and Transgender Youth. Brighton: Faculty of Health, School of Applied Social Science, University of Brighton; 2006.

12. **Abramovich A.** No fixed address: young, queer, and restless. In: **Gaetz S, O'Grady B, Buccieri K, Karabanow J, Marsolais A** (Eds), Youth Homelessness in Canada: Implications for Policy and Practice. Toronto: Canadian Homelessness Research Network; 2013:387–403.

13. **Australian Institute of Health and Welfare.** Homelessness Among Indigenous Australians. Canberra: Australian Institute of Health and Welfare; 2014.

14. **Lawson D, Dutertre S.** Finding Home in Victoria: Refugee and Migrant Young People Who Are Homeless or at Risk of Homelessness. Victoria: The Centre for Multicultural Youth; 2010.

15. **Gaetz S, Gulliver T, Richter T.** The State of Homelessness in Canada: 2014. Toronto: The Homeless Hub Press; 2014.

16. **Karabanow J, Naylor T.** Pathways towards stability: young people's transitions off of the streets. In: **Gaetz S, O'Grady B, Buccieri K, Karabanow J, Marsolais A** (Eds), In: Youth Homelessness in Canada: Implications for Policy and Practice. Toronto: Canadian Homelessness Research Network; 2013:39–52.

17. **Gaetz S, O'Grady B.** Making money: exploring the economy of young homessless workers. Work Employ Soc. 2002;**16**(3):433–456.

18. **Braitstein P, Li K, Tyndall M,** et al. Sexual violence among a cohort of injection drug users. Soc Sci Med. 2003;**57**(3):561–569.

19. **Ballon BC, Courbasson CMA, Smith PD.** Physical and sexual abuse issues among youths with substance use problems. Can J Psychiatry. 2001;**46**(7):617–621.

20. **Tyler KA, Cauce AM.** Perpetrators of early physical and sexual abuse among homeless and runaway adolescents. Child Abuse Negl. 2002;**2002**(26):1261–1274.

21. **Thrane LE, Hoyt DR, Whitbeck LB, Yoder KA.** Impact of family abuse on running away, deviance, and street victimization among homeless rural and urban youth. Child Abuse Negl. 2006;**30**(10):1117–1128.

22. **Tyler KA, Schmitz RM.** Family histories and multiple transitions among homeless young adults: pathways to homelessness. Child Youth Serv Rev. 2013;**35**(10):1719–1726.

23. **Karabanow J.** How young people get off the street: exploring paths and processes. In: **Hulchanski JD, Campsie P, Chau S, Hwang S, Paradis E** (Eds), Finding Home: Policy Options for Addressing Homelessness in Canada. Toronto: Cities Centre, University of Toronto; 2009: Chapter 3.6. Available from: https://www.homelesshub.ca/resource/36-how-young-people-get-street-exploring-paths-processes.

24. **Janus MD, Archambault FX, Brown SW, Welsh LA.** Physical abuse in Canadian runaway adolescents. Child Abuse Negl. 1995;**19**(4):433–447.

25. **Winland D.** Reconnecting with family and community: pathways out of youth homelessness. In: **Gaetz S, O'Grady B, Buccieri K, Karabanow J, Marsolais A** (Eds),

Youth Homelessness in Canada: Implications for Policy and Practice. Toronto: Canadian Homelessness Research Network; 2013:15–38.

26. **Mallet S, Rosenthal D, Keys D.** Young people, drug use and family conflict: pathways into homelessness. J Adolesc. 2005;**28**(2):185–199.

27. **McMorris BJ, Tyler KA, Whitbeck LB, Hoyt DR.** Familial and 'on-the-street' risk factors associated with alcohol use among homeless and runaway adolescents. J Stud Alcohol. 2002;**63**(1):34–43.

28. **Andres-Lemay VJ, Jamieson E, MacMillan HL.** Child abuse, psychiatric disorder, and running away in a community sample of women. Can J Psychiatry. 2005;**50**(11):684–689.

29. **Karabanow J, Hugues J, Ticknor J, Kidd S, Patterson D.** The economics of being young and poor: how homeless youth survive in neo-liberal times. J Sociol Soc Welf. 2010;**37**(4):39–63.

30. **Boivin J-F, Roy É, Haley N, Galbaud du Fort G.** The health of street youth: a Canadian perspective. Can J Public Health. 2005;**96**(6):432–437.

31. **Dachner N, Tarasuk V.** Homeless youth, nutritional vulnerability, and community food assistance programs. In: **Gaetz S, O'Grady B, Buccieri K, Karabanow J, Marsolais A** (Eds), Youth Homelessness in Canada: Implications for Policy and Practice. Toronto: Canadian Homelessness Research Network; 2013:131–145.

32. **Saewyc EM, Drozda C, Rivers R, MacKay L, Peled M.** Which comes first: sexual exploitation or other risk exposures among street-involved youth? In: **Gaetz S, O'Grady B, Buccieri K, Karabanow J, Marsolais A** (Eds), Youth Homelessness in Canada: Implications for Policy and Practice. Toronto: Canadian Homelessness Research Network; 2013:147–160.

33. **Tyler KA, Hoyt DR, Whitbeck LB.** The effects of early sexual abuse on later sexual victimization among female homeless and runaway adolescents. J Interpers Violence. 2000;**15**(3):235–250.

34. **Gaetz S, O'Grady B, Buccieri K.** Surviving Crime and Violence: Street Youth and Victimization in Toronto. Toronto: Justice for Children and Youth, Homeless Hub; 2010.

35. **Baron S.** Why street youth become involved in crime. In: **Gaetz S, O'Grady B, Buccieri K, Karabanow J, Marsolais A** (Eds), Youth Homelessness in Canada: Implications for Policy and Practice. Toronto: Canadian Homelessness Research Network; 2013:353–368.

36. **Hagan J, McCarthy B, Parker P, Climenhage JA.** Mean Streets: Youth Crime and Homelessness. New York: Cambridge University Press; 1997.

37. **Gaetz S.** Whose safety counts? Street youth, social exclusion, and criminal victimization. In: **Hulchanski JD, Campsie P, Chau S, Hwang S, Paradis E** (Eds), Finding Home: Policy Options for Addressing Homelessness in Canada. Toronto: Homeless Hub; 2009: Chapter 3.2. Available from: https://www.homelesshub.ca/resou rce/32-whose-safety-counts-street-youth-social-exclusion-criminal-victimization.

38. **Ford Shah M, Black C, Felver B, Albrecht C, Beall K.** Impact of Homelessness on Youth Recently Released from Juvenile Rehabilitation Facilities. Olympia: Washington State Department of Commerce, Community Services and Housing Division; 2013.

39. **Kidd SA, Gaetz S, O'Grady B.** The 2015 National Canadian Homeless Youth Survey: mental health and addiction findings. Can J Psychiatry. 2017;**62**(7):493–500.

40. **Martijn C, Sharpe L.** Pathways to youth homelessness. Soc Sci Med. 2006;**62**(1):1–12.

41. **Narendorf S, Bowen E, Santa Maria D, Thibaudeau E.** Risk and resilience among youth adults experiencing homelessness: a typology for service planning. Child Youth Serv Rev. 2018;**86**:157–165.

42. **Spatz Widom C, Marmorstein NR, Raskin White H.** Childhood victimization and illicit drug use in middle adulthood. Psychol Addict Behav. 2006;**20**(4):394–403.

43. **Bebbington PE, Bhugra D, Brugha T, et al.** Psychosis, victimisation and childhood disadvantage. Br J Psychiatry. 2004;**185**(3):220–226.

44. **Bebbington PE, Jonas S, Kuipers E, et al.** Childhood sexual abuse and psychosis: data from a cross-sectional national psychiatric survey in England. Br J Psychiatry. 2011;**199**(1):29–37.

45. **Folsom DP, Hawthorne W, Lindamer L, et al.** Prevalence and risk factors for homelessness and utilization of mental health services among 10,340 patients with serious mental illness in a large public mental health system. Am J Psychiatry. 2005;**162**(2):370–376.

46. **Martijn C, Sharpe L.** Pathways to youth homelessness. Soc Sci Med. 2006;**62**(1):1–12.

47. **Coates J, McKenzie-Mohr S.** Out of the frying pan, into the fire: trauma in the lives of homeless youth prior to and during homelessness. J Sociol Soc Welf. 2010;**37**(4):65–96.

48. **Craig TK, Hodson S.** Homeless youth in London: I. Childhood antecedents and psychiatric disorder. Psychol Med. 1998;**28**(6):1379–1388.

49. **Hodgson KJ, Shelton KH, van den Bree MBM, Los FJ.** Psychopathology in young people experiencing homelessness: a systematic review. Am J Public Health. 2013;**103**(6):24–37.

50. **Bender K, Ferguson K, Thompson S, Langenderfer L.** Mental health correlates of victimization classes among homeless youth. Child Abuse Negl. 2014;**38**(10):1628–1635.

51. **Narendorf SC.** Intersection of homelessness and mental health: a mixed methods study of young adults who accessed psychiatric emergency services. Child Youth Serv Rev. 2017;**81**:54–62.

52. **Whitbeck LB, Johnson KD, Hoyt DR, Cauce AM.** Mental disorder and comorbidity among runaway and homeless adolescents. J Adolesc Health. 2004;**35**(2):132–140.

53. **Hodgson KJ, Shelton KH, van den Bree MBM.** Psychopathology among young homeless people: longitudinal mental health outcomes for different subgroups. Br J Clin Psychol. 2015;**54**(3):307–325.

54. **Chen X, Thrane L, Whitbeck LB, Johnson K.** Mental disorders, comorbidity, and postrunaway arrests among homeless and runaway adolescents. J Res Adolesc. 2006;**16**(3):379–402.

55. **Martin I, Lampinen TM, McGhee D.** Methamphetamine use among marginalized youth in British Columbia. Can J Public Health. 2006;**97**(4):320–324.

56. **Roy É, Haley N, Leclerc P.** Mortality in a cohort of street youth in Montreal. JAMA. 2004;**292**(5):569–574.

57. **Slesnick N, Prestopnik J.** Dual and multiple diagnosis among substance using runaway youth. Am J Drug Alcohol Abuse. 2005;**31**(1):179–201.

58. **Kidd S, Slesnick N, Frederick T, Karabanow J, Gaetz S.** Mental Health and Addiction Interventions for Youth Experiencing Homelessness: Practical Strategies for Front-line Providers. Toronto: Canadian Observatory on Homelessness Press; 2018.

59. **Ouellet-Plamondon C, Rousseau C, Nicole L, Abdel-Baki A.** Engaging immigrants in early psychosis treatment: a clinical challenge. Psychiatr Serv. 2015;**66**(7):757–759.

60. **Levesque IS, Abdel-Baki A.** What do we know about homelessness in first episode psychosis? Early Interv Psychiatry. 2014;**8**(Suppl 1):82.

61. **Abdel-Baki A, Levesque I-S, Ouellet-Plamondon C, Nicole L.** Should we care about homelessness in first episode psychosis? International Conference on Early Psychosis, 17 November 2014; Tokyo, Japan.

62. **Abdel-Baki A, Ouellet-Plamondon C, Salvat É, Grar K, Potvin S.** Symptomatic and functional outcomes of substance use disorder persistence 2 years after admission to a first-episode psychosis program. Psychiatry Res. 2017;**247**:113–119.

63. **Muir-Cochrane E, Fereday J, Jureidini J, Drummond A, Darbyshire P.** Self-management of medication for mental health problems by homeless young people. Int J Ment Health Nurs. 2006;**15**(3):163–170.

64. **Kort-Butler L, Tyler K.** A cluster analysis of service utilization and incarceration among homeless youth. Soc Sci Res. 2012;**41**(3):612–623.

65. **National Learning Community on Youth Homelessness.** Mental Health of Homeless Youth National Survey. 2012. Available from: http://learningcommunity.ca/mental-health-of-homeless-youth-national-survey-results/.

66. **Baker Collins SD.** From homeless teen to chronically homeless adult: a qualitative study of the impact of childhood events on adult homelessness. Crit Soc Work. 2013;**14**(2):61–81.

67. **Lethby M.** Homeless Employment Access; Niagara Region. St. Catharines: Start Me Up Niagara; 2006.

68. **Díaz-Caneja CM, Pina-Camacho L, Rodríguez-Quiroga A, Fraguas D, Parellada M, Arango C.** Predictors of outcome in early-onset psychosis: a systematic review. NPJ Schizophr. 2015;**4**(1):14005.

69. **MacKenzie D, Flatau P, Steen A, Thielking M.** The Cost of Youth Homelessness in Australia. Melbourne: Swinburne University; 2016.

70. **Duval J, René JF.** Les pratiques d'affiliation dans les Auberges du cœur au Québec: partir de soi pour s'inscrire dans le monde. Sociétés et jeunesses en difficulté. 2009;**6**:1–21.

71. **Baer JS, Rosengren DB, Dunn CW, Wells EA, Ogle RL, Hartzler B.** An evaluation of workshop training in motivational interviewing for addiction and mental health clinicians. Drug Alcohol Depend. 2004;**73**(1):99–106.

72. **Welch M, Mooney J.** Managing services that manage people with a coexisting mental health and substance use disorders. Australas Psychiatry. 2001;**9**(4):345–349.

73. **Lombrail P.** Accès aux soins. In: **Leclerc A, Fassin D, Grandjean H,** et al. (Eds), Les inégalités sociales de santé. Paris: La Découverte, Recherches; 2000:403–418.

74. **Gaetz S.** Street Justice: The Legal and Justice Issues of Homeless Youth in Toronto. Toronto: Justice for Children and Youth; 2002.

75. **Gaetz S, O'Grady B.** Making money: exploring the economy of young homeless workers. Work Employ Soc. 2002;**16**(3):433–456.

76. **Gaetz S, O'Grady B, Buccieri K.** Surviving Crime and Violence Street Youth and Victimization in Toronto. Toronto: Canadian Observatory on Homelessness; 2010.

77. **Dore-Gauthier V, Miron JP, Jutras-Aswad D, Ouellet-Plamondon C, Abdel-Baki A.** Specialized assertive community treatment intervention for homeless youth with first episode psychosis and substance use disorder: a 2-year follow-up study. Early Interv Psychiatry. 2020;**14**(2):203–210.

78. **Courtney M, Heuring DH.** The transition to adulthood for youth 'aging out' of the foster care system. In: **Osgood DW, Foster EM, Flanagan C, Ruth GR** (Eds), On Your Own Without a Net: The Transition to Adulthood for Vulnerable Populations. Chicago, IL: University of Chicago Press; 2005:27–67.

79. **Baker Collins S.** Childhood stress and mobility among rural homeless youth. In: **Gaetz S, O'Grady B, Buccieri K, Karabanow J, Marsolais A** (Eds), Youth Homelessness in Canada: Implications for Policy and Practice. Toronto: Canadian Homelessness Research Network; 2013:53–74.

80. **Gaetz S, O'Grady B, Buccieri K, Karabanow J, Marsolais A** (Eds). Youth Homelessness in Canada: Implications for Policy and Practice. Toronto: Canadian Homelessness Research Network; 2013.

81. **Gaetz S, Marsolais A, Gulliver T**, et al. Le rond-point de l'itinérance. Toronto: The Homeless Hub Press; 2014.

82. **Karabanow J.** Being Young and Homeless: Understanding How Youth Enter and Exit Street Life. New York: Peter Lang; 2004.

83. **Kidd S.** Social Stigma and Homeless Youth. Finding Home: Policy Options for Addressing Homelessness in Canada. Toronto: Cities Centre Press, University of Toronto; 2009.

84. **Kidd S.** Mental health and youth homelessness: a critical review. In: **Gaetz S, O'Grady B, Buccieri K, Karabanow J, Marsolais A** (Eds), Youth Homelessness in Canada: Implications for Policy and Practice. Toronto: Canadian Homelessness Research Network; 2013:217–228.

85. **Milburn NG, Liang LJ, Lee SJ, Rotheram-Borus MJ.** Trajectories of risk behaviors and exiting homelessness among newly homeless adolescents. Vulnerable Child Youth Stud. 2009;**4**(4):346–352.

86. **Dworsky A, Napolitano L, Courtney M.** Homelessness during the transition from foster care to adulthood. Am J Public Health. 2013;**103**(2):318–323.

87. **Mendes P, Moslehuddin B.** From dependence to interdependence: towards better outcomes for young people leaving state care. Child Abuse Rev. 2006;**15**(2):110–126.

88. **Lemon Osterling K, Hines AM.** Mentoring adolescent foster youth: promoting resilience during developmental transitions. Child Fam Soc Work. 2006;**11**(3):242–253.

89. **Bickley H, Kapur N, Hunt IM**, et al. Suicide in the homeless within 12 months of contact with mental health services: a national clinical survey in the UK. Soc Psychiatry Psychiatr Epidemiol. 2006;**41**(9):686–691.

90. **Caton CL.** Mental health service use among homeless and never-homeless men with schizophrenia. Psychiatr Serv. 1995;**46**(11):1139–1143.

91. **French R, Reardon M, Smith P.** Engaging with a mental health service: perspectives of at-risk youth. Child Adolesc Soc Work J. 2003;**20**(6):529–548.

92. **Nicol R, Stretch D, Whitney I**, et al. Mental health needs and services for severely troubled and troubling young people including young offenders in an N.H.S. region. J Adolesc. 2000;**23**(3):243–261.

93. McGorry PD, Tanti C, Stokes R, et al. Headspace: Australia's National Youth Mental Health Foundation—where young minds come first. Med J Aust. 2007;**187**(S7):S68–S70.

94. Illback RJ, Bates T. Transforming youth mental health services and supports in Ireland. Early Interv Psychiatry. 2011;5(Suppl 1):22–27.

95. National Institute for Health and Care Excellence. Transition from children's to adults' services for young people using health or social care services (NICE Guideline NG43). 2016. Available from: https://www.nice.org.uk/guidance/ng43.

96. NHS England. Future in Mind: Promoting, Protecting and Improving our Children and Young People's Mental Health and Wellbeing. NHS England Publication Gateway Ref. No 02939. London: NHS England; 2015.

97. Solorio MR, Milburn NG, Andersen RM, Trifskin S, Rodríguez MA. Emotional distress and mental health service use among urban homeless adolescents. J Behav Health Serv Res. 2006;**33**(4):381–393.

98. Jorm AF, Korten AE, Jacomb PA, Christensen H, Rodgers B, Pollitt P. 'Mental health literacy': a survey of the public's ability to recognise mental disorders and their beliefs about the effectiveness of treatment. Med Aust. 1997;**166**(4):182–186.

99. Brown A, Rice SM, Rickwood DJ, Parker AG. Systematic review of barriers and facilitators to accessing and engaging with mental health care among at-risk young people. Asia Pac Psychiatry. 2016(1):3–22.

100. Munson MR, Jaccard J, Smalling SE, Kim H, Werner JJ, Scott LD. Static, dynamic, integrated, and contextualized: a framework for understanding mental health service utilization among young adults. Soc Sci Med. 2012;**75**(8):1441–1449.

101. O'Reilly M, Taylor HC, Vostanis P. 'Nuts, schiz, psycho': an exploration of young homeless people's perceptions and dilemmas of defining mental health. Soc Sci Med. 2009;**68**(9):1737–1744.

102. Biddle L, Donovan J, Sharp D, Gunnell D. Explaining non-help-seeking amongst young adults with mental distress: a dynamic interpretive model of illness behaviour. Sociol Health Illn. 2007;**29**(7):983–1002.

103. Artaud L. Observance en début de psychose: acceptation, refus ou processus? Montréal: Université de Montréal; 2014.

104. Barnaby L, Penn R, Erikson P. Drugs, Homelessness & Health: Homeless Youth Speak Out About Harm Reduction. The Shout Clinic Harm Reduction Report, 2010. Toronto: Shout Clinic and Central Toronto Community Health Centres; 2010.

105. Center for Behavioral Health Statistics and Quality. Behavioral health trends in the United States: results from the 2014 National Survey on Drug Use and Health. HHS Publication No SMA 15-4927, NSDUH Series H-50. 2015. Available from: https://www.samhsa.gov/data/report/behavioral-health-trends-united-states-results-2014-national-survey-drug-use-and-health.

106. Wilson CJ, Deane FP, Ciarrochi J. Can hopelessness and adolescents' beliefs and attitudes about seeking help account for help negation? J Clin Psychol. 2005;**61**(12):1525–1539.

107. Andrews G, Henderson S, Hall W. Prevalence, comorbidity, disability and service utilisation: overview of the Australian National Mental Health Survey. Br J Psychiatry. 2001;**178**(2):145–153.

108. Gharabaghi K, Stuart C. Voices from the periphery: prospects and challenges for the homeless youth service sector. Child Youth Serv Rev. 2010;**32**(12):1683–1689.

109. **Kozloff N, Cheung AH, Ross LE,** et al. Factors influencing service use among homeless youths with co-occurring disorders. Psychiatr Serv. 2013;**64**(9):925–928.

110. **Craig TK, Hodson S.** Homeless youth in London: II. Accommodation, employment and health outcomes at 1 year. Psychol Med. 2000;**30**(1):187–194.

111. **Wong CF, Clark LF, Marlotte L.** The impact of specific and complex trauma on the mental health of homeless youth. J Interpers Violence. 2016;**31**(5):831–854.

112. **Anda RF, Felitti VJ, Bremner JD,** et al. The enduring effects of abuse and related adverse experiences in childhood. A convergence of evidence from neurobiology and epidemiology. Eur Arch Psychiatry Clin Neurosci. 2006;**256**(3):174–186.

113. **Keys D, Mallett S, Edwards J, Rosenthal D.** Who Can Help Me? Homeless Young Persons Perceptions of Services: A Report of Selected Results from Project I: Homeless Young People in Melbourne and Los Angeles (2000–2005). Victoria: University of Melbourne; 2004.

114. **Lloyd S, Dixon M, Hodges C, Sanci L, Bond L.** Attitudes Towards and Pathways to and from the Young People's Health Service Mental Health Services. Melbourne: Young People's Health Service, Beyond Blue; 2004.

115. **Garrett SB, Higa DH, Phares MM, Peterson PL, Wells EA, Baer JS.** Homeless youths' perceptions of services and transitions to stable housing. Eval Program Plann. 2008;**31**(4):436–444.

116. **Hudson AL, Nyamathi A, Greengold B,** et al. Health-seeking challenges among homeless youth. Nurs Res. 2010;**59**(3):212–218.

117. **Hudson AL, Nyamathi A, Sweat J.** Homeless youths' interpersonal perspectives of health care providers. Issues Ment Health Nurs. 2008;**29**(12):1277–1289.

118. **Christiani A, Hudson AL, Nyamathi A, Mutere M, Sweat J.** Attitudes of homeless and drug-using youth regarding barriers and facilitators in delivery of quality and culturally sensitive health care. J Child Adolesc Psychiatr Nurs. 2008;**21**(3):154–163.

119. **De Rosa CJ, Montgomery SB, Kipke MD,** et al. Service utilization among homeless and runaway youth in Los Angeles, California: rates and reasons. J Adolesc Health. 1999;**24**(3):190–200.

120. **Booth ML, Bernard D, Quine S,** et al. Access to health care among Australian adolescents young people's perspectives and their sociodemographic distribution. J Adolesc Health. 2004;**34**(1):97–103.

121. **Crowley A.** Making It Matter: Improving the Health of Young Homeless People. London: DePaul UK; 2012.

122. **Skott-Myhre HA, Raby R, Nikolaou J.** Towards a delivery system of services for rural homeless youth: a literature review and case study. Child Youth Care Forum. 2008;**37**(2):87–102.

123. **Baker Collins S.** Sofas, Shelters and Strangers: A Report on Youth Homelessness in Niagara. Niagara Region: Niagara Region Community Services; 2010.

124. **McManus HH, Thompson SJ.** Trauma among unaccompanied homeless youth: the integration of street culture into a model of intervention. J Aggress Maltreat Trauma. 2008;**16**(1):92–109.

125. **Black EB, Fedyszyn IE, Mildred H,** et al. Homeless youth: barriers and facilitators for service referrals. Eval Program Plann. 2018;**68**:7–12.

126. **Kelly TM, Daley DC, Douaihy AB.** Treatment of substance abusing patients with comorbid psychiatric disorders. Addict Behav. 2012;**37**(1):11–24.

127. **Drake RE, Yovetich NA, Bebout RR, Harris M, McHugo GJ.** Integrated treatment for dually diagnosed homeless adults. J Nerv Ment Dis. 1997;**185**(5):298–305.

128. **Calsyn RJ, Morse GA, Klinkenberg WD, Trusty ML, Allen G.** The impact of assertive community treatment on the social relationships of people who are homeless and mentally ill. Community Mental Health J. 1998;**34**(6):579–593.

129. **Calsyn RJ, Winter JP, Morse GA.** Do consumers who have a choice of treatment have better outcomes? Community Ment Health J. 2000;**36**(2):149–160.

130. **Coldwell CM, Bender WS.** The effectiveness of assertive community treatment for homeless populations with severe mental illness: a meta-analysis. Am J Psychiatry. 2007;**164**(3):393–399.

131. **Dixon L, Weiden P, Torres M, Lehman A.** Assertive community treatment and medication compliance in the homeless mentally ill. Am J Psychiatry. 1997;**154**(9):1302–1304.

132. **Korr WS, Joseph A.** Housing the homeless mentally ill: findings from Chicago. J Soc Serv Res. 1996;**21**(1):53–68.

133. **Shern DL, Tsemberis S, Anthony W,** et al. Serving street-dwelling individuals with psychiatric disabilities: outcomes of a psychiatric rehabilitation clinical trial. Am J Public Health. 2000;**90**(12):1873–1878.

134. **Herman DB.** Randomized trial of critical time intervention to prevent homelessness after hospital discharge. Psychiatr Serv. 2011;**62**(7):713–719.

135. **Susser E, Valencia E, Conover S, Felix A, Tsai WY, Wyatt RJ.** Preventing recurrent homelessness among mentally ill men: a 'critical time' intervention after discharge from a shelter. Am J Public Health. 1997;**87**(2):256–262.

136. **Clark C, Rich AR.** Outcomes of homeless adults with mental illness in a housing program and in case management only. Psychiatr Serv. 2003;**54**(1):78–83.

137. **Forchuk C, MacClure SK, Van Beers M,** et al. Developing and testing an intervention to prevent homelessness among individuals discharged from psychiatric wards to shelters and 'no fixed address'. J Psychiatr Ment Health Nurs. 2008;**15**(7):569–575.

138. **Goering P, Veldhuizen S, Watson A,** et al. National At Home/Chez Soi Final Report. Calgary: Mental Health Commission of Canada; 2014.

139. **Greenwood RM, Schaefer-McDaniel NJ, Winkel G, Tsemberis SJ.** Decreasing psychiatric symptoms by increasing choice in services for adults with histories of homelessness. Am J Community Psychol. 2005;**36**(3-4):223–238.

140. **McHugo GJ, Bebout RR, Harris M,** et al. A randomized controlled trial of integrated versus parallel housing services for homeless adults with severe mental illness. Schizophr Bull. 2004;**30**(4):969–982.

141. **Padgett DK.** Housing first services for people who are homeless with co-occurring serious mental illness and substance abuse. Res Soc Work Pract. 2006;**16**(1):74–83.

142. **Tsemberis SJ, Moran L, Shinn M, Asmussen SM, Shern DL.** Consumer preference programs for individuals who are homeless and have psychiatric disabilities: a drop-in center and a supported housing program. Am J Community Psychol. 2003;**32**(3-4):305–317.

143. **Wagner V, Sy J, Weeden K,** et al. Effectiveness of intensive case management for homeless adolescents: results of a 3-month follow-up. J Emot Behav Disord. 1994;**2**(4):219–227.

144. **Correll CU, Galling B, Pawar A**, et al. Comparison of early intervention services vs treatment as usual for early-phase psychosis: a systematic review, meta-analysis, and meta-regression. JAMA Psychiatry. 2018;**75**(6):555–565.

145. **Boonstra N, Klaassen R, Sytema S**, et al. Duration of untreated psychosis and negative symptoms—a systematic review and meta-analysis of individual patient data. Schizophr Res. 2012;**142**(1–3):12–19.

146. **Marshall M, Lewis S, Lockwood A, Drake R, Jones P, Croudace T.** Association between duration of untreated psychosis and outcome in cohorts of first-episode patients: a systematic review. Arch Gen Psychiatry. 2005;**62**(9):975–983.

147. **Perkins DO, Gu H, Boteva K, Lieberman JA.** Relationship between duration of untreated psychosis and outcome in first-episode schizophrenia: a critical review and meta-analysis. Am J Psychiatry. 2005;**162**(10):1785–1804.

148. **Iyer SN, Malla AK.** [Early intervention in psychosis: concepts, current knowledge and future directions]. Sante Ment Que. 2014;**39**(2):201–229.

149. **Darbyshire P, Muir-Cochrane E, Fereday J**, et al. Engagement with health and social care services: perceptions of homeless young people with mental health problems. Health Soc Care Community. 2006;**14**(6):553–562.

150. **Slesnick N, Kang MJ, Bonomi AE, Prestopnik JL.** Six- and twelve-month outcomes among homeless youth accessing therapy and case management services through an urban drop-in center. Health Serv Res. 2008;**43**(1 Pt 1):211–229.

151. **Malla A, Iyer S, Shah J**, et al. Canadian response to need for transformation of youth mental health services: ACCESS Open Minds (Esprits ouverts). Early Interv Psychiatry. 2019;**13**(3):697–706.

152. **McGorry PD.** Youth mental health: building beyond the brand. Med J Aust. 2017;**207**(10):428–429.

153. **Abdel-Baki A, Aubin D, Morisseau-Guillot R**, et al. Improving mental health services for homeless youth in downtown Montreal, Canada: partnership between a local network and ACCESS Esprits ouverts (Open Minds), a National Services Transformation Research Initiative. Early Interv Psychiatry. 2019;**13**(Suppl 1):20–28.

154. **Morisseau-Guillot R, Aubin D, Deschenes JM**, et al. A promising route towards improvement of homeless young people's access to mental health services: the creation and evolution of an outreach service network in Montreal. Community Ment Health J. 2020;**56**(2):258–270.

155. **Black EB, Fedyszyn IE, Mildred H**, et al. Homeless youth: barriers and facilitators for service referrals. Eval Program Plann. 2018;**68**:7–12.

156. **Deslandes R, Bertrand R.** Une meilleure harmonisation des services offerts aux jeunes à risque et à leur famille: que savons-nous? Sante Ment Que. 2002;**27**(2):136–153.

157. **Doré-Gauthier V, Côté H, Jutras-Aswad D, Ouellet-Plamondon C, Abdel-Baki A.** How to help homeless youth suffering from first episode psychosis and substance use disorders? The creation of a new intensive outreach intervention team. Psychiatry Res. 2019;**273**:603–612.

Chapter 25

Homelessness among intellectual and developmental disability populations: Implications for practice developments

Michael J. Brown and Edward McCann

Definitions

The World Health Organization defines homelessness as living in housing that is below the minimum standard or lacks secure tenure. People can be categorized as homeless if they are living on the streets; moving between temporary shelters including houses of friends, family, and emergency accommodation; or living in private boarding houses without a private bathroom and/or security of tenure (1). The definition of homelessness has been developed further by the charity Crisis who state that 'a home is not just a physical space: it also provides roots, identity, security and a sense of belonging and a place of emotional well-being' (2). It is recognized that people with cognitive impairment are over-represented among the homeless, a situation affected by a range of psychosocial problems. People with intellectual and developmental disabilities (IDD) are a subgroup of the homeless and have distinct and unique issues and concerns that contribute to their homeless situation.

Internationally, the term IDD is used to describe a range of limitations in intellectual impairment and developmental delay. Globally, different terms are used to describe people with IDD, including mental retardation, mental handicap, and learning disability. Intellectual disability is characterized by limitations in adaptive behaviour and level of intellectual functioning. Intellectual disability starts before the age of 18 years. Adaptive behaviour refers to conceptual skills including language, literacy, concept of time, and self-direction; social skills including self-esteem, social problem-solving, interpersonal skills, and gullibility; and practical skills including personal care, activities of daily living, personal safety, occupational skills, and healthcare utilization. In some jurisdictions, intellectual functioning is assessed by intelligent quotient testing with a score less than 70 indicating limitations in intellectual functioning. IDD is sometimes referred to as mild, moderate, severe, or profound impairment. Developmental disability refers to a range of conditions that are usually identified at an early age and are characterized by delays in developmental functioning with limitations in communication, language development, learning, cognition, behaviour, and socialization. Developmental disability includes, for example, autism spectrum disorder, fetal alcohol spectrum disorder, and attention deficit hyperactivity disorder. Some people with IDD may also have significant physical impairments associated with conditions such as cerebral palsy, sensory impairments, and genetic disorders. An IDD condition is lifelong with a need for access to ongoing supports from a diverse range of services.

Demographic picture

A systematic review identified 30–40% of homeless adults as having a cognitive impairment (3). The number of people with IDD who are homeless is difficult to determine due to the paucity of comprehensive prevalence studies. However, four studies have attempted to address this issue (4–7). One of the studies, conducted in Canada, reported 34% of homeless people had IDD (5). In several of the studies, IDD was identified by a participant self-report screening test rather than a standardized test such as the Wechsler Adult Intelligence Scale (WAIS). Another study, involving a small sample ($n = 7$) using the WAIS, identified 40% of homeless people with an IDD (7).

From a wider population perspective, the number of children and young people with IDD is increasing. This phenomenon is due to a range of factors including improved maternal healthcare, improved health and social care services, and developments in neonatal intensive care. Life expectancy for people with IDD is increasing, yet remains shorter when compared to the typically developing population. The more severe and complex the IDD, the shorter the life expectancy (8). For people with mild IDD, their life expectancy is now similar to the typically developing population. At the other end of the age continuum, the number of older people with IDD is increasing with more living into old age, many with a range of comorbid health and social care support needs (9). An international picture is emerging of an IDD population with an increasing number of young people with severe cognitive and physical impairments who are dependent on all aspects of their care and support. However, the current evidence is suggestive of the tendency of males, of older age, following relationship or family breakdown to be more predisposed to homelessness (10).

Clinical issues

People with IDD present with a diverse range of physical and mental health conditions (11). Physical health conditions are particularly common with epilepsy being the most prevalent neurological disorder. Respiratory disorders are the leading cause of death for people with IDD (12). Chest infections and pneumonia are common and increase with the severity of IDD and also contribute to avoidable and premature death (13). Asthma is prevalent in people with IDD who are obese and smoke, with a need for effective management to avoid unnecessary hospitalization (14,15). Significant levels of smoking were found in one study involving homeless IDD people at 71% (16). Across the IDD population, the prevalence of epilepsy is approximately 18% compared to 1% in the general population (17), and in older adults, the figure is 31% (18). Cardiovascular disease is the second most common cause of premature death in the IDD population and is experienced at a younger age. Cardiac and circulatory system disorders affect some 21% of adults with IDD and contribute to their premature death (19). People with IDD are more likely to experience hypertension, be overweight and obese, and be physically inactive (20,21). As a consequence of the number of their physical health conditions, people with IDD require access to health screening that identifies their unmet physical health needs. Additionally, support is required to facilitate access to and through the healthcare system for many people with IDD, thereby ensuring that they have equality of access and better health outcomes.

Mental health issues

As with the general population, many people with IDD experience mental ill health. While the exact prevalence rates remain unknown, the reported rates of anxiety and depression are similar to the general population and are higher in people with Down's syndrome (22). People with IDD appear at greater risk of developing mental ill health due to adverse life events and environmental stressors such as sexual abuse, violence, and poverty (23). Diagnosing mental illness in people with IDD can be difficult due to communication deficits, physical health conditions, and diagnostic overshadowing (24). People with IDD experience interrelated physical and mental health conditions for which medication is frequently prescribed (25). Medication is often prescribed for the treatment of mental illness. However, there are concerns around the overprescribing of mood stabilizers, antidepressants, tranquillisers, sedatives, and antipsychotics for the management of challenging behaviours (26). A 2016 systematic review identified that despite the prevalence of mental illness in people with IDD, there is limited evidence of the provision and possible benefits of psychological interventions (27). However, the evidence is evolving of the potential attributes of modified cognitive behavioural therapy for the treatment of anger, and depression (28). Studies have also reported the effectiveness of group cognitive behavioural therapy for the treatment of depression (29). The National Institute for Health and Clinical Excellence in the UK recommends trauma-focused cognitive behavioural therapy and eye movement desensitization and reprocessing (30).

Current evidence suggests that mental illness is a contributing factor in pathways into homelessness for people with IDD (10). In some studies, involving homeless people with IDD, the presenting mental health issues were PTSD, mood disorders, psychosis, and alcohol and substance misuse. The most common issue at 18% was mood disorder. Substance-related concerns were 14% and major mental illness, such as psychosis, was 4% (7,31). To ensure effective assessment, diagnosis, treatment, and support for homeless people with IDD and mental illness, there is a need for practitioners to recognize and respond to the full extent of the mental health and psychosocial needs of this population.

Physical health conditions

People with IDD experience a range of physical health conditions that, if untreated, impact their health and well-being. For example, in one study, conducted in the Netherlands, that included a subsample of homeless adults with IDD, the most common physical issues identified were musculoskeletal and connective tissue complaints (31%), respiratory disorders including asthma and chronic obstructive pulmonary disease (20%), gastrointestinal disorders (14%), cardiovascular disorders including hypertension (11%), visual impairments (24%), dental conditions (24%), and podiatry issues (13%) (32). These physical health conditions are relatively amenable to assessment and treatments such as visual and podiatry interventions, with others requiring more sustained and longer-term medical management such as hypertension and chronic obstructive pulmonary disease. Therefore, access to effective primary care services is indicated for this population. Given the clearly established evidence base of the significant physical health conditions experienced by many people with IDD, with the appropriate access to assessment treatments, there can be a marked improvement in physical health outcomes. Specific areas included nutrition and dental care (10). The care needs of homeless people with IDD need to be recognized as enduring rather than temporary.

Social aspects

The majority of people with IDD have generally always lived at home with their family. However, congregated care is still evident in some countries. There has been a move away from institutional models of care and support to the locus of care being provided in the community where people with IDD can live independently and are often gainfully employed. Others, as the level of IDD increases, may require greater access to care services that will include housing, education, social welfare, and healthcare. The currently available research literature regarding homelessness and people with IDD highlights key issues around family breakdown, the presence of mental illness, and challenging behaviour. Further research is required to more fully understand the differences between women with IDD who appear to have shorter periods of homelessness compared to men with IDD (5). Men with IDD who become homeless are older when compared to typically developing men (7). More males than females with IDD were found in homeless services (6). Other related homeless risk factors include poor education attainment (4) and a tendency to be unemployed (33).

The changing profile of complexity of need for many young people with IDD, including behaviours that challenge, mental illness, impulsivity, and hyperactivity, are possible new factors that may contribute to increasing homelessness in the future. All can lead to insurmountable stressors on the family that can result in family breakdown and, ultimately, homelessness for the individual (31). The current evidence suggests that where people with IDD become homeless, they are less likely to be reintegrated back into the family home, with implications for service delivery and supports (34). In some countries, people with IDD continue to be considered burdensome, and shame and stigma are significant factors in whether people with IDD will get the necessary supports from their families (35). If people with IDD are unable to achieve functional independence through targeted interventions, they are unlikely to be effectively reintegrated back within their family. In one study, the death of a significant adult was a primary factor precipitating homelessness (5). Homelessness services and support agencies may provide opportunities for skills development, confidence, and self-esteem development that will be beneficial for the pathways from homelessness. In one study, volunteering within the homeless service, while seen as potentially beneficial, needs to be carried out within the context of facilitating the move out of homelessness (36).

Policy

There is a need to recognize the factors that can lead to homelessness for people with IDD. These issues are similar for the non-IDD population while appreciating the distinct circumstances related to those people with IDD, for example, relationship breakdown. When people with IDD are within homeless services, some issues need to be addressed regarding their physical and mental healthcare requirements. In terms of physical concerns, people with IDD need access and support within primary care services to ensure that their needs are assessed and investigated, and treatment and management plans implemented. For mental health, policy needs to be reflective of the significant mental ill health that exists within the IDD homeless population and ensure that their needs are effectively identified and met. It is already recognized from a policy perspective that people with IDD remain disadvantaged regarding healthcare access and service utilization, with significant implications for the provision of responsive services and adequate supports. What is required is a seamless and coordinated policy response that addresses the comprehensive needs of the population, including those who are homeless.

Implications for practice

Practitioners need to recognize that people with IDD do become homeless and have specific support needs. They need to have greater knowledge and a better grasp of IDD issues, and the differing and distinct factors that lead to homelessness. It is important to recognize that people with IDD are not a heterogeneous population and will, therefore, have unique experiences and support needs. The current evidence suggests that men with IDD who are older are more likely to become homeless than women with IDD. Men with IDD appear to spend longer in homeless services than women with IDD. Practitioners need to be aware that identifying people with IDD who are homeless can be challenging as the intellectual and developmental impairments may not initially be apparent when presenting at homeless services. It is, therefore, critical that they appreciate the potential existence of the IDD and respond appropriately. For example, education and preparation of health and social care practitioners should include theories, skills development, and practice learning that take account of and reflect this population's unique needs.

Furthermore, surveillance and prevention strategies are needed to identify early detection of risks of homelessness in people with IDD, when they are at their most vulnerable to becoming homeless, in order to develop and provide responsive supports and services to rapidly and effectively address individual needs. Many live at home with families; however, should the person with IDD become bereaved due to the death of the main family member or carer, then the changes in social circumstances can lead to homelessness, if not effectively addressed (37). Given the evidence of mental ill health and challenging behaviours in the IDD population, it is necessary to have in place services provided by professionals such as psychiatrists, clinical psychologists, occupational therapists, dieticians, nurses, and social workers to enable coordinated and responsive care. As a result of the range of physical health conditions, it is necessary to provide additional support to enable access to primary care services and general hospitals. Such access is required to ensure the effective assessment, investigation, treatment, and management of their conditions. Due to the number of physical and psychosocial issues and concerns, it is necessary for people with IDD to access specific coordinated supports including housing, day care, employment, education, mental health, and primary care services. Evidence highlights that fully supporting people with IDD when homeless can bring about improvements in their health, well-being, and social circumstances (10,32).

Suggestions for future research

From the current research evidence, it is apparent that there exist multifactorial issues that lead to homelessness for people with IDD. Further, there are issues around population identification within homeless groups and of gaining informed consent from people with IDD that can be time-consuming (38). Given the apparent higher prevalence of mental illness, substance misuse, sexually transmitted diseases, HIV, and other vulnerabilities, it is important that people with IDD are included in homelessness research. Researchers need to identify and understand the range of factors that lead into homelessness and whether they are amenable to prevention, supports, and interventions. They need to comprehend the issues and concerns once people with IDD become homeless and to identify their specific support needs. Leading out of homelessness, there is a need to conceptualize the needs and supports that may influence and impact the individual's trajectory from homelessness and provide the necessary and appropriate service responses. There is a distinct lack of qualitative studies investigating the unique views and experiences through the lens of homeless people with IDD. This could include their perceptions of the issues that led to homelessness, the circumstances and experiences within homeless services, and the help and supports necessary to exit homelessness successfully. Future studies could address the factors that maintain their newly established housing and support situation.

The existing research evidence base has understandably focused on utilizing quantitative research designs in an attempt to quantify the prevalence of IDD homelessness. This evidence has begun to develop a picture and understanding of the unique issues of people with IDD by attempting to capture the numbers of people with IDD who are homeless in particular jurisdictions and of their particular health and social care needs. However, the evidence base in this area is evolving, with significant gaps remaining. Future researchers need to ensure that the subpopulation of people with IDD are included within their study sample. To date, the existing research studies have understandably adopted convenience snowball sampling techniques with self-reporting, in an attempt to identify people with IDD who are homeless. In order to more fully develop the evidence base in this area and understand what works for people with IDD, there is a need to undertake larger multicentre research studies that incorporate larger samples of people with IDD. This is an important next step as much of the available research has attempted to identify people with IDD as a subpopulation of the general homeless population. The current research evidence suggests that men with IDD can remain homeless for prolonged periods, and there is a need to understand their situation and the interventions more fully and the supports necessary to effect change. Therefore, multicentre longitudinal studies would be beneficial in informing policy, service developments, and evidence-based practice.

Conclusion

People with IDD can and do become homeless for a diverse range of reasons. Yet, they continue to be a marginalized and relatively invisible population within the context of homelessness. This chapter has set out specific factors and concerns regarding people with IDD and the issues that can lead to homelessness, the circumstances that exist while homeless, and the supports necessary to enable people with IDD to exit homelessness. Homelessness for people with IDD results from a unique set of personal situations that need to be recognized, understood, and responded to. There is a clear and well-established international evidence base regarding the scope and extent of the physical and mental health needs experienced by many people with IDD. These health priorities need to be appropriately assessed and managed to reduce health inequalities and improve health and quality of life outcomes within a homelessness context.

The mental health and challenging behaviours experienced by some people with IDD can have a direct influence on their becoming homeless. Therefore, a key strategic policy focus must include proactive responses to address individual needs. A significant challenge facing service providers relates to the identification of people with IDD after they have become homeless. This is important because it may not be initially apparent to practitioners in homelessness services that IDD is present. As a result, housing and homelessness services have to be aware of the fact that people with IDD can and do become homeless and have specific support and care needs that need to be addressed. Specialist intellectual disability services have an important role to play in working collaboratively with primary care and other health services, housing and homeless services, social work, criminal justice, and education services. This is necessary to ensure that people with IDD have access to the full range of services and supports that may guide their journey from homelessness. It should, therefore, be a policy priority to ensure that the distinct needs of people with IDD are fully reflected and integrated within homelessness policy initiatives. There is also scope for shared continuing professional development opportunities that bring together the key stakeholders involved in the care and support of people with IDD. In order to more fully respond to the distinct needs of people with IDD who are homeless, there is a need and opportunity to develop new national and international research collaborations that can grow and develop the research evidence base in this area.

References

1. **World Health Organization**. WHO Housing and Health Guidelines. Geneva: World Health Organization; 2018.
2. **Crisis.** Homeless knowledge hub. Available from: https://www.crisis.org.uk/ending-homelessness/homelessness-knowledge-hub/.
3. **Spence S, Stevens R, Parks R.** Cognitive dysfunction in homeless adults: a systematic review. J R Soc Med. 2004;97(8):375–379.
4. **Oakes PM, Davies RC.** Intellectual disability in homeless adults: a prevalence study. J Intellect Disabil. 2008;12(4):325–334.
5. **Mercier C, Picard S.** Intellectual disability and homelessness. J Intellect Disabil Res. 2011;55(4):441–449.
6. **Van Straaten B, Schrijvers CT, Van der Laan J,** et al. Intellectual disability among Dutch homeless people: prevalence and related psychosocial problems. PLoS One. 2014;9(1):e86112.
7. **Nishio A, Yamamoto M, Horita R,** et al. Prevalence of mental illness, cognitive disability, and their overlap among the homeless in Nagoya, Japan. PLoS One. 2015;10(9):e0138052.
8. **Hosking FJ, Carey IM, Shah SM,** et al. Mortality among adults with intellectual disability in England: comparisons with the general population. Am J Public Health. 2016;106(8):1483–1490.
9. **Emerson E, Hatton C.** Estimating Future Need for Social Care Among Adults with Learning Disabilities in England: An Update. Durham: Improving Health and Lives Learning Disability Observatory; 2011.
10. **Van Straaten B, Rodenburg G, Van der Laan J, Boersma SN, Wolf JR, Van de Mheen D.** Self-reported care needs of Dutch homeless people with and without a suspected intellectual disability: a 1.5-year follow-up study. Health Soc Care Community. 2017;25(1):123–136.

11. **Truesdale M, Brown M.** People with Learning Disabilities in Scotland: Health Needs Assessment Update Report 2017. Glasgow: NHS Health Scotland; 2017.

12. **Trollor J, Srasuebkul P, Xu H, Howlett S.** Cause of death and potentially avoidable deaths in Australian adults with intellectual disability using retrospective linked data. BMJ Open. 2017;**7**(2):e013489.

13. **Tyrer F, McGrother C.** Cause-specific mortality and death certificate reporting in adults with moderate to profound intellectual disability. J Intellect Disabil Res. 2009;**53**(11):898–904.

14. **Dunn K, Hughes-McCormack L, Cooper SA.** Hospital admissions for physical health conditions for people with intellectual disabilities: systematic review. J Appl Res Intellect Disabil. 2018;**31**:1–10.

15. **Gale L, Naqvi H, Russ L.** Asthma, smoking and BMI in adults with intellectual disabilities: a community-based survey. J Intellect Disabil Res. 2009;**53**(9):787–796.

16. **Nishio A, Yamamoto M, Ueki H, et al.** Prevalence of mental illness, intellectual disability, and developmental disability among homeless people in Nagoya, Japan: a case series study. Psychiatry Clin Neurosci. 2015;**69**(9):534–542.

17. **Matthews T, Weston N, Baxter H, Felce D, Kerr M.** A general practice-based prevalence study of epilepsy among adults with intellectual disabilities and of its association with psychiatric disorder, behaviour disturbance and carer stress. J Intellect Disabil Res. 2008;**52**(2):163–173.

18. **McCarron M, O'Dwyer M, Burke E, McGlinchey E, McCallion P.** Epidemiology of epilepsy in older adults with an intellectual disability in Ireland: associations and service implications. Am J Intellect Dev Disabil. 2014;**119**(3):253–260.

19. **Heslop P, Blair PS, Fleming P, Hoghton M, Marriott A, Russ L.** The Confidential Inquiry into premature deaths of people with intellectual disabilities in the UK: a population-based study. Lancet. 2014;**383**(9920):889–895.

20. **Haveman M, Heller T, Lee L, Maaskant M, Shooshtari S, Strydom A.** Major health risks in aging persons with intellectual disabilities: an overview of recent studies. J Policy Pract Intellect Disabil. 2010;**7**(1):59–69.

21. **Cooper SA, McLean G, Guthrie B, et al.** Multiple physical and mental health comorbidity in adults with intellectual disabilities: population-based cross-sectional analysis. BMC Fam Pract. 2015;**16**(1):110.

22. **Mantry D, Cooper SA, Smiley E, et al.** The prevalence and incidence of mental ill-health in adults with Down syndrome. J Intellect Disabil Res. 2008;**52**(2):141–155.

23. **Emerson E, Brigham P.** Exposure of children with developmental delay to social determinants of poor health: cross-sectional study. J Appl Res Intellect Disabil. 2014;**27**:4.

24. **Cooper SA, Smiley E, Morrison J, Williamson A, Allan L.** Mental ill-health in adults with intellectual disabilities: prevalence and associated factors. Br J Psychiatry. 2007;**190**(1):27–35.

25. **Carey IM, Shah SM, Hosking FJ, et al.** Health characteristics and consultation patterns of people with intellectual disability: a cross-sectional database study in English general practice. Br J Gen Pract. 2016;**66**(645):e264–e270.

26. **Ali A, Blickwedel J, Hassiotis A.** Interventions for challenging behaviour in intellectual disability. Adv Psychiatr Treat. 2014;**20**(3):184–192.

27. **Osugo M, Cooper SA.** Interventions for adults with mild intellectual disabilities and mental ill-health: a systematic review. J Intellect Disabil Res. 2016;**60**(6):615–622.

28. **Vereenooghe L, Langdon PE.** Psychological therapies for people with intellectual disabilities: a systematic review and meta-analysis. *Res Dev Disabil.* 2013;**34**(11):4085–4102.

29. **McGillivray JA, Kershaw M.** Do we need both cognitive and behavioural components in interventions for depressed mood in people with mild intellectual disability? J Intellect Disabil Res. 2015;**59**(2):105–115.

30. **National Collaborating Centre for Mental Health UK.** Post-Traumatic Stress Disorder: The Management of PTSD in Adults and Children in Primary and Secondary Care. London: Gaskell, 2005.

31. **Nishio A, Horita R, Sado T,** et al. Causes of homelessness prevalence: relationship between homelessness and disability. Psychiatry Clin Neurosci. 2017;**71**(3):180–188.

32. **Van der Laan J, Van Straaten B, Boersma SN, Rodenburg G, Van de Mheen D, Wolf JR.** Predicting homeless people's perceived health after entering the social relief system in The Netherlands. Int J Public Health. 2018;**63**(2):203–211.

33. **McCarthy J, Chaplin E, Underwood L,** et al. Characteristics of prisoners with neurodevelopmental disorders and difficulties. J Intellect Disabil Res. 2016;**60**(3):201–206.

34. **Gowda GS, Gopika G, Kumar CN,** et al. Clinical outcome and rehabilitation of homeless mentally ill patients admitted in mental health institute of South India: 'Know the Unknown' project. Asian J Psychiatry. 2017;**30**:49–53.

35. **Gouveia L, Massanganhe H, Mandlate F,** et al. Family reintegration of homeless in Maputo and Matola: a descriptive study. Int J Ment Health Syst. 2017;**11**(1):25.

36. **Morton LG, Cunningham-Williams RM, Gardiner G.** Volunteerism among homeless persons with developmental disabilities. Soc Work Disabil Rehabil. 2010;**9**(1):12–26.

37. **Brown M, McCann E.** The views and experiences of families and direct care support workers regarding the expression of sexuality by adults with intellectual disabilities: a narrative review of the international research evidence. Res Dev Disabil. 2019;**90**:80–91.

38. **Morton LG, Cunningham-Williams RM.** The capacity to give informed consent in a homeless population with developmental disabilities. Community Ment Health J. 2009;**45**(5):341–348.

Chapter 26

Homelessness among youth who identify as LGBTQ+

Edward McCann and Michael J. Brown

Definitions

To be more fully inclusive of the range of sexual and gender identities, including groups such as asexual, intersex, questioning, and queer, the contemporary umbrella term lesbian, gay, bisexual, transgender, and questioning plus (LGBTQ+) is now being more widely adopted (1). However, the subgroups within this conceptualization are not homogeneous and, as a result, have unique and distinct experiences and needs. Homelessness can involve individuals who are dwelling on the streets, staying in emergency shelters, or in temporary accommodation such as couch surfing, a vehicle, or squatting. A home can offer more than just a physical space; it is a place that may provide roots, identity, security, and a sense of belonging and emotional well-being (2). According to Gaetz et al. (3), youth homelessness can be understood as:

> Youth aged 13–24 who are living independently of parents and/or caregivers and lack social supports necessary for transition from childhood to adulthood. They do not have a stable or consistent source of income or place of residence, nor do they necessarily have adequate access to support networks to foster a safe and nurturing transition into the responsibilities of adulthood.

Demographic picture

Worldwide, there is a growing concern and focus on the issue of homelessness. Further, there are issues regarding the phenomena of homelessness in youth populations (4). Also attracting attention are the concerns around the prevalence of homelessness as experienced by LGBTQ+ youth. The exact prevalence of LGBTQ+ youth experiencing homelessness is unknown and there is a distinct absence of national and international data that identify and collate this information. There are no prevalence research studies that comprehensively sets out the scope and extent of the population (5). However, it has been estimated across studies undertaken in different locations that between 25% and 40% of homeless youth identify as LGBTQ+ (6). The pathways to homelessness are multifarious. Some youth may inevitably become homeless due to factors unrelated to their LGBTQ+ identity and it is essential to recognize this. However, there is some evidence that supports the view that 'coming out' as LGBTQ+ may receive a negative response, sometimes from within families, thereby resulting in rejection and ejection from the family home. In one UK study, it was identified that 'coming out' led to 77% of LGBTQ+ youth becoming homeless. Further, abuse within the family (69%) and family aggression and violence (69%) were significant factors leading to homelessness (7).

Clinical issues

Homeless LGBTQ+ youth present as high risk for a multitude of clinically relevant issues and concerns related to events that led up to their homeless situation and the direct consequences of homelessness (6). Presenting physical problems include, for example, sexually transmitted infections, poorly controlled asthma, tuberculosis, trauma, and dermatological infestations. Mental health issues can include significant rates of drug and alcohol use, depression, anxiety, suicidality, and post-traumatic stress disorder. Due to their health needs, some LGBTQ+ youth may have difficulties accessing and using public health services with health conditions remaining untreated and individuals becoming socially excluded and increasingly vulnerable (8). Young people remain reticent about accessing supports due to barriers and factors related to their lack of experience, knowledge, and life skills; their fears and concerns not being taken seriously; confidentiality and trust issues; and anxieties around potential police and social welfare services involvement. Therefore, improved access is necessary for all homeless youth if service providers are to make available appropriate and responsive supports tailored to their specific needs. These responses must also include the specific and distinct needs of youth who identify as LGBTQ+. Clinical assessments provide the starting point for initial screening. Through the use of open and non-judgemental approaches to history taking, a clear picture of individual circumstances such as family dynamics, home circumstances, social supports, self-care abilities, financial situation, social networks, health behaviours, and physical and mental health can be established (9). By obtaining this essential information, it is possible to start to plan and deliver appropriate treatment packages and provide supports that begin to address concerns related to fear and isolation, vulnerability, exploitation, and sexual abuse issues that are common in LGBTQ+ homeless youth. In this regard, practitioners must be self-aware, culturally competent, and skilled in utilizing affirmative approaches within their practice when working with young people who identify as LGBTQ+. In order to support and encourage positive, socially inclusive, and rights-based approaches to working with diverse groups, much of the current evidence suggests that education and training initiatives should be made available to all clinicians and practitioners who may be working with patients and clients who identify as LGBTQ+ (10).

Mental health issues

The experiences of living in a heteronormative society and environments whereby individuals may be subjected to negative reactions can contribute adversely to mental health. Stigma, discrimination, and victimization experiences can lead to increases in mental health issues, physical health concerns, as well as social challenges (11). While it is well documented that LGBTQ+ people are subjected to discriminatory experiences and the associated consequences of victimization, many have developed positive coping strategies and resilience. Building on resilience can be achieved through effective social networks, thereby minimizing the potential for isolation, loneliness, and limited community participation (12). The concept of *minority stress* has been developed to support the understanding of the discriminatory experiences described by some LGBTQ+ people, and the recognition that minority stress in LGBTQ+ youth can potentially lead to internalized shame, emotional trauma, and, in some cases, abuse and violence (13).

Additionally, the findings from US research, for example, suggest that family responses to LGBTQ+ disclosure may lead to increased homelessness (14,15). Therefore, social welfare services need to be alert to the specific needs of LGBTQ+ youth when they access, for example, housing support, health services, social care services, education provision, and employment agencies. The societal stigma of mental illness per se is slowly being addressed through, for example, education programmes, policy initiatives, and anti-stigma campaigns, where individuals are actively encouraged and supported to discuss their mental health concerns and needs (16). This positive work is encouraged and needs to continue and be further developed. These developments also need to take account of and reflect the mental health profile and experiences of LGBTQ+ youth that is demonstrably more prevalent in this population (11). This is necessary as there is evidence that points to specific mental health conditions such as depression, anxiety, post-traumatic stress disorder, substance use, self-harm, and eating disorders (17). In US studies, for example, significant mental health issues have been identified with substance use being more prevalent and experienced at a younger age by LGB youth who were homeless compared with non-LGB homeless youth (18).

There continue to be some organized and evangelical religions that hold un-shakeable and immovable beliefs towards diverse groups, based on their inter-pretation of the bible. Such attitudes have resulted in homelessness for some LGBTQ+ youth when they have disclosed their sexuality, leading to further exclusion and marginalization. Another related issue that is receiving attention from the media and mental health organizations is 'reparative' or conversion 'therapy'. Fortunately, many jurisdictions have taken active steps to prohibit the promotion and practice of 'conversion therapy' towards LGBTQ+ people, with critics describing the approaches used as 'cruel', damaging, and counter-thera-peutic, often leading to depression, anxiety, drug use, suicidality, and home-lessness. The practice has been prohibited in Brazil since 1999, the first country in the world to ban the use of conversion techniques (19). Many countries worldwide are following suit by legislating against its use (20) (for example, see https://www.oireachtas.ie/en/debates/debate/seanad/2018-05-02/12/).

Physical health concerns

Homelessness and issues related to physical health are common. This is per-haps unsurprising as individuals often have to endure sleeping on the streets, in hostels, and in overcrowded or substandard conditions. Recent research evi-dence showed that homeless people are 17 times more likely to be subjected to violence and victimization (2). Overall, youth in general tend to be healthy, while it is recognized that some might experience everyday health conditions such as type 1 diabetes and asthma (21). From the perspective of LGBTQ+ homelessness, there is limited research evidence focusing specifically on the wider physical health conditions that may be experienced by this population. However, higher rates and greater risks for cardiovascular disease have been found in LGBT homeless attributable to the enduring effects of *minority stress*, including stigma, discrimination, and victimization experiences (22). To date, much of the health research focus is on mental health and sexual health con-cerns. Homeless LGBTQ+ youth were found to be participating in unpro-tected sex and, due to their homelessness, stayed with strangers. In a study by Gangamma et al. (23), it was identified that sex health risks increased as a result of 'survival sex'. 'Survival sex' is where a young person participates in sexual activities in exchange for shelter, food, money, or drugs. It has been reported that amphetamine use and increased alcohol consumption played a significant part in survival sex (24). The existing research evidence also highlights that LGBTQ+ youth who are homeless, when compared with non-homeless youth, engage in sexually risky behaviours and are exposed to sexually transmitted in-fections (25). Homeless individuals can have difficulties accessing appropriate healthcare supports and services. LGBTQ+ people have reported experiencing discrimination, heteronormativity, homophobia, biphobia, and transphobia (26–28). They may present at the emergency department having experienced family hostility and violence and abuse, culminating in being kicked out of the family home. They have an increased risk of victimization experiences while living on the streets and being subjected to traumatic circumstances and events, leading to greater physical and psychosocial issues.

Social aspects

The causes of homelessness are multifactorial and often complex. The consequences for LGBTQ+ youth can be particularly challenging and can be lifelong. What is known is that being homeless is stressful and has a detrimental effect on health and well-being. It may be attributed to wider social policy 'structural' factors such as lack of affordable housing, unemployment, poverty, and inadequate health and social services. Unemployment and the inability to pay rent can result in homelessness. It may also be due to 'personal' factors related to substance use, mental health concerns, family rejection, and risky sexual behaviours. Mental ill health can also be the precursor to people losing their home. Poor housing conditions or living on the street can have a profound effect on a person's physical health. Excessive alcohol or drug use can lead to homelessness and some turn to addictions while living on the streets. Homeless individuals experience barriers to accessing health services and treatments and health recovery is challenging without somewhere safe to stay.

LGBTQ+ youth are at increased risk to sexual abuse and exploitation, social stigma, and discrimination. They may also be subjected to bullying, harassment, and abuse at schools and colleges and can be the recipients of online bullying and cyberbullying. The UK government plans to ensure that support is available to LGBTQ+ students who are subjected to hate crime and online bullying (29). From an education perspective, many experience lower levels of educational attainment, thus increasing their disadvantages in potential work opportunities. To try and address these experiences, the UK government has recently introduced and funded a homophobic, biphobic, and transphobic anti-bullying programme to be initiated throughout the UK and which aims to reach 1200 schools. They have also financed programmes in colleges and higher education institutions to tackle bullying and abuse. Furthermore, the Crown Prosecution Service will review their Hate Crime Schools Initiative in collaboration with LGBTQ+ youth and further develop anti-bullying strategies.

All of these factors compound the stressors that individuals may face as they express and come to terms with their sexual and/or gender identities. The endured distress can have adverse consequences on familial relationships and the home environment. Without adequate family and social supports, LGBTQ+ youth can face significant obstacles in meeting their physical, emotional, and social needs (30). It is therefore important to provide parents and families with access to resources that enable them to support their family member in 'coming out', including individual transgender experiences. For LGBTQ+ youth preparing to enter the workforce, it is necessary to ensure that all employers have in place policies that reflect their obligations regarding antidiscrimination and equality legislation. Employers, therefore, need to have in place supportive and conducive working conditions and environments for LGBTQ+ people, particularly those who are transgender. There is also an opportunity to develop further education opportunities to facilitate LGBTQ+ youth back into education and training. From a leisure perspective, there is a need to provide inclusive and supportive recreational environments where LGBTQ+ people can flourish and fully participate in events related to culture, society, and sport, thereby reducing LGBTQ+ stigma and promoting inclusion. This can in part be achieved by providing supports that promote diversity, inclusion, and visible representation through sports clubs, cultural bodies, youth groups, and businesses. Such developments need to be underpinned by policy and communication campaigns that reflect and promote the diversity that exists within families, strategies focusing on promoting positive mental health that improves health and well-being, and the public presentation of positive images of LGBTQ+ people thereby challenging and changing negative stereotypes, by highlighting the positive representations of LGBTQ+ people in sport, culture, and within wider society.

The importance of social and support networks for LGBTQ+ youth who are homeless has been identified. There are well-established gay and transgender national networks which have developed different programmes to support LGBTQ+ clientele to openly talk about health matters, sexual identity, and sexual behaviours. Individuals need access to supportive networks that are supportive and reduce isolation, stressful life events, and negative social relationships, thereby enhancing opportunities to expand friendships. This can, in part, be achieved by encouraging participation in and attendance at LGBTQ+ centres and gay–straight alliance groups to establish new and more supportive friendships and relationships.

Policy

Once any legislation is enacted, it must be supported by a policy that sets out how the implementation is to be taken forward. An integral part of policy implementation is the need to ensure that welfare systems fully recognize and effectively respond to LGBTQ+ youth needs and their requirements. Where welfare services are responsive and well developed, as in some European countries, the housing needs of people are often provided for (31). In other countries, however, current evidence demonstrates, particularly in some parts of the US, this may not be the case. Therefore, housing, health, social care, and other support services need to review and define the concept of 'priority need' and identify those most vulnerable and at risk, putting in place appropriate and responsive services. Services may be unavailable or underdeveloped, thereby reducing responsiveness to the needs of LGBTQ+ people, notably young people (5). Therefore, assumptions should not be made that welfare systems, where they do exist, effectively meet the needs of LGBTQ+ youth, and this is an issue that needs to be recognized and addressed. To enable accurate policy responses, governments need to work collaboratively with local service providers to collect data on the LGBTQ+ identity of people who use their services and their distinct needs. To improve practice, best practice guidelines should be developed in partnership with LGBTQ+ youth that reflect their needs and concerns.

Implications for practice

Professionals need to have greater knowledge and a better grasp of LGBTQ+ and trans-specific issues, supported by culturally competent education and transparent policies to guide supports and interventions (32). The needs and experiences of LGBTQ+ people are unique and distinct to each individual. While they are possibly helpful in focusing the attention on a particular community, the requirements and supports are wide and diverse. It is, therefore, critical that practitioners appreciate and respond appropriately (5). For example, education and preparation of health and social care practitioners should include theories, skills development, and practice learning that takes account of and reflects this population's needs (32). Within that, it is also necessary to recognize the distinct needs of lesbians, gay men, bisexuals, transgender people, or the people who do not identify with any of the groupings. Furthermore, surveillance strategies are needed to identify early detection of risks of homelessness to develop and provide responsive supports and services to rapidly and effectively address individual needs (33).

Suggestions for future research

There is a shortage of data regarding the prevalence, needs, and concerns of LGBTQ+ youth. The evidence that does exist has been predominantly conducted in the US. Therefore, caution needs to be exercised when considering their implications and transferability to other jurisdictions (5). This is important as legislation, policy, welfare systems, and access to services, networks, and supports vary significantly on a global context. For example, countries who have proactively enacted legislation, protecting the rights of LGBTQ+ people, in areas such as marriage equality and trans rights, while others continue to discriminate actively. There is, therefore, an opportunity and a need for an increased research focus on LGBTQ+ homeless youth and subpopulations such as bisexuals and trans individuals. Furthermore, there is scope for national and international research networks and collaborations that work together to undertake multicentre studies involving diverse populations under the umbrella of LGBTQ+. Research initiatives need to be fully informed by theoretical models, including *minority stress theory* and *queer theory* (31).

Conclusion

Homeless youth who identify as LGBTQ+ are considered to be one of the most marginalized and disenfranchised groups in society. This chapter has identified specific factors and experiences related to LGBTQ+ homeless youth, including pathways into homelessness and the psychosocial and physical effects of homelessness. What remains are considerations of potential routes out of homelessness and particular facets that may influence individual LGBTQ+ youth trajectories. There are concerns that individuals are more susceptible to being rejected, disowned, and ejected from the family home, and as a result, experience significantly higher incidences of vulnerability and risky behaviours. Most of the current research evidence originates in the US, where the welfare supports are variable across different states and may be poor or non-existent (6).

In contrast, in the UK and many northern European countries, there is access to supported housing, services, and support networks for the general homeless population, including physical and psychosocial care. Still, it remains unclear the extent to which homeless services are tailored to the distinct needs and requirements of LGBTQ+ people. To improve the situation, there needs to be clearly defined and focused legislation, policies, and practice guidelines to steer service developments and supports. Human rights and equality legislation needs to be used to ensure that the necessary supports are in place that enable social inclusion, challenge discrimination, and reduce health inequalities.

There needs to be sustained investment, whereby necessary resources are provided, that adequately supports initiatives and developments in housing and service provision and education and practice. There must be consistent monitoring of LGBTQ+ service use to ensure the provision of accessible, safe, and affordable housing accommodation for all. This is necessary to ensure that housing, health, social care, and other agencies are accessible, non-discriminatory, affirming, and inclusive. To address individual needs, assistance should be provided by culturally competent, skilled, and knowledgeable practitioners who appreciate the experiences and needs of LGBTQ+ youth. Necessary supports should also be available to families to enable them to connect or reconnect with family members. To improve care and support for this population, all developments must be informed and driven by the most recent research evidence. To improve the situation of LGBTQ+ homeless youth, solutions require to be coordinated and supported by strategic, collaborative working across housing, health, social care, and specialist LGBTQ+ organizations. From an educational perspective, there is the need to fully integrate the requirements of LGBTQ+ homeless youth within undergraduate, postgraduate, and continuing professional development programmes. Practice development champions roles could be developed to provide guidance and leadership in driving forward policy, education, and practice initiatives that are interprofessional and interagency. Only by having in place a strong and effective focus by way of developments in legislation, policy, service provision, and practice can we fully focus on and meet the unique holistic needs of LGBTQ+ youth who are at risk of becoming, or are currently, homeless.

References

1. **Fredriksen-Goldsen KI.** The future of LGBT+ aging: a blueprint for action in services, policies, and research. Generations. 2016;**40**(2):6–15.
2. **Crisis.** Homeless knowledge hub. 2021. Available from: https://www.crisis.org.uk/ending-homelessness/homelessness-knowledge-hub/.
3. **Gaetz S, O'Grady B, Buccieri K, Karabanow J, Marsolais A.** Youth Homelessness in Canada: Implications for Policy and Practice. Ontario: Canadian Homeless Research Network, The Homeless Hub; 2013.
4. **Embleton L, Lee H, Gunn J, Ayuku D, Braitstein P.** Causes of child and youth homelessness in developed and developing countries: a systematic review and meta-analysis. JAMA Pediatr. 2016;**170**(5):435–444.
5. **McCann E, Brown M.** Homelessness among youth who identify as LGBTQ+: a systematic review. J Clin Nurs. 2019;**28**(11–12):2061–2072.
6. **Ecker J.** Queer, young, and homeless: a review of the literature. Child Youth Serv. 2016;**37**(4):325–361.
7. **Albert Kennedy Trust.** Strategy 2018–2021: Preventing LGBTQ+ Youth Homelessness: Because no Young Person Should Have to Choose Between a Safe Home and Being Who They Are. London: Albert Kennedy Trust; 2018.
8. **Morton MH, Dworsky A, Matjasko JL,** et al. Prevalence and correlates of youth homelessness in the United States. J Adolesc Health. 2018;**62**(1):14–21.

9. **Makadon HJ, Mayer KH, Potter J, Goldhammer H.** The Fenway Guide to Lesbian, Gay, Bisexual, and Transgender Health. Philadelphia, PA: American College of Physicians; 2015.

10. **Fadus M.** Mental health disparities and medical student education: teaching in psychiatry for LGBTQ care, communication, and advocacy. Acad Psychiatry. 2019;**43**(3):306–310.

11. **Painter KR, Scannapieco M, Blau G, Andre A, Kohn K.** Improving the mental health outcomes of LGBTQ youth and young adults: a longitudinal study. J Soc Serv Res. 2018;**44**(2):223–235.

12. **Toomey RB, Ryan C, Diaz RM, Russell ST.** Coping with sexual orientation-related minority stress. J Homosex. 2018;**65**(4):484–500.

13. **Meyer IH.** Resilience in the study of minority stress and health of sexual and gender minorities. Psychol Sex Orient Gend Divers. 2015;**2**(3):209–213.

14. **Bruce D, Stall R, Fata A, Campbell RT.** Modelling minority stress effects on homelessness and health disparities among young men who have sex with men. J Urban Health. 2014;**91**(3):568–580.

15. **Bruce D, Harper GW, Bauermeister JA.** Minority stress, positive identity development, and depressive symptoms: implications for resilience among sexual minority male youth. Psychol Sex Orient Gend Divers. 2015;**2**(3):287–296.

16. **Clement S, Schauman O, Graham T,** et al. What is the impact of mental health-related stigma on help-seeking? A systematic review of quantitative and qualitative studies. Psychol Med. 2015;**45**(1):11–27.

17. **Russell ST, Fish JN.** Mental health in lesbian, gay, bisexual, and transgender (LGBT) youth. Annu Rev Clin Psychol. 2016;**12**:465–487.

18. **Rosario M, Schrimshaw EW, Hunter J.** Risk factors for homelessness among lesbian, gay, and bisexual youths: a developmental milestone approach. Child Youth Serv Rev. 2012;**34**(1):186–193.

19. **Macedo CMRD, Sívori HF** The sexual diversity debate in Brazilian psychology: professional regulation at stake. Psicol Cienc Prof. 2019;**39**(SPE3):88–102.

20. **Department of Children and Youth Affairs.** LGBTI+ National Youth Strategy 2018–2020: LGBTI+ Young People: Visible, Valued and Included. Dublin: Department of Children and Youth Affairs; 2018.

21. **Edidin JP, Ganim Z, Hunter SJ, Karnik NS.** The mental and physical health of homeless youth: a literature review. Child Psychiatry Hum Dev. 2012;**43**(3):354–375.

22. **Flentje A, Leon A, Carrico A, Zheng D, Dilley J.** Mental and physical health among homeless sexual and gender minorities in a major urban US city. J Urban Health. 2016;**93**(6):997–1009.

23. **Gangamma R, Slesnick N, Toviessi P, Serovich J.** Comparison of HIV risks among gay, lesbian, bisexual and heterosexual homeless youth. J Youth Adolesc. 2008;**37**(4):456–464.

24. **Walls NE, Bell S.** Correlates of engaging in survival sex among homeless youth and young adults. J Sex Res. 2011;**48**(5):423–436.

25. **Tyler KA.** Homeless youths' HIV risk behaviors with strangers: investigating the importance of social networks. Arch Sex Behav. 2013;**42**(8):1583–1591.

26. **Sellers MD.** Absent inclusion polices: problems facing homeless transgender youth. Public Integr. 2018;**20**(6):625–639.

27. **Andrews C, Shelton J, McNair R.** Developments in responding to LGBTQ+ homelessness in Australia and the United States. Parity. 2019;**32**(3):21.

28. **Moore E, Warf C.** Providing clinical care to youth experiencing homelessness. In: **Warf C, Charles G** (Eds), *Clinical Care for Homeless, Runaway and Refugee Youth*. Cham: Springer; 2020:187–209.

29. **Government Equalities Office.** LGBT Action Plan: Improving the Lives of Lesbian, Gay, Bisexual and Transgender People. London: HMSO; 2018.

30. **Sharek D, Huntley-Moore S, McCann E.** Education needs of families of transgender young people: a narrative review of international literature. Issues Ment Health Nurs. 2018;**39**(1):59–72.

31. **Matthews P, Poyner C, Kjellgren R.** Lesbian, gay, bisexual, transgender and queer experiences of homelessness and identity: insecurity and home(o)normativity. Int J Hous Policy. 2019;**19**(2):232–253.

32. **McCann E, Brown M.** The inclusion of LGBT+ health issues within undergraduate healthcare education and professional training programmes: a systematic review. Nurse Educ Today. 2018;**64**:204–214.

33. **Rice E, Petering R, Rhoades H,** et al. Homelessness and sexual identity among middle school students. J Sch Health. 2015;**85**(8):552–557.

Section 7

Conclusions

Chapter 27

Conclusions

João Mauricio Castaldelli-Maia,
Antonio Ventriglio, and Dinesh Bhugra

Background

The close and cruel relationship between homelessness and mental illnesses needs to be approached both at clinical and policy levels in a joined-up manner. Enabling homeless individuals with mental illness to have easy and appropriate access to mental health services is of utmost importance. Through the establishment of research networks, delivery of psychiatric care and outcomes need to be developed and measured so that interventions are evidence based (1). Although early interventions and therapies are incredibly effective, these can only succeed if people have an element of protection in their housing (2) which is a basic human need. Current mental healthcare must also consider psychosocial factors that may lead to homelessness and poverty among the psychiatric population, and psychiatrists must advocate for change in social strategy via the lens of equity and equality (2).

There is evidence that secure housing can contribute to better cognitive functioning and this deserves more robust evaluation (3). In psychiatric practice, accommodation and social welfare must be part of ambitious, inclusive campaigns and programmes truly sticking to biopsychosocial models of intervention. In order to deliver these, an element of advocacy is required on the part of the psychiatric profession and hence this needs to be included in the training curricula. Closer partnerships with non-governmental organizations and housing associations will lead to collaborative research and interventions. Such an approach is likely to increase the potential to raise sufficient resources to provide effective and affordable services to vulnerable people who are mentally ill and homeless (4). While precise reports are scarce, through particular pieces of legislation and the recorded history of the organizations developed to deal with the issue, we can obtain some understanding of what happens to homeless people with mental illness (4) so that lessons can be learnt and examples of good practice shared widely. In psychiatric clinical practice, the tension between forced treatment and personal freedoms has always been evident over the centuries (5).

Research

Although levels of homelessness and definitions of insecure accommodation may vary and change across nations, there are similarities in the impact these have on individuals' well-being and functioning. We propose that the researchers should agree on criteria for homelessness and also for insecure accommodation and these findings should be reported separately rather than aggregated, as these two subgroups are likely to have different needs, including their experiences with mental ill health (6). Sampling techniques should be recorded, and a representative sample should be collected using sophisticated probability sampling procedures. To identify mental illness among the homeless, researchers can use clear and multimethod approaches with proven psychometric properties sensitive to those specific cultures. Diagnostic interviews such as the Diagnostic Interview Schedule, for example, show reasonably reliable estimates across the US and fairly stable estimates across countries (7). Research would also benefit from having other composite figures, including a count of symptoms and a history of hospitalizations, rather than relying on one single metric. Thus, when comparing rates of mental illness across research, a common battery of interventions, translated for implementations across various nations, is important. These recommendations would enable people to investigate commonalities and dissimilarities among the homeless in terms of features of mental ill-health, which would help increase our capacity to spot reasonable reasons for proper global disparities (6,7).

Clinical care

The rates of mental disorders among the homeless are known to vary across countries. For example, Germany reports a higher prevalence of alcohol use disorders compared with other Western countries (8). Therefore, the country reports problems related to psychiatric disorders as well as complicated administrative procedures, language gaps, and barriers to mental healthcare (8) related to increased morbidity and mortality. Similarly, in Hungary, poor engagement of the homeless into mental healthcare confirms that the conventional model of treatment may not be entirely suitable for this specific population (9). Therefore, one possible solution is to have multidisciplinary teams who are specially trained and fully resourced.

Homelessness and inadequate housing are very prevalent in Latin America as well (10). An innovative approach for improving mental healthcare in this population has been the development of Brazilian psychosocial care centres (Centros de Atenção Psicossocial (CAPS)) (11,12) which are freely available to all citizens living in Brazil. There is no doubt that more appropriate policy interventions to avoid deleterious, almost unchanging, long-term outcomes in this disadvantaged group (11,12) have to be at the core of design, development, and delivery of services. As in many countries, Latin American nations also illustrate the phenomena of street youth, particularly associations with mental illness and substance abuse as well as belonging to gangs (13). Many such street kids are living on the streets whereas others may have homes to go to but may be either unemployed or in insecure employment. They may be exposed to traumatic events thereby contributing to further distress (13).

Even though some Asian countries offer free public-sector medical services for people who are unable to afford healthcare, the rates of undertreatment for both physical and mental disorders remain outrageously high (14). In Hong Kong, a non-profit organization and volunteer medical workers have recently partnered to develop a medical outreach service for mentally ill people who are homeless (14). One of the at-risk and vulnerable groups is women (15). As described in this volume, India has many non-governmental organizations working with homeless people and has a policy to ensure care for homeless people with mental disorders (16).

In preserving the present nature of homeless people, cognition seems to play a crucial role, which is frequently overlooked in light of more urgent and immediate medical problems. Studies have started to examine cognitive skills training with an emphasis on social abilities training in order to approach cognition explicitly (17). Therefore, particular areas to be targeted are to help people use skills to help with memory or strategies that specifically aid with adherence to medication in this group. The same refers to risk factors for homelessness and their relation to cognitive impairment, such as intellectual disability, malnutrition, drug usage, traumatic brain injury, and childhood trauma. In order to identify the cognitive disability and allow for more homogeneous results, future studies must include widely agreed diagnostic assessment.

Services

While many homeless programmes began as services for psychosis, it has become apparent that there are many other homeless people who may benefit from a broader variety of services (4). And to satisfy this need, several novel psychological measures have emerged—pioneers in multiple behavioural health research styles, including assertive outreach styles and more open therapeutic counselling models. And, by their much greater levels of cooperation with non-medical and therapeutic agencies, since they are leaders of numerous forms of coordinating mental healthcare as part of a wider community, they are ideally able to address the needs of a person in a systematic and organized manner (4,15). Psychiatric provision has been used in all successful recovery programmes as a standardized aspect of the more general provision of accommodation and social services (5). They also predicted, in several ways, the needs-led appraisal, case management, and collaboration developed as part of group psychiatry services (4,5).

It is also necessary to recognize and respect their perspectives and opinions in order to strengthen the provision of services to people experiencing homelessness (18). Important questions can then be posed from this vantage point about the degree to which programmes are planned and delivered with service users in mind. It is possible to find the potential for incremental improvements that can have major impacts by recognizing how programmes can make life more difficult for people experiencing homelessness. It will also be beneficial to improve the capacity of homeless sector providers to perform structured programmes that directly involve the homeless to maximize the provision of person-centred treatment and care (18).

Special vulnerable groups

For refugees and migrants, homelessness and mental health issues are quite prevalent and are primarily instigated by pre-migration stressful events and mid-migration and post-migration sources of stress (19). There is an immediate need for new nations to provide comprehensive mental health services for this vulnerable population. This will help the new countries benefit from the positive aspects of migration and avoid the looming burdens on future social, political, and economic lives caused by untreated mental illnesses among refugees and migrants (19).

Homeless or street youth as mentioned previously, are another special group. There are several obstacles to mental healthcare due to the suboptimal usage of established facilities and deficiencies in accessing them for serious mental disorder (20). It is also important to identify factors that promote access and measures to overcome these obstacles by rethinking the organization of programmes and introducing unique strategies targeted at homeless young people and related communities with significant mental illnesses (20).

Some persons with intellectual and developmental disabilities have additional mental illnesses and troubling habits that can lead to homelessness (21). Other factors which may cause mental illnesses include the dissolution of marriages and families and bereavements. Further research is also needed to establish data in this field and, in particular, on the perceptions and experiences of homeless people with intellectual and developmental disabilities.

As a result of this social marginalization process to which they are exposed, mental health issues arise more often in lesbian, gay, bisexual, and transgender (LGBT) people than in homeless people in general or in LGBT people who have somewhere to live (22). In addition to the intersectionality with race, the specifics of segments within the homeless LGBT category should be further researched, especially regarding transgender people. For care practices in institutions that seek to provide care for this category, there are key elements required. These concern critical reflection on heterosexism, cisgenderism, and structural racism, along with recognition by these individuals of the multiplicity of constructs of subjectivities, thereby allowing dialogue-based care responses to be developed (22).

Conclusion

It is of paramount importance to enable homeless people with mental illness to easily access mental health services, and this is a global challenge.

A significant improvement is through early detection of psychiatric disorders in homeless individuals. In view of their greater vulnerability, the special psychological treatment needs are obvious. The high incidence of mental disorders also means that this group may not have appropriate care for these diseases. Each nation needs to develop optimal models of social care and rehabilitation that rely on the particular research-driven needs of homeless people with mental illnesses. In order to improve the availability of services to the homeless, it is also important to consider and value their experiences and opinions. Refugees and migrants, youth, those with intellectual and developmental disabilities, and LGBT people represent some special subgroups for focus prevention, specialized care, and research.

References

1. **Ventriglio A, Mari M, Bellomo A, Bhugra D.** Homelessness and mental health: a challenge. Int J Soc Psychiatry. 2015;**61**(7):621–622.
2. **Bhugra D, Ventriglio A.** Home is where hearth is. Acta Psychiatr Scand. 2015;**131**(4):235–236.
3. **Stergiopoulos V, Cusi A, Bekele T,** et al. Neurocognitive impairment in a large sample of homeless adults with mental illness. Acta Psychiatr Scand. 2015;**131**(4):256–268.
4. **Timms PW, Fry AH.** Homelessness and mental illness. Health Trends. 1989;**21**(3):70–71.
5. **Timms PW, Craig TK.** Deinstitutionalisation, imprisonment and homelessness. Br J Psychiatry. 2016;**209**(4):349–350.

6. Toro PA, Hobden KL, Wyszacki Durham K, Oko-Riebau M, Bokszczanin A. Comparing the characteristics of homeless adults in Poland and the United States. Am J Community Psychol. 2014;53(1–2):134–145.

7. Toro PA. Homelessness. In: Bellack AS, Hersen M (Eds), Comprehensive Clinical Psychology. Vol. 9: Applications in Diverse Populations. New York: Pergamon; 1998:119–135.

8. Schreiter S, Bermpohl F, Krausz M, et al. The prevalence of mental illness in homeless people in Germany. Dtsch Arztebl Int. 2017;114(40):665–672.

9. Braun E, Gazdag G. Pszichiátriai zavarok előfordulása hajléktalanok között. Psychiatr Hung. 2015;30:60–67.

10. Torales J, Villalba-Arias J, Ruiz-Díaz C, Chávez E, Riego V. The right to health in Paraguay. Int Rev Psychiatry. 2014;26(4):524–529.

11. Castaldelli-Maia JM, Ventriglio A. The impact of Basaglia on Brazilian psychiatry. Int J Soc Psychiatry. 2016;62(5):411–414.

12. Castaldelli-Maia JM, da Silva NR, Campos MR, et al. Implementing evidence-based smoking cessation treatment in psychosocial care units (CAPS) in Brazil. Int J Soc Psychiatry. 2017;63(8):669–673.

13. Pluck G, Banda-Cruz DR, Andrade-Guimaraes MV, Trueba AF. Socioeconomic deprivation and the development of neuropsychological functions: a study with 'street children' in Ecuador. Child Neuropsychol. 2018;24(4):510–523.

14. Yim LC, Leung HC, Chan WC, Lam MH, Lim VW. Prevalence of mental illness among homeless people in Hong Kong. PLoS One. 2015;10(10):e0140940.

15. Gowda GS, Gopika G, Kumar CN, et al. Clinical outcome and rehabilitation of homeless mentally ill patients admitted in mental health institute of South India: 'Know the Unknown' project. Asian J Psychiatr. 2017;30:49–53.

16. Swaminath G, Enara A, Rao R, Kumar KVK, Kumar CN. Mental Healthcare Act, 2017 and homeless persons with mental illness in India. Indian J Psychiatry. 2019;61(Suppl 4):S768–S772.

17. Medalia A, Saperstein AM, Huang Y, Lee S, Ronan EJ. Cognitive skills training for homeless transition-age youth: feasibility and pilot efficacy of a community based randomized controlled trial. J Nerv Ment Dis. 2017;205(11):859–866.

18. Kerman N, Gran-Ruaz S, Lawrence M, Sylvestre J. Perceptions of service use among currently and formerly homeless adults with mental health problems. Community Ment Health J. 2019;55(5):777–783.

19. Idemudia ES. Trauma and PTSS of Zimbabwean refugees in South Africa: a summary of published studies. Psychol Trauma. 2017;9(3):252–257.

20. Abdel-Baki A, Aubin D, Morisseau-Guillot R, et al. Improving mental health services for homeless youth in downtown Montreal, Canada: partnership between a local network and ACCESS Esprits ouverts (Open Minds), a National Services Transformation Research Initiative. Early Interv Psychiatry. 2019;13(Suppl 1):20–28.

21. Brown M, McCann E. Homelessness and people with intellectual disabilities: a systematic review of the international research evidence. J Appl Res Intellect Disabil. 2021;34(2):390–401.

22. Garcia MR. LGBT homeless people, nomadism and contexts of vulnerability to HIV/ AIDS. Temas Psicol. 2013;21(3):1005–1019.

Index

For the benefit of digital users, indexed terms that span two pages (e.g., 52–53) may, on occasion, appear on only one of those pages.

Notes
As the subject of this book concerns the homeless, the use of this term has been kept to a minimum in the index.

Tables and figures are indicated by *t* and *f* following the page number
vs. indicates a comparison